COMMUNICATION SCIENCES

AND DISORDERS

From Science to Clinical Practice

SECOND EDITION

Ronald B. Gillam, PhD
Raymond L. and Eloise H. Lillywhite Professor
Utah State University
Logan, Utah

Thomas P. Marquardt, PhD
Ben H. Love Regents Professor
The University of Texas at Austin
Austin, Texas

Frederick N. Martin, PhD
Jamail Centennial Professor Emeritus
The University of Texas at Austin
Austin, Texas

JONES AND BARTLETT PUBLISHERS
Sudbury, Massachusetts
BOSTON   TORONTO   LONDON   SINGAPORE

World Headquarters

Jones and Bartlett Publishers
40 Tall Pine Drive
Sudbury, MA 01776
978-443-5000
info@jbpub.com
www.jbpub.com

Jones and Bartlett Publishers
Canada
6339 Ormindale Way
Mississauga, Ontario L5V 1J2
Canada

Jones and Bartlett Publishers
International
Barb House, Barb Mews
London W6 7PA
United Kingdom

Jones and Bartlett's books and products are available through most bookstores and online booksellers. To contact Jones and Bartlett Publishers directly, call 800-832-0034, fax 978-443-8000, or visit our website www.jbpub.com.

Substantial discounts on bulk quantities of Jones and Bartlett's publications are available to corporations, professional associations, and other qualified organizations. For details and specific discount information, contact the special sales department at Jones and Bartlett via the above contact information or send an email to specialsales@jbpub.com.

The authors, editor, and publisher have made every effort to provide accurate information. However, they are not responsible for errors, omissions, or for any outcomes related to the use of the contents of this book and take no responsibility for the use of the products and procedures described. Treatments and side effects described in this book may not be applicable to all people; likewise, some people may require a dose or experience a side effect that is not described herein. Drugs and medical devices are discussed that may have limited availability controlled by the Food and Drug Administration (FDA) for use only in a research study or clinical trial. Research, clinical practice, and government regulations often change the accepted standard in this field. When consideration is being given to use of any drug in the clinical setting, the health care provider or reader is responsible for determining FDA status of the drug, reading the package insert, and reviewing prescribing information for the most up-to-date recommendations on dose, precautions, and contraindications, and determining the appropriate usage for the product. This is especially important in the case of drugs that are new or seldom used.

Production Credits

Publisher: David Cella
Associate Editor: Maro Gartside
Editorial Assistant: Teresa Reilly
Production Editor: Amanda Clerkin
Marketing Manager: Grace Richards
Manufacturing and Inventory Control
  Supervisor: Amy Bacus

Composition: Shawn Girsberger
Cover Design: Kristin E. Parker
Cover Image Credit: © zhuda/
  ShutterStock, Inc.
Photo Researcher: Carolyn Arcabascio
Printing and Binding: Malloy, Inc.
Cover Printing: Malloy, Inc.

Library of Congress Cataloging-in-Publication Data

Communication sciences and disorders : from science to clinical practice / [edited by] Ronald B. Gillam, Thomas Marquardt, and Frederick Martin. — 2nd ed.
    p. ; cm.
Includes bibliographical references and index.
ISBN-13: 978-0-7637-7975-7 (alk. paper)
ISBN-10: 0-7637-7975-X (alk. paper)
1. Communicative disorders. I. Gillam, Ronald B. (Ronald Bradley), 1955- II. Marquardt, Thomas P. III. Martin, Frederick N.
[DNLM: 1. Communication Disorders. 2. Communication. 3. Speech--physiology. WL 340.2 C7344 2011]
RC423.C647 2011
616.85'5--dc22

                       2009038822

6048

Printed in the United States of America
14 13 12 11 10   10 9 8 7 6 5 4 3 2 1

To Sandi, whose love and encouragement means everything to me.
—Ronald B. Gillam

To Barbara.
—Thomas P. Marquardt

To my many students who made mine a wonderful career.
—Frederick N. Martin

Contents

chapter three

The Social and Cultural Bases of Communication   **51**
Elizabeth D. Peña and Janice E. Jackson

section II

INDIVIDUALS WITH SPEECH DISORDERS   **71**

chapter four

Speech Science   **73**
Thomas P. Marquardt and Christine L. Matyear

chapter five

chapter six

chapter seven

chapter eight

chapter nine

section III

chapter ten

chapter eleven

chapter twelve

section IV

chapter thirteen

chapter fourteen

chapter fifteen

chapter sixteen

Preface

This book was written for undergraduate students who are enrolled in their first course in communication sciences and disorders. We wrote it with two important assumptions in mind. First, we assumed that the students who read this book would have relatively little prior knowledge about the scientific study of communication, the nature of communication disorders, or the professions of audiology and speech-language pathology. Second, we assumed that if students found the content of this book to be interesting, they would be likely to enroll in courses that would examine most of the topics that are included in this book in much greater detail.

Given these assumptions, we focused on providing the reader with a wide-angle view of communication sciences and disorders. We wanted to show the considerable forest that is communication sciences and disorders without having to focus on too many individual trees. Whenever possible, we selected a wide-angle lens rather than a narrow lens. Readers should get a sense of the variety of topics that speech, language, and hearing scientists study and the variety of individuals that audiologists and speech-language pathologists treat.

Like many introductory texts, the book contains basic information about speech disorders that are related to impairments in articulation, voice, and fluency; language disorders in children and adults; and hearing disorders that cause conductive and sensorineural hearing losses. We also include basic information on the speech, language, and hearing sciences and practical information about assessment and intervention practices. Finally, readers will be happy to note that this book includes chapters on multicultural issues, deafness, dysarthria, and dysphagia.

We do not want to tell readers everything we know about each topic. To this end, we describe only the most critical concepts in detail, provide many examples, and cite only seminal works. If we have selected our topics wisely and have explained them well, the content of this book will provide students with the background knowledge they need to get the most out of subsequent undergraduate and graduate courses.

Finally, we have provided students with a means for seeing and hearing the human communication disorders they are reading about. The CD-ROM that accompanies the book enables professors to provide information about common or unusual cases in a single, highly accessible format, and it enables students to watch the segments many times over to make the most of the enhanced learning opportunities they provide.

This second edition of this book includes a number of changes. We reorganized the sections so that they follow the way many instructors sequence their introductory classes. The text begins with overviews of the professions, the nature of communication across the life span, and social-cultural issues that affect communication and communication disorders. The second section examines the variety of speech disorders. We begin with a summary of basic principles of speech science, and then we provide chapters that focus on speech sound disorders in children, laryngeal and resonance disorders (combined into one chapter), fluency disorders, dysarthria, and dysphagia. The third section of the book concerns language disorders across the life span. We begin with language disorders in infants, toddlers, and preschoolers; move to a discussion of language disorders in school-age children; and then end the section with a discussion of acquired neurogenic language disorders. The last section of the book concerns hearing and hearing disorders. We begin with a summary of basic principles of hearing science, and then we provide a survey of hearing disorders and hearing testing, a summary of audiologic rehabilitation (hearing aids and cochlear implants), and a description of the education of students who are deaf or hard of hearing.

We want students in introductory courses to begin to understand what it means to have a communication disorder. We have added personal stories about events in our careers and case studies to the chapters to highlight the human side of the professions of speech-language pathology, audiology, and deaf education. We want these vignettes, together with the video segments on the CD-ROM, to demonstrate that the concepts and principles in the chapters relate to real people who have real needs that can be addressed by caring and well-educated professionals. We hope the students who read this book will find this subject matter to be both interesting and uplifting.

Acknowledgments

Many people contributed to the creation of this book. We would like to thank Shannon Davenport, Tanja Jensen, Jennifer Gillam, Emily Swatner, Amy Montuoro, Bonnie Lindgren, Kristy Price, and Brittany Atwood for their helpful assistance in preparing the revised manuscript. At Jones and Bartlett Publishers, Maro Gartside provided a great deal of advice and encouragement at the most critical times.

A number of people assisted us in creating the CD-ROM. First, and foremost, LaVae Hoffman endured the hardship of working for many masters, none of whom understood the intricacies of multimedia development. Without her loyalty, ingenuity, and hard work, this project would not have been possible. We thank many of our colleagues and students who agreed to appear in the video segments. Grateful appreciation is extended to Mr. Chad Smiddy who created the embryologic morphing sequence of the human face.

Finally, the editors and authors thank those individuals with communication disorders and their family members who allowed their images and words to be included on the CD-ROM. We applaud their continuing struggle to compensate for or overcome their communication disorders, and we share their hope that their appearance on the CD-ROM will contribute to the education of the next generation of speech-language pathologists, audiologists, and deaf educators.

Contributors

Lisa Bedore, PhD (CCC-SLP), is an associate professor in the Department of Communication Sciences and Disorders at the University of Texas at Austin. She teaches courses on language development, language disorders, and bilingualism. Her research interests are in the areas of language and phonological development in Spanish-English bilingual children with typically developing language skills and language disorders.

Mark E. Bernstein, EdD, is the associate dean for Student Affairs in the College of Communication at the University of Texas at Austin and the coordinator of the Deafness Studies/Deaf Education major in the Department of Communication Sciences and Disorders. His scholarly interests range from techniques for speech development in the deaf, to working with parents of children with hearing impairments, to descriptive studies of the use of simultaneous communication, to issues surrounding bilingual/bicultural (ASL/English) approaches to deaf education.

Courtney Byrd, PhD (CCC-SLP), is an assistant professor at the University of Texas at Austin and is the founder and director of the Austin Center for Stuttering Intervention and Research. She teaches courses in the Department of Communication Sciences and Disorders in assessment and treatment of child speech and language disorders, fluency disorders, and voice disorders. Her primary research focus is the contribution of linguistic and motor planning to developmental stuttering with a secondary focus on evidence-based practice for young children who stutter.

Craig A. Champlin, PhD (CCC-A), is the Lillie Hage Jamail Centennial Professor of Communication at the University of Texas at Austin. He has published research articles in the areas of psychoacoustics, auditory electrophysiology, and diagnostic audiology. Craig has served as the editor of the *Journal of Speech, Language, and Hearing Research*, chair of the Bioacoustics section of the American National Standards Institute and is a fellow of American Academy of Audiology and the American Speech-Language-Hearing Association.

Rodger Dalston, PhD (CCC-SP), is an emeritus professor in the Department of Communication Sciences and Disorders at the University of Texas at Austin. He taught courses in voice disorders, craniofacial anomalies, and research design. His primary research interest concerned oral-facial clefts and their impact upon speech and language development.

Barbara Davis, PhD (CCC-SLP), is the Houston Harte Centennial Professor of Communication at the University of Texas at Austin. She teaches courses in the Department of Communication Sciences and Disorders in infant–toddler intervention, developmental speech disorders, and speech science. Her research interests focus on the interactive influences of production and perception on speech acquisition in typically developing children, children with speech disorders, and children with early identified hearing impairment.

Margaret Dean, PhD (CCC-A), is chief of Audiology and assistant professor at Texas A&M University at Scott & White Hospital in Temple, Texas, where she works as a clinical audiologist specializing in the areas of behavioral and electrophysiological diagnostic testing, hearing aids, cochlear implants, and central auditory processing testing. She has conducted research and published articles in the areas of bone conduction testing and the occlusion effect.

Ronald Gillam, PhD (CCC-SLP), holds the Raymond L. and Eloise H. Lillywhite chair in the Department of Communicative Disorders and Deaf Education at Utah State University, where he teaches courses on research methods and evidence-based practices. His research primarily concerns information processing, diagnostic markers of language impairments, language intervention procedures, and narrative development in school-age children and adults. He is a fellow of the American Speech-Language-Hearing Association.

Sandra Laing Gillam, PhD (CCC-SLP), is an associate professor in Communication Disorders and Deaf Education at Utah State University. She teaches courses in language development and disorders, phonological development and disorders, and literacy in school-age children. Her research interests include assessment and intervention for language and literacy impairments, multicultural populations, and processes involved in text comprehension.

Dena Granof, PhD (CCC-SLP), is a senior lecturer in Communication Sciences and Disorders at the University of Texas. She teaches courses in dysphagia and language disorders in children and adults. Her primary clinical interests are in assessment and treatment of communication and swallowing disorders in children with multiple handicaps.

Janice E. Jackson, PhD (CCC-SLP), is an assistant professor of Special Education and Speech-Language Pathology at the University of West Georgia. She teaches courses in language acquisition, language disorders, and literacy. Her research interests are related to language development, distinguishing language impairment from linguistic difference, and the use of psycholinguistics to develop nonbiased language assessment.

Swathi Kiran, PhD (CCC-SLP), is an associate professor in the Department of Speech and Hearing Sciences at Boston University. Her research interests focus around lexical semantic treatment for individuals with aphasia, bilingual aphasia, and neuroimaging of brain plasticity following a stroke. Her papers have appeared in journals such as *Brain and Language, Aphasiology, Journal of Speech Language and Hearing Research,* and the *American Journal of Speech Language Pathology.*

Thomas Marquardt, PhD (CCC-SLP), is the Ben F. Love Regents professor in the Department of Communication Sciences and Disorders at The University of Texas. He conducts research on speech motor control disorders in children and adults and teaches courses on acquired neurogenic speech and language disorders in addition to introduction to communication disorders. He is a fellow of the American Speech-Language-Hearing Association.

Frederick N. Martin, PhD (CCC-A), is the Jamail Centennial Professor Emeritus in Communication Sciences and Disorders at The University of Texas at Austin. His research concerns diagnostic audiology, pediatric diagnosis, and counseling. He is a fellow of the American Academy of Audiology and the American Speech-Language-Hearing Association, has received the Career Award in Hearing from the American Academy of Audiology, and was the first to receive the Lifetime Achievement Award from the Texas Academy of Audiology.

Christine L. Matyear, PhD, is a senior lecturer in Communication Sciences and Disorders at the University of Texas at Austin. She teaches courses in phonetics, speech science, hearing science, anatomy and physiology, deafness, and research. Her research interests include speech acquisition in infants and the acoustic analysis of speech sounds.

John A. Nelson, PhD (CCC-A), is the director of Copenhagen Audiology, Research and Development for ReSound Group and resides in Denmark. His research focuses on psychoacoustics, amplification, and digital signal processing.

Elizabeth Peña, PhD (CCC-SLP), is a professor of Communication Sciences and Disorders at the University of Texas at Austin. She teaches courses in language development, language disorders, psychometrics, and bilingualism. Her research interests are in the areas of language development and assessment of Spanish English bilingual children with typically developing language skills and language disorders.

Douglas Petersen, PhD (CCC-SLP), is an assistant professor at the University of Wyoming. His clinical and research interests include the assessment and intervention of childhood language disorders, with a specific focus on narrative assessment and intervention, assessment and prevention of early literacy difficulties in bilingual children, and cultural/linguistic diversity.

I section *I*

General Considerations

one

chapter one

An Introduction to the Discipline of Communication Sciences and Disorders

RONALD B. GILLAM AND SANDRA LAING GILLAM

LEARNING OBJECTIVES

1. To understand the discipline of communication sciences and disorders.

2. To understand how disorders of hearing, speech, and language adversely affect communication.

3. To compare and contrast the meaning of the following terms: *impairment*, *disability*, *handicap*, *disorder*, and *difference*.

4. To learn about the major types of speech, language, and hearing disorders.

5. To learn about the educational background and professional activities of speech, language, and hearing scientists, audiologists, and speech-language pathologists.

6. To understand the regulation of the professions of audiology and speech-language pathology by state agencies and professional organizations.

THE DISCIPLINE

Many children and adults have difficulties speaking and hearing. In fact, in the United States today, there are approximately 46 million people who have some type of a communication disorder (National Institute on Deafness and Other Communication Disorders, 1995). Some of these individuals were born with conditions such as deafness (an inability to hear sounds) or cleft palate (a large opening in the roof of the mouth). Others acquired their difficulties as a result of diseases (such as meningitis) or accidents (traumatic brain injury). Fortunately, specialists can offer help to people with communication disorders and their families. These specialists are called speech, language, and hearing scientists, audiologists, and speech-language pathologists (SLPs). These are *professions* within the *discipline* of **communication sciences and disorders (CSD)**.

A **discipline** is a unique area of study, but a **profession** is an area of practice. The discipline of CSD encompasses the study of human communication processes, breakdowns in those processes (referred to as communication disorders), and the **efficacy** of practices involved in assessing and assisting individuals with communication differences and disorders. The major components of the discipline are speech, language, and hearing sciences, audiology, and speech-language pathology. **Deaf education** (education and rehabilitation of individuals with severe to profound hearing impairments) is a related profession. Speech, language, and hearing science, audiology, speech-language pathology, and deaf education are not mutually exclusive professions because some professionals may be engaged in activities related to one, two, or even all four of these areas of practice.

There are many factors that justify the need for CSD, and there are many beneficiaries of the research and practices that occur within the discipline. Research in human communication processes can add greatly to our understanding of how people interact with one another, solve problems, and process information. Individuals with impairments in speech, language, or hearing and their families can benefit substantially from the research and clinical services provided by speech, language, and hearing scientists, audiologists, SLPs, and deaf educators.

CSD is a relatively new discipline. The term *communication sciences and disorders* has been used for only the last 15 or 20 years. The terms *speech pathology* and *audiology* have longer histories. For example, Lee Edward Travis first used the term *speech pathology* in 1924 in a course description for clinical psychology of speech (Moeller, 1976). The word *language* was added to form the term *speech-language pathology* when it became obvious that professionals were dealing with much more than just the process of speech production. Drs. Ray Carhart and Norton Canfield coined the term *audiology* during World War II to describe a new science that focused on the aural (hearing) rehabilitation of individuals who suffered war-related hearing loss (Newby, 1958). World War II was a catalyst for the advancement of the field of audiology and fostered a union among the fields of audiology and speech pathology.

Early leaders in CSD stressed the importance of basing treatment on sound research. The emphasis on scientific problem solving in the laboratory, the clinical setting (hospitals and private practices), and the classroom (schools) is a hallmark of the discipline of CSD. We believe it is critical that all assessment and treatment decisions be based on sound scientific principles and research findings. Today, we use the term

evidence-based practice to describe how decisions that professionals make about clinical service delivery are guided by high-quality clinical research. In fact, federal guidelines related to Medicare, No Child Left Behind, and the Individuals with Disabilities Education Act mandate that SLPs and audiologists provide treatment that is based on sound scientific evidence.

The next sections of this chapter focus on the nature of communication, types of communication disorders and the roles that speech, language, and hearing scientists, SLPs, audiologists, and deaf educators play in studying, assessing, and treating individuals with communication disorders.

INDIVIDUALS WITH COMMUNICATION DISORDERS

Communication involves an exchange of meaning between a sender and a receiver. Most of the time, meanings are exchanged via a code, called language, that can be written or signed, but that is most often spoken. A simple way to differentiate between language and speech is to remember that language is what you say (i.e., the meanings of words and sentences) and speech is how you say it (i.e., the sounds that make up the words and sentences).

Speakers articulate a series of programmed movements to form sequences of sounds that represent words, phrases, and sentences. Then, listeners interpret the message by converting the acoustic (sound) energy that reaches their ears into mental representations of words and sentences. Through communication, the individual can influence society at large. At the same time, social and cultural experiences play an important role in shaping the way individuals think and communicate.

Most people communicate pretty effectively by the time they are 3 or 4 years old, and most children are relatively expert at this process by the time they are 9 years old. Unfortunately, there are many ways that the processes involved in communication can break down. When they do, people routinely turn to SLPs and audiologists for help.

This chapter presents a systematic classification of communication differences and disorders and the kinds of communicative disruptions that individuals experience when they have difficulties with one or more of the processes that contribute to speech, language, and hearing. It is important to realize that communication is a system with many reciprocal relationships. A problem with one aspect of the communication process often affects many of the other processes that are related to it. For example, children who have a hearing loss receive limited acoustic input, which adversely affects the development of their language and speech. The language and speech problems experienced by children who have a hearing loss often have an adverse impact on their social and academic development.

Communication Disorders

There are appropriate and inappropriate ways to refer to people who have unusual difficulties with communication. According to the World Health Organization (Wood, 1980), the word **impairment** should be used to refer to any loss or abnormality of psychological, physiological, or anatomic structure or function. This is a relatively neutral term with respect to a person's ability to function in society. For example, a hearing impairment means only that someone has unusually poor hearing. It doesn't mean that the individual cannot function well in daily living and working situations. With hearing aids, the person with a hearing impairment might live life as completely and fully as people who hear well. The concept of impairment leads us to ask questions such as, "What is wrong with the person, and can it be fixed? What does this person do well? What skills and abilities can be used to compensate for this person's impairment?"

The word **disability** refers to a reduced competence in meeting daily living needs. The person with a disability might not be able to perform a particular life activity in a particular context. For example, a person with hearing impairment might not be able to communicate well on the telephone, even when he or she is wearing a hearing aid. In this case, the hearing impairment led to a disability. The concept of a disability leads us to ask, "What are the communication requirements of the environments that the individual functions in every day, and to what extent can the person access important daily living activities if some sort of compensation (such as a hearing aid) is provided?"

The word **handicap** refers to a social, educational, or occupational disadvantage that results from an impairment or disability. This disadvantage is often affected by the nature of the person's impairment and by the attitudes and biases that may be present in the person's environment. For example, a child with a hearing loss may have a hearing aid that allows him or her to hear most speech sounds without difficulties. However, he or she might not be able to hear very well in a noisy classroom. Unless the classroom teacher undertakes measures to lessen the extent of classroom noise, the child might not hear important classroom instructions, resulting in an educational handicap. The concept of a handicap leads us to ask, "Does this person experience social, educational, and vocational penalties? To what extent can we lessen these penalties by compensating for the person's impairment and by educating important people in the environment about ways that they can modify the environment?" The term *handicap* is considered to be pejorative by many people and is not used often.

The term **communication disorder** is sometimes used as a synonym for impairment and other times as a synonym for disability. In this book, we use the term *communication disorder* to refer to any communication structure or function that is diminished to a significant degree. In essence, a communication disorder interferes with the exchange of meaning and is apparent to the communication partners. Unless specifically stated, we do not imply any cultural, educational, or vocational disadvantage. Unfortunately, many people with communication disorders experience communication disabilities and handicaps, although this is not necessarily so.

Communication Differences

Some people communicate in ways that differ from that of the mainstream culture. We use the term **communication difference** to mean communication abilities that differ from those usually encountered in the mainstream culture even though there is no evidence of impairment. For example, when they begin school, children who have spoken Spanish for most of their lives will not communicate like their monolingual

English-speaking classmates. Children who learn Spanish without any difficulty do not have a communication disorder. Unfortunately, these children's communication differences may contribute to periodic social and educational disadvantages within the school environment. These children may need extra assistance in learning English as a second language. However, unless children present communication impairments (characterized by loss or decline in communicative structures or functions that adversely affects their communication in all the languages they speak), they should not be diagnosed with a communication disorder, and should not be treated by SLPs or audiologists. There is much more information about communication differences in Chapter 3.

Person-First Language

It is important to recognize that the problems that individuals experience do not define who they are. For example, a person who stutters is not just a stutterer. That person may be a caring parent, a good friend, a successful business owner, or even a good communicator. For this reason, most researchers and clinicians use **person-first language** to refer to individuals with communication disorders. By "person-first," we mean that the communication disorder is a descriptor of the individual and not a person's primary attribute. We follow that convention as much as possible in this book by using such phrases as "children with language disorders" instead of "language-disordered children." When we refer to groups of individuals who present a particular disorder, we might sometimes use the name of the disorder alone (i.e., "aphasics"). When we use the name of a communication disorder to refer to the group of individuals who present that disorder, readers should know that we do not mean to imply that the disorder is the sole defining characteristic of individuals who happen to present that kind of problem. As a matter of fact, many of the people we work with tell us that they do not like to be defined by their disabilities.

TYPES OF COMMUNICATION DISORDERS

Communication disorders typically are categorized into speech disorders, language disorders, and hearing disorders. Additional parameters of classification include the etiological basis (cause) of the disorder and the point during the maturation of the individual that the disorder occurred. **Organic** disorders have a physical cause. For example, an adult with difficulty retrieving words after a stroke and a child who has problems producing speech sounds as a result of inadequate closure between the nose and mouth after the repair of a cleft palate have a physical problem that can account for the communication problem. In contrast, there are communication disorders termed **functional** for which a physical cause cannot be found. For example, a man may continue to speak at the same pitch as a child even though the vocal folds are normal. In this case, there is no physical basis for the problem. For some communication disorders, it is difficult to determine whether the cause of the disorder would best be described as organic or functional. A young child may have difficulty producing speech sounds in comparison to peers, but it is not known with surety whether the disorder is organic in nature (e.g., a result of delayed maturation of the nervous system) or functional (e.g., a result of poor speech models or lack of environmental opportunity for speaking).

When the disorder occurs is also an important consideration. **Developmental disorders**, such as delays in speech and language development, occur early in the maturation of the individual but may continue into adulthood. **Acquired disorders**, such as speech and language disorders resulting from brain trauma following an accident, occur after communication skills have been fully developed.

With these distinctions in mind we provide a brief overview of hearing, speech, and language disorders. We make some reference to the **incidence** (percentage of the population that experienced a disorder during their lifetime) and **prevalence** (number of individuals with a disorder at some point in time). More detailed information about each disorder is provided in later chapters.

Speech Disorders

Speech disorders (Table 1-1) result from an interruption in the process of speech production. This process starts with the programming of motor movements and ends with the acoustic signal that carries the sound to the listener. By historical convention, speech disorders are categorized on the basis of the aspect of speech production (articulation, fluency, voice, etc.) that is affected.

Articulation and Phonological Disorders

Individuals with **articulation and phonological disorders** have problems with the production of speech sounds. Such problems result from deviations in anatomic structures, physiological functions, and learning. When the problem is thought to be related to the way sounds are represented in the brain, it is commonly referred to as a phonological disorder. The problem may be minimal at one extreme (interfering with the way that one or two speech sounds, like /s/ or /r/ are produced) or severe, rendering speech unintelligible. Included in this category are developmental speech disorders,

Table 1-1 Speech Disorders

Disorder	Characteristics
Articulation and phonological disorders	Problems producing speech sounds correctly as a result of differences in anatomic structures, physiological functions, or learning.
Cleft palate	Nasal loss of air during consonant production; abnormal resonance, speech sound production errors
Cerebral palsy	Articulation and voice disorders associated with abnormal muscle function in children.
Fluency disorder	Unusual disruptions in the rhythm and rate of speech. These disruptions are often characterized by repetitions or prolongations of sounds or syllables plus excessive tension.

neuromuscular speech disorders in adults and children, and articulation disorders resulting from orofacial anomalies such as cleft palate. Approximately 10% of preschool and school-age children present articulatory or phonological disorders (National Institute on Deafness and Other Communication Disorders, 2007).

Fluency Disorders

A **fluency disorder** is an unusual interruption in the flow of speaking. Individuals with fluency disorders have an atypical rhythm and rate and an unusual number of sound and syllable repetitions. Their disruptions in fluency are often accompanied by excessive tension, and they may struggle visibly to produce the words they want to say. The most common fluency disorder is stuttering. Approximately 1% of the general population stutters, but as many as 5% of all adults report they stuttered at some point in their lives.

Voice Disorders

The category of voice disorders is usually divided into two parts: phonation and resonation. **Phonatory disorder**s result from abnormalities in vocal fold vibration that yield changes in loudness, pitch, or quality (e.g., breathiness, harshness, or hoarseness). Problems closing the opening between the nose and the mouth during production of speech sounds are termed **resonance disorders**. It has been estimated that between 3% and 9% of the total population of the United States has some type of a voice disorder (National Institute on Deafness and Other Communication Disorders, 2007).

Language Disorders

Language refers to the words and sentences that are used to represent objects, thoughts, and feelings. A language disorder is a significant deficiency in understanding or in creating messages. There are three main types of language disorders: developmental (or functional) language disorders that occur during childhood, acquired language disorders that can occur during childhood but most often occur in older adults, and dementia, which nearly always occurs in older adults. It has been estimated that between 6 million and 8 million individuals in the United States have some form of language disorder (National Institute on Deafness and Other Communication Disorders, 2007).

Language Delay

During the preschool years, some children have delayed language development that is not associated with a known etiology. That is, children have difficulties using and understanding language for no apparent reason. These children have smaller vocabularies, shorter sentences, and they may not say as much as most other children their age. Approximately half of the children who have significant early language delays (i.e., vocabularies less than 50 words) at 2 years of age will have language growth spurts that enable them to catch up to their same-age peers by the time they are 5 years old (Paul, Hernandez, Taylor, & Johnson, 1996). Unfortunately, we do not yet know how to predict which children with early language delays will outgrow them and which children will not.

Developmental Language Disorder

Some children have impaired language comprehension and/or production problems that significantly interfere with socialization and educational success. These children might have a variety of problems including difficulty formulating sentences that express what they want to say, an unusual number of grammatical errors, difficulties thinking of words they know at the moment they need them, and/or difficulties with the social use of language (they tend to say the wrong thing at the wrong time). As with language delay, language disorder is not associated with a specific cause. Until children are in the late preschool and early school-age years, it is difficult to distinguish a language delay from a language disorder. A language disorder may be differentiated from language delay when the impairment persists beyond age 5 and children do not catch up with their peers. Between 6% and 8% of all children have language disorders. The primary types of childhood language disorders are presented in Table 1-2.

Acquired Language Disorders

Acquired language disorders are caused by brain lesions, which are specific areas of damage to the brain. The most common type of an acquired language disorder is aphasia, which typically occurs in older adults after they have suffered a cerebrovascular accident or stroke. Individuals with aphasia frequently have trouble remembering words they once knew or using sentence structures they once used without any problems. It has been estimated that about 1 million Americans have aphasia, and

Table 1-2 Common Developmental Language Disorders

Disorder	Characteristics
Intellectual disability	Significantly subaverage mental function with associated difficulties in communication, self-help skills, independence, and motor development.
Specific language impairment	Significant deficits in language abilities that cannot be attributed to deficits in hearing, intelligence, or motor functioning.
Autism spectrum disorders	Unusual disturbances in social interaction, communication, behaviors, interests, and activities that affect the capacity to relate appropriately to people, events, and objects.
Central auditory processing disorder	Difficulty identifying, interpreting, or organizing auditory information despite normal auditory acuity.
Learning disability	Difficulties in the acquisition and use of listening, speaking, reading, writing, reasoning, or mathematical abilities.
Dyslexia	A specific reading disorder that results from difficulties with phonological representation and phonological analysis.

approximately 80,000 individuals acquire aphasia each year (American Speech-Language-Hearing Association [ASHA], 2000).

Traumatic injury to the brain results in a syndrome of cognitive and language disturbances. The communication deficits associated with the injury are primarily a consequence of impaired cognitive processes related to memory, orientation, and organization and include problems more apparent in communication than in speech and language functioning. Most cases of brain trauma are caused by motor vehicle accidents with an incidence of approximately 7 million new cases each year.

Dementia

Dementia is a general mental deterioration resulting from a pathological deterioration of the brain. Dementia is characterized by disorientation; impaired memory, judgment, and intellect; and shallow affect. It is most often seen in individuals who have Alzheimer's disease. Many of the estimated 2 million Americans with dementing diseases such as Alzheimer's disease and Parkinson's disease also have significant language impairments.

Hearing Disorders

People with hearing disorders have a deficiency in their ability to detect sounds. This deficiency can vary in terms of how loud sounds need to be presented before they can be heard. Hearing can also vary with respect to the pitch level of the sounds that are heard. Some individuals can hear low-frequency sounds such as the notes from a bass guitar better than they can hear high-frequency sounds such as a small bell. Other individuals do not hear sounds at any frequency very well. According to the ASHA (ASHA, 2000), of the estimated 46 million citizens with a communication disorder, more than 28 million have some kind of hearing disorder.

Hearing loss can have a large or small effect on communication depending on the degree of loss and the type of sounds that are affected (see Table 1-3).

People with mild degrees of hearing loss that affect only their ability to hear high-pitched sounds will miss out on final sounds of words like *bath*, but they will hear most other sounds reasonably well enough so that they can usually fill in the missing pieces. For example, you can probably read the following sentence even though the letters representing the final sounds are missing, "Joh_ wen_ upstair_ to ta_ a ba_ ." However, people with a hearing loss that affects their ability to hear high- and low-pitched sounds produced at conversational speech levels will be at a significant disadvantage in communication. Imagine what you might think this sentence means if you could hear only the following sounds, "_o__ we_ u__air_ _o _a_ a _a_ ."

If you could not hear conversations, it would be difficult for you to interact with your friends, to take notes in your classes, or to perform the duties associated with most jobs. Thus, there can be serious social, educational, and vocational consequences of moderate to severe hearing losses. Other important factors that influence the degree of the impact that a hearing loss has on communication include whether the hearing loss is **unilateral** (one ear) or **bilateral** (two ears), the kind of amplification that is

Table 1-3 The Impact of Hearing Loss on Communication

Degree of Loss	Severity	Impact on Communication
15–30 dB	Mild	Can hear all vowels and most consonants spoken at conversational loudness levels. Children with this degree of loss typically experience some difficulties with communication development until they receive appropriate amplification. Adults with this degree of loss have some difficulty understanding women and children with high-pitched voices, and they may struggle with conversation in noisy environments such as restaurants.
30–50 dB	Moderate	Can hear most vowels and some consonants spoken at conversational loudness levels. People with this degree of hearing loss find it difficult to hear unstressed words and word endings. Children with this degree of loss experience significant delays in communication development. Adults with this degree of loss have some difficulty understanding others during conversations.
50–70 dB	Severe	Can hear most loud noises in the environment (car horns) but not speech unless it is spoken very loudly. Children usually have marked communication difficulties and delays. Adults miss a significant amount of information spoken in conversations.
70+ dB	Profound	Can hear extremely loud noises (jet planes landing) but cannot hear language spoken at conversational levels. Without suitable amplification, individuals with this degree of hearing loss are not able to communicate through speech.

provided, the length of time the individual has had amplification, and the attitudes of the individual and his or her family members.

The age of the person with a hearing loss also plays an important role in the degree of impact that a hearing loss has on communication. A moderate hearing loss that is present from birth is much more problematic than a moderate hearing loss that is contracted when an individual is 40 years old. That is because good hearing is critical for communicative development. Children who do not hear well have considerable difficulties understanding language that is spoken to them, learning to produce speech sounds clearly, and developing the words and sentence structures necessary for expressing complex ideas. Early detection of hearing loss is absolutely critical so that children can receive intervention as soon as possible. Some children can profit a great deal from being fitted with a hearing aid. The sooner they receive appropriate amplification, the better it is for speech and language development. Other children are able to not hear much even with amplification. These children need to be exposed to sign language or specialized speech training to develop language.

Many people believe that people who have a hearing loss simply cannot hear sounds as loud as others hear them. If this were the case, the obvious solution to any hearing loss would be to simply make sounds louder to make them audible. Although this conception of hearing loss is sometimes accurate, more often the ability to hear speech is more complicated. Not only do people with hearing impairments perceive sounds as being less loud, but they also perceive sounds as less clear. So, even when speech is amplified so that it is louder, individuals with some kinds of hearing losses may still have difficulty with **discrimination** (hearing differences between sounds) as a result of a loss of the clarity of sounds. For example, they may confuse the word *ball* for the word *doll*. In effect, they hear but do not understand because the auditory information is distorted. The degree of deterioration of the auditory image is often directly related to the degree of the hearing loss. The result is that it can be difficult to find the kind of hearing aid that will assist some people with hearing loss. Fortunately, in its short life (about 50 years), audiology has advanced to the point where diagnosis and rehabilitation measures can assist the majority of children and adults.

THE PROFESSIONS

The remainder of this chapter provides a brief overview of the professionals who serve individuals with speech, language, or hearing disorders. More information about the specific disorders is also provided.

Speech, Language, and Hearing Scientists

For our purposes, we consider speech, language, and hearing sciences as the investigation of anatomic, physiological, and perceptual factors that form the bases of and contribute to the production and comprehension of speech and language. Some of the research conducted in this area is directed toward the exploration of other human processes (e.g., visual processes) that may help us understand how we communicate.

Speech, language, and hearing scientists come from a variety of educational backgrounds. These professionals often hold advanced degrees, most often a Doctor of Philosophy. Their degrees may be awarded in areas such as engineering, anatomy and physiology, biological sciences, CSD, education, linguistics, physics, psychology, or speech communication.

Speech, language, and hearing scientists most often engage in research and teaching in university settings. However, some work for governmental agencies such as the Veterans Administration or for independent operations such as Bell Telephone and Haskins Laboratories. The primary goal of the speech, language, and/or hearing scientist is to discover and better understand human communication processes. Some scientists are engaged in research that deals exclusively with the normal processes of communication. We need information on normal communication to determine whether a patient's performance on measures of speech and language functioning is within the normal range or not. Other scientists focus on the processes that are different in disordered communication. Regardless of the underlying objectives, however, basic research about communication will undoubtedly be of value to professionals in speech-language pathology and audiology and individuals with communication differences and disorders.

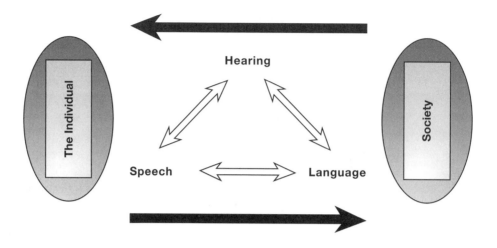

Figure 1-1 Hearing, speech, and language as links between the individual and society.

Some speech scientists contribute to criminal investigations. For example, speech scientists have the ability to identify characteristics in the voice that can be used to identify specific speakers. These acoustic characteristics can be as distinctive as the human fingerprint. Speech scientists can assist law enforcement personnel in identifying speakers whose voices have been recorded as part of an investigation of a crime.

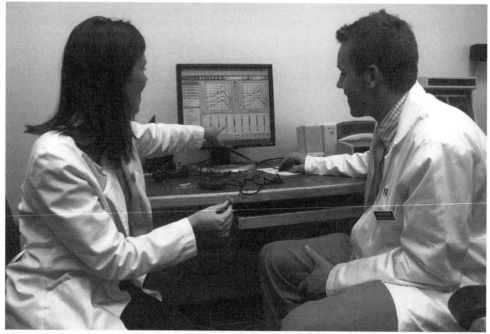

Figure 1-2 Two hearing scientists preparing stimuli for a study of speech perception. Courtesy of Ronald Gillam, Utah State University

It is vital that the practicing professional stay abreast of current research results to provide the best possible services. Some of the measurements we can obtain through speech, language, and hearing science are useful in measuring the effectiveness of treatment programs that we implement with our patients. For example, certain measures that we can obtain from the human voice can help us to determine whether a particular approach for treating cancer of the larynx is effective.

A firm grounding in normal communication processes is necessary to pursue any of the professions in our discipline. As a result, a course of study emphasizing science is an integral part of the curriculum in CSD. Course work with titles such as hearing science, speech science, language science, language acquisition, neurolinguistics, psychoacoustics, and psycholinguistics are regular offerings in CSD departments and programs. Many of these courses occur early in the academic program so that students will have the prerequisite knowledge they need to understand breakdowns in communication, ways to analyze those breakdowns, and ways to help individuals with communication breakdowns.

Speech-Language Pathologists

Approximately 200,000 professional SLPs work in various settings today. It is amazing that there were fewer than 5,000 such practitioners 50 years ago. These professionals assess and treat a variety of individuals with speech and/or language disorders.

Speech-language pathology developed from interests in disorders of speech, particularly stuttering. Much of the early research was aimed at discovering the causes of stuttering, but soon attention was directed to providing remedial services to individuals with various types of speech problems. As early as the 1920s, academic courses in "speech correction" were offered at some universities. Clinical sites for providing services to individuals with problems in speech and language, however, were limited. Initially, the vast majority of such services were provided at college and university clinics that were developed primarily as training facilities. Increasingly, however, service programs were developed in medical settings and the public schools.

Speech-language pathology professionals who practiced in the medical environment were usually called speech therapists; those who practiced in the public school setting were often called speech correctionists or speech teachers. Although the term *speech pathologist* was introduced early in the development of the field and was widely used by those in the profession for many years, the term *speech therapist* is probably the title that is most often used by the general public. The ASHA adopted the title *speech-language pathologist* in 1976. The term *language* was added to the official title because much of the work being done by CSD professionals concerned both speech production (how words and sentences are spoken) and symbolic language (the form and content of what is said and understood). The term *pathologist* was selected to emphasize that CSD professionals prescribe and deliver their own treatment. They do not work under doctor's orders. Thus, although it is rather cumbersome, the designator of choice for the profession has become the speech-language pathologist, which is often shortened to SLP.

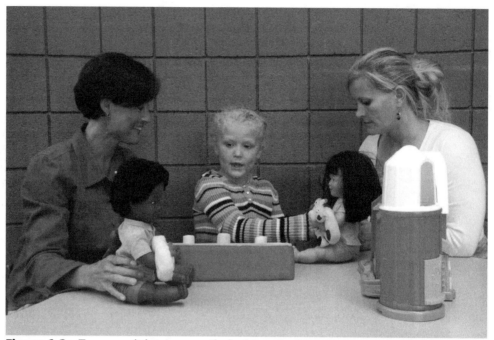

Figure 1-3 Two speech-language pathologists collecting a language sample from a child. Courtesy of Ronald Gillam, Utah State University

Speech-language pathology services are provided in schools, hospitals, rehabilitation centers, nursing homes, and private clinical practices. Increasingly, speech-language pathology services are also being provided in infant and early childhood programs housed in state agencies and private schools. Thus, the SLP provides assessment and rehabilitation services to patients from birth to old age. The kinds of activities that SLPs are engaged in depends largely on the setting in which they work.

It is ASHA's official policy that a master's degree should be the minimum qualification for working as an SLP. Many states have licensure laws that make it illegal for individuals who do not have a master's degree to provide services as an SLP.

Audiologists

Audiology is a widely recognized profession that is practiced in many different work environments. Audiologists are professionals who study, assess, and treat individuals who have hearing impairments. Some audiologists are engaged in the evaluation and diagnosis of hearing loss; others provide educational and/or rehabilitative services. The number of professional audiologists has increased significantly in the past 50 years, but there are far fewer audiologists than there are SLPs. It has been estimated that between 20,000 and 25,000 audiologists practice in the United States today.

Audiology was first identified as an area of scientific study and professional practice during World War II. This area of study grew out of a merger between audiology and *otology* services provided to soldiers and veterans in aural rehabilitation centers (Newby, 1958). **Otology** is the medical specialty that deals with ear disease and the peripheral hearing mechanism. Although professionals worked with persons who were hearing impaired prior to the 1940s, the professional field of audiology was not in existence before that time.

Since the beginning of the profession, many audiologists have been employed in medical environments such as physicians' offices, hospitals, and rehabilitation centers. Other audiologists, sometimes referred to as educational or habilitative audiologists, are employed in educational facilities such as public schools or schools for the deaf or hearing impaired. Increasing numbers of audiologists own private practices where they dispense hearing aids and other devices.

Audiologists have traditionally been engaged in the evaluation of the extent and type of hearing loss, assessment of the benefits of amplification, and habilitation and rehabilitation of those who exhibit hearing impairments. Primarily, their employment setting influences the kinds of activities they are engaged in. For example, audiologists employed by physicians spend most of their time evaluating patients to determine the nature and extent of a hearing loss and the potential benefits of amplification (hearing aids). Audiologists employed in educational or rehabilitation centers are more likely to provide both assessment and rehabilitative services.

Audiologists may work with newborn children providing hearing screenings in the neonatal intensive care unit or the newborn nursery. They also work with children in schools, patients in hospitals and doctors' offices, and with older adults in nursing

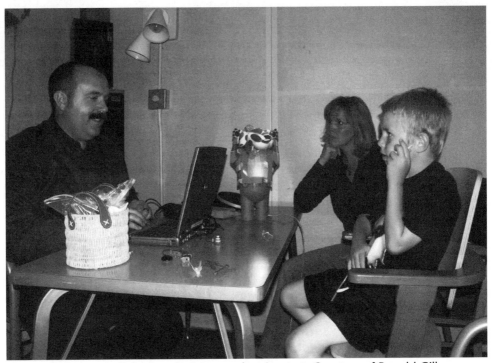

Figure 1-4 An audiologist administers a hearing test. Courtesy of Ronald Gillam, Utah State University

homes. Audiologists assess how well individuals hear tones, words, and sentences. Based on these assessments, audiologists make recommendations to parents, patients, physicians, and school personnel about how a hearing loss should be managed and what the ramifications of the loss will be. Most children are screened for hearing problems early in their school years. You have probably received a hearing test at some point in your life, and the examiner may well have been an audiologist. Some audiologists also provide assessments for balance disorders caused by inner ear problems or program cochlear implants. The scope of practice for audiologists is always changing and expanding, making it a very exciting profession to be a part of.

The current policy of the ASHA is that a doctorate of audiology (commonly referred to as an AuD) is the minimal level of education for an individual to practice as an independent professional. Satisfactory completion of specified course work and clinical practice as part of the degree is also necessary. Other requirements to qualify for professional credentials exist, and we consider them in later chapters.

PROFESSIONAL AND SCHOLARLY ASSOCIATIONS

There are a number of associations that speech, language, and hearing scientists, SLPs, and audiologists can join. Some of these associations are discussed in this section.

American Speech-Language-Hearing Association

ASHA serves as the primary professional and scholarly home for speech, language, and hearing scientists, SLPs, and audiologists. ASHA is a large organization (approximately 120,000 members and growing) with headquarters in Rockville, Maryland, near the nation's capital. ASHA engages in numerous activities designed to serve the needs of its members as well as individuals with communication disorders. Some of these activities include research dissemination, public relations, and lobbying for CSD professionals and the public they serve.

Another useful function of ASHA is making information available to its members and other interested individuals, including students. There is a toll-free number, 1-888-321-2724, for all kinds of information about the organization, the discipline, and the professions. ASHA also maintains a Web site, www.asha.org, with a vast amount of data that are continually updated. ASHA also sponsors an annual convention and many local workshops that provide members and students with important information about new research results and clinical procedures.

Publications

One of the important functions of ASHA is to provide information to its members through research and professional publications. ASHA publishes several scholarly and professional journals on a regular basis. These include the *Journal of Speech, Language, and Hearing Research*, the *American Journal of Audiology*, the *American Journal of Speech-Language Pathology*, and *Language, Speech, and Hearing Services in Schools*. In addition, ASHA regularly publishes a number of newsletters that address many important issues, such as the *ASHA Leader*.

American Academy of Audiology

Several associations comprise almost exclusively audiologists, whereas other organizations include subgroups of audiologists. Examples of those organizations are the Academy of Dispensing Audiologists, the Academy of Rehabilitative Audiologists, and the Educational Audiology Association. The American Academy of Audiology (AAA) was created to address the needs of all audiologists. The academy has grown rapidly to 5,000 members since it was founded in 1994. The goal of the academy is to provide an organization specifically for audiologists (Hood, 1994). Some of the activities in place or planned by AAA are also carried out by ASHA. Examples include approving and monitoring continuing education experiences for members and certifying audiologists. AAA also sponsors annual conventions and various publications.

REGULATION

Consumers want to know that persons who present themselves as physicians, lawyers, SLPs, or audiologists (to name just a few service-oriented professions) have received an appropriate level of training in their area. Just as you would not want to be operated on by a physician who failed medical school, you would not want to be fitted for a hearing aid by someone whose education and training consisted of a 10-page correspondence course on hearing aids from the Quickie School of Easy Degrees. Poor services by SLPs and audiologists can cause real harm. To protect the public interest, audiology and speech-language pathology must be regulated.

There are basically two ways in which individual professionals are regulated: **licensure** and **certification**. For the purposes of this discussion, *licensure* refers to fully credentialed SLPs and audiologists as defined by an individual state. In the case of licensure, a state government passes an act (a law) that creates a set of minimum criteria for practicing as a professional in that state. Most licensure acts also create state-funded licensure boards of examiners who manage the law through writing implementation rules and monitoring the process and the licensees.

State licensure of speech-language pathology and audiology is relatively new. Florida adopted the first licensure act for speech-language pathology and audiology in 1969. Since that time the number of states that regulate speech-language pathology and audiology has steadily increased. Presently, 46 states license both SLPs and audiologists. The other four states regulate speech-language pathology or audiology, but not both.

Certification is somewhat different from licensure in that the standards are developed and administered by professional organizations or state agencies. In the case of speech-language pathology and audiology, this function is assumed by standards boards that are affiliated with ASHA. These boards also set criteria and monitor **accreditation** of academic programs and facilities providing clinical services in CSD.

Licensure and Certification Standards

ASHA developed a standards program to certify individuals in speech-language pathology and audiology at a time when there were no state regulations and no licensure laws related to these professions. A person may be certified by ASHA and licensed in a state (or multiple states) in either speech-language pathology or audiology or both.

SLPs can obtain the **Certificate of Clinical Competence (CCC)** in either profession from ASHA. To obtain the CCC, the applicant must have earned a master's degree or a higher degree with a major emphasis in speech-language pathology or a professional AuD degree. The academic content areas that the course work must include are specified, and it is further required that students satisfactorily complete supervised clinical practice during their education. During their graduate education, students in speech-language pathology and audiology must have met the academic and clinical competencies specified on the Knowledge and Skills Acquisition summary form. Finally, applicants must obtain a passing score on a national, standardized examination and complete an internship known as a clinical fellowship year (CFY).

It is important for practicing SLPs and audiologists to have the CCC as well as a state license. These credentials assure the consumer that the professional has met minimum educational and practical prerequisites. In addition, professionals who provide speech-language pathology or audiology services often need to have the CCC to be reimbursed for their services. Federal laws and regulations have been adopted that require that all Medicare or Medicaid speech-language pathology or audiology services must be provided or supervised by a person holding the CCC. A number of insurance carriers who reimburse for speech-language pathology or audiology services have adopted similar requirements. Agencies, including public school programs that receive reimbursement for these services, must ensure that qualified personnel as defined by the regulations provide them. These regulations have a major impact on funding and are a strong incentive for agencies to hire qualified personnel.

Professional education doesn't end after completing a graduate degree and qualifying for the CCC. ASHA now requires that professionals complete 30 hours of continuing education, or 3.0 **continuing education units (CEUs)** in a 36-month cycle to maintain the CCC. Similarly, 41 states require continuing education for license renewal. Most state licenses are issued on an annual basis and thus must be renewed each year. In those states that require continuing education, the renewal application must include evidence of the satisfactory completion of CEUs.

ETHICS

The principles of conduct governing an individual or a group are called **ethics**. Generally, we think of ethics as a measure of what is the moral or "right thing to do" whether or not it is legal. One overriding consideration for professionals (providers) who serve the public is that their activities be in the best interest of the consumer and not themselves. For example, an audiologist may recommend a hearing aid that he or she thinks is the most appropriate for the type and degree of hearing loss the patient is experiencing. An audiologist may not recommend a particular hearing aid for a patient based on the knowledge that one more sale of a certain brand of hearing aid will result in a free trip to Aruba for the audiologist. Although this is an obvious breach of ethical principles, it is often the case that professionals disagree about what constitutes ethical behavior. Therefore, most professional groups, including ASHA, have developed official codes of ethics (ASHA, 2007). Table 1-4 summarizes the principles of ethics that have been adopted by ASHA.

Table 1-4 Principles of Ethics and Representative Rules of Ethics from the Code of Ethics of the American Speech-Language-Hearing Association

PRINCIPLE I   Individuals shall honor their responsibility to hold paramount the welfare of persons they serve professionally.
- Individuals shall provide all services competently.
- Individuals shall use every resource, including referral, to ensure that high-quality services are provided.
- Individuals shall not discriminate in the delivery of professional services on the basis of race, sex, age, religion, national origin, sexual orientation, or handicapping condition.
- Individuals shall not reveal, without authorization, any professional or personal information about the person served professionally, unless required by law to do so or unless doing so is necessary to protect the welfare of the person or of the community.

PRINCIPLE II   Individuals shall honor their responsibility to achieve and maintain the highest level of professional competence.
- Individuals shall engage in only those aspects of the professions that are within the scope of their competence considering their level of education, training, and experience.
- Individuals shall continue their professional development throughout their careers.

PRINCIPLE III   Individuals shall honor their responsibility to the public by promoting public understanding of the professions, by supporting the development of services designed to fulfill the unmet needs of the public, and by providing accurate information in all communications involving any aspect of the professions.
- Individuals shall not misrepresent their credentials, competence, education, training, or experience.
- Individuals shall not misrepresent diagnostic information, services rendered, or products dispensed or engage in any scheme or artifice to defraud in connection with obtaining payment or reimbursement for such services or products.

PRINCIPLE IV   Individuals shall honor their responsibilities to the professions and their relationships with colleagues, students, and members of allied professions. Individuals shall uphold the dignity and autonomy of the profession, maintain harmonious interprofessional and intraprofessional relationships, and accept the professions' self-imposed standards.
- Individuals shall not engage in dishonesty, fraud, deceit, misrepresentation, or any form of conduct that adversely reflects on the professions or on the individual's fitness to serve persons professionally.
- Individuals' statements to colleagues about professional services, research results, and products shall adhere to prevailing professional standards and shall contain no misrepresentations.
- Individuals who have reason to believe that the Code of Ethics has been violated shall inform the Ethical Practice Board.

Source: Reprinted with permission from *Code of Ethics* [Ethics]. Available from www.asha.org/policy. Copyright 2003 by American Speech-Language-Hearing Association.

Codes of ethics are subject to change as new issues arise or as views as to what constitutes ethical behavior are modified. For example, at one time it was considered unethical for speech and language therapy to be provided solely by correspondence (over the phone, with written documents only). Today, speech language pathology services are frequently provided via telecommunication (computer/Internet based) in areas of the country where SLPs are in short supply. Ethical considerations regarding the extent to which services may be provided over the Internet are still being developed. For example, is it ethical to provide all assessment and intervention services to patients who demonstrate significant swallowing difficulties (dysphagia) over the Internet? Some would argue that there is a safety issue with regard to choking (aspiration) that precludes SLPs from providing dysphagia services except in face-to-face contexts. Others would disagree.

Because people have different beliefs as to what constitutes ethical and unethical behavior, enforcement of ethical practices may be problematic. Among professional organizations, including ASHA, once a code of ethics has been adopted by the membership, the organization must assume the responsibility of enforcing the code. The Ethical Practices Board (EPB) of ASHA is charged with enforcing the ASHA code of ethics. If an individual member has been judged to be in violation of the code, a number of disciplinary actions are available to the EPB. These include reprimands, censures, or revocation of licenses (Irwin, Pannbacker, Powell, & Vekovius, 2007).

Most states that have adopted licensure laws have also drafted codes of ethics and have the authority to enforce them legally. Sharing of information among the states and with ASHA is critical to protect the public from unethical practitioners.

SUMMARY

CSD is a discipline that consists of three professions: speech, language, and hearing sciences, speech-language pathology, and audiology. Professionals in this discipline study and treat individuals with a variety of disorders that affect speech, language, and hearing abilities.

This chapter provides information about the professions in terms of scopes of practice, academic preparation, work settings, and populations served. Speech, language, and hearing scientists study basic communication processes and the nature of speech, language, and/or hearing disorders. Most scientists work in university settings, although some work in hospitals as well. SLPs assess and treat speech and language disorders in infants, toddlers, preschoolers, school-age children, and adults. They may work in medical or educational settings. Audiologists primarily test hearing and prescribe and fit hearing aids. Most audiologists work in medical settings, although many have established their own private practices.

This chapter introduces some of the differences and disorders encountered by individuals that interfere with their abilities to communicate. These disorders are discussed in greater detail in the sections that follow this chapter. We want readers to have a general sense of the breadth of the field of CSD before we review specific types of disorders in greater detail. Some communication disorders relate to the way individuals receive information. These disorders involve various degrees and kinds of hearing abnormalities. Other communication disorders involve the way information is processed after it is received. These disorders involve various degrees and kinds of language difficulties. Finally, some communication disorders affect output, including difficulties related to speech articulation, voice, and fluency. As with any difficulty, speech, language, and hearing impairments exist on a continuum.

ASHA is the primary scholarly and professional home for the discipline. It publishes journals that disseminate research findings, promotes the professions in the media, and lobbies for CSD professionals and the public they serve. The association also operates a standards program that certifies individuals within the professions, accredits academic programs and clinical facilities, and maintains a code of ethics. Students can also join other professional organizations such as the AAA and the National Student Speech Language Hearing Association.

SLPs and audiologists are regulated through certification by ASHA and by state agencies. Professionals who obtain a master's degree (SLPs) and/or AuD (audiologists), pass a national examination, and complete a CFY are eligible for the CCC from ASHA. These same kinds of experiences are often required for obtaining a state license.

As you read the rest of this book, we hope you will remember that there are reciprocal relationships between input, processing, and output systems. A disorder in hearing, speech, or language will have negative consequences for the other two. The specific consequences vary somewhat from person to person. This is why SLPs and audiologists need to work closely with individuals with communication disorders, their families, and with other professionals. This is also why any type of a communication disorder requires careful analysis and description before therapy begins.

BOX 1-1 Personal Story by Ron Gillam

I am a person who stutters. Fortunately, with the help of a number of influential speech-language pathologists, I have learned how to control my fluency and to minimize my speaking fears and my feelings of shame about stuttering to the point that stuttering plays a relatively minor role in my life. I give speeches to large audiences several times each year; I serve on or chair a number of professional committees; I teach university classes; and I spend too much time talking on the phone each day—all with relatively little concern about my speech. It's not that I never stutter, it's that my stuttering rarely interferes with my ability to communicate effectively. It wasn't always that way.

I struggled with and against stuttering during my childhood. Throughout my elementary school and middle school years, my parents took me to many speech-language pathologists, but I didn't seem to improve much. When I was a junior in high school, I started to worry about how I could possibly get along in college if I continued to stutter badly. We lived in the Denver area, and my parents suggested that I might like to see someone they had heard about at the University of Denver. I agreed, reluctantly, and we scheduled an evaluation. Dr. Jim Aten and some of his students observed me as I conversed with my parents, had me read aloud, had me tell them about some of my favorite activities, and had me make a couple of phone calls to local businesses. I remember stuttering very badly. I also remember a feeling of relief immediately after the evaluation when Dr. Aten met with me and laid out a therapy plan. Near the end of our meeting, Dr. Aten told me that he was a stutterer, that he had learned how to manage his stuttering to the point that it didn't interfere with his life in any way, and that one of the graduate students who assisted him with the evaluation was also a stutterer. I enrolled in therapy that semester and spent the next 2 years working on my feelings about my stuttering and ways to stutter more easily. Dr. Aten didn't "cure" my stuttering. I continued to receive stuttering therapy from other outstanding clinicians for another 5 years. However, Dr. Aten was an inspiration to me, and his therapy laid a firm foundation for successes that would follow. I felt better about myself as a person and as a speaker after working with him. As a result, I left for college with a positive outlook on life, and I changed my major from engineering to speech-language pathology.

During the past 30 years, I have worked as a public school speech-language clinician, a researcher, and a university professor. I look ahead with anticipation to teaching the next generation of speech-language pathologists and conducting research that could have a positive impact on the lives of children with communication disorders. Thank you, Dr. Aten, for giving me hope at a time that I was really struggling with my speech, for empathizing with me, and for being a great role model of a productive, happy, and influential person who just happened to stutter a little.

STUDY QUESTIONS

1. How does a discipline differ from a profession?

2. A hallmark of the discipline of communication sciences and disorders is that it is based on sound scientific principles and research findings. What term do we use today to describe how decisions professionals make about clinical service delivery are guided?

3. How did World War II affect communication sciences and disorders?

4. How can you differentiate between a communication disorder and a communication difference?

5. What are some common speech disorders in children and/or adults?

6. How can you differentiate between language delay, developmental language disorder, and acquired language disorder?

7. What are the different ways of regulating the professions of speech-language pathology and audiology?

8. What are the differences between certification and licensure?

9. What are the important functions of the American Speech-Language-Hearing Association?

KEY TERMS

Accreditation
Acquired disorders
Articulation and phonological
  disorders
Bilateral hearing loss
Certificate of Clinical
  Competence (CCC)
Certification
Communication difference
Communication disorder
Communication sciences and
  disorders (CSD)
Continuing education units
  (CEUs)

Deaf education
Developmental disorders
Disability
Discipline
Discrimination
Efficacy
Ethics
Evidence-based practice
Fluency disorder
Functional
Handicap
Impairment

Incidence
Licensure
Organic
Otology
Person-first language
Phonatory disorders
Prevalence
Profession
Resonance disorders
Unilateral hearing loss

REFERENCES

American Speech-Language-Hearing Association. (2000). *Communication facts*. Rockville, MD: Author.

American Speech-Language-Hearing Association. (2007). *Code of Ethics*. Retrieved August 4, 2009, from http://www.asha.org/docs/html/ET2003-00166.html

Hood, L. J. (1994). The American Academy of Audiology: Unifying and working for the profession of audiology. *Audiology Today, 6*(3), 15.

Irwin, D., Pannbacker, M., Powell, M., & Vekovius, G. (2007). *Ethics for speech-language pathologists and audiologists. An illustrative casebook*. Austin, TX: Thomson Delmar Learning.

Moeller, D. (1976). *Speech pathology and audiology: Iowa origins of a discipline*. Iowa City: University of Iowa Press.

National Institute on Deafness and Other Communication Disorders. (1995). *Research on human communication*. Bethesda, MD: Author.

National Institute on Deafness and Other Communication Disorders. (2007). *Research on human communication*. Bethesda, MD: Author.

Newby, H. (1958). *Audiology: Principles and practice*. New York: Appleton-Century Crofts.

Paul, R., Hernandez, R., Taylor, L., & Johnson, K. (1996). Narrative development in late talkers: Early school age. *Journal of Speech and Hearing Research, 39*, 1295–1303.

Travis, L. E. (1931). *Speech pathology*. New York: D. Appleton-Century.

Wood, P. (1980). Appreciating the consequences of disease: The classification of impairments, disabilities, and handicaps. *World Health Organization Chronicle, 34*, 376–380.

SUGGESTED READINGS

American Speech-Language Hearing Association. (2007). Explore the Professions. Retrieved August 4, 2009, from http://www.asha.org/students/professions/

American Speech-Language-Hearing Association. (2007). State Licensure Trends. Retrieved August 4, 2009, from http://www.asha.org/advocacy/state/StateLicensureTrends.htm

Martin, F. N., & Clark, J. G. (2006). *Introduction to audiology* (8th ed.). Needham Heights, MA: Allyn & Bacon.

National Student Speech Language Hearing Association. (2007). Welcome to NSSLHA. Retrieved August 4, 2009, from http://www.nsslha.org/nsslha/

chapter two

Communication Across the Life Span

RONALD B. GILLAM, LISA M. BEDORE, AND BARBARA L. DAVIS

LEARNING OBJECTIVES

1. To learn about the major processes in communication.

2. To know the definition of language.

3. To understand the processes and systems that underlie speech and language development.

4. To differentiate between language form, content, and use.

5. To learn about important changes in language development that occur during four major periods of development: infancy, the preschool years, the school-age years, and adulthood.

This is a book about communication and the ways that it can be disrupted. **Communication** is any exchange of meaning between a sender and a receiver. This seemingly simple exchange is important because it is the primary means by which humans share their thoughts and feelings, express their identity, build relationships, pass on traditions, conduct business, teach, and learn. Some communication is intentional, as when you tell your friend about your course schedule. Some communication is unintentional, as when your friend interprets your facial expressions or your body language that indicate how you are feeling. Sometimes, a message that you intend to be understood in one way is actually understood differently. Such miscommunication can have negative consequences, such as when a friend takes an offhand comment or an e-mail message as a personal insult even though you did not intend it in that way.

Most of the time, meaning is exchanged via a code, called language. **Language** is best defined as a standardized set of symbols and the knowledge about how to combine those symbols into words, sentences, and texts to convey ideas and feelings. Let's consider the parts of that definition more carefully.

Language is composed of a set of symbols. This means that one thing (a combination of sounds, letters, or hand movements) represents or stands for something else (ideas, feelings, or objects). Groups of sounds, printed letters, or hand movements (as in the case of **American Sign Language**) do not have very much intrinsic meaning in and of themselves. For example, all speakers of English agree that the group of sounds, *t – r – ee*, spoken in succession, represents a tall object with a trunk and leaves. We may not all have exactly the same type of tree in our minds when we hear the three sounds *t – r – ee*, but nearly all speakers of English share the same general concept. This is because language is standardized. The speakers of any particular language share reasonably similar meanings for certain groups of sounds, letters, or hand movements.

Languages need more than just words. Many of our thoughts are so complex that we cannot express them adequately with single words; groups of words are needed. Another important aspect of language is the conventions for grouping words together. For there to be meaningful communication, speakers need to agree not only on word meanings, but also on meanings that are inherent in word order. For example, if I said, "Mary helped Billy." We would all agree that Mary was the helper and Billy was the person who was helped. That isn't the same thing as, "Billy helped Mary" even though

BOX 2-1   CD-ROM Summary

The CD-ROM that accompanies this book contains a folder named Chapter 02. Three movies are in this folder. The first movie (Ch.02.01) shows children of various ages telling a story. We refer to various segments of this movie to demonstrate changes in language development over time. The second and third movies (Ch.02.02 and Ch.02.03) show a 2-year-old boy playing with a graduate student in speech-language pathology. These segments illustrate preverbal and early verbal communication.

the words themselves did not change. Our knowledge of the word-order conventions of our language makes it possible for us to use word sequences to express precise ideas about our environment.

THE PROCESS OF LANGUAGE PRODUCTION AND COMPREHENSION

Figure 2-1 depicts the primary processes that are involved in spoken language. In language production, senders encode their thoughts into some form of a language code. This code is usually spoken or written, but it can also be signed. In speech, which is the most common means of expressing language, the sounds, words, and sentences that express the speaker's thoughts are formed by sending commands to the muscles responsible for respiration (primarily the diaphragm), phonation (primarily the larynx), and articulation (primarily the tongue, lips, and jaw). Sequences of spoken sounds leave the oral cavity in the form of sound waves.

In listening and comprehension, the sound waves enter the receiver's ear, where they are turned into electrical impulses. These impulses are carried to the brain, where they are recognized as speech and then decoded into words and sentences. Listeners interpret the words and sentences based on their understanding of the meaning of the words in relationship to the other words that were spoken and the speaking context.

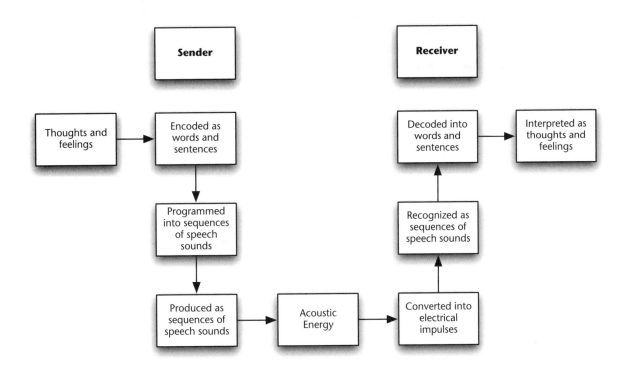

Figure 2-1   A Basic Model of Speech Communication Processes

THE BUILDING BLOCKS OF SPEECH

Speech production depends on two critical components: phonemes and syllables. The next section explains the roles that phonemes and syllables play in creating spoken words.

Phonemes

Languages have two basic types of sounds: consonants and vowels. Think about the words *bee*, *key*, and *tea*. Each word ends with the same vowel, the long [ee] sound. They are spelled differently because, in English, sounds in words can be represented by many different letters. But, let's put spelling aside for the moment. In English, these are three words with different meanings because the first consonant in each one differs. The sounds /b/, /k/, and /t/ differ in the way they are produced, and that difference results in a change in meaning. Sounds of a language that cause changes in meaning are called **phonemes**. It is worth noting however, that not all changes in the way a sound is produced result in a change in meaning. The phoneme /l/ has several variants. For example, the "light" /l/ produced in a word such as lip is a little different from the "dark" /l/ produced in a word such as dull. These variants of a sound are called **allophones**. Try saying *light* with both a light and a dark /l/. It's still the same word even though the /l/ at the beginning is not produced quite the same way.

Consonants and vowels differ in their basic manner of production. Vowels are produced with no constriction in the vocal tract, whereas consonants are produced with a significant blockage in the vocal tract. The vowels of English, listed in Table 2-1, are classified by jaw height and placement of the tongue in the mouth. The tongue can move in the front–back dimension (represented across the top of the table) or in the high to low dimension (listed in the left-hand column of Table 2-1). Lip position is associated with the front–back dimension in English. Front vowels are produced with spread lips (i.e., feel how your lips are positioned when you say the word *eat*). Back vowels, such as the /u/ sound in *boot*, are produced with the lips rounded. English also makes use of diphthongs, which are two vowels produced in close proximity to one another. The difference is that the tongue is moving in diphthongs. Some diphthongs that are contrastive or phonemic in English are /ɔɪ/ (e.g., boy), /aʊ/ (e.g., cow), and /aɪ/ (e.g., bye).

The consonants of English are listed in Table 2-2. Notice in Tables 2-1 and 2-2 that many of the symbols for sounds correspond to the English alphabet. Some symbols look unfamiliar. These symbols are from the International Phonetic Alphabet. This alphabet is a special set of symbols that we use to represent the sounds of speech in phonetic transcription. This is useful because there are many written letters that correspond to more than one speech sound. For example the word *garage* begins and ends with two different sounds, even though they are both spelled with the letter *g*. If you look ahead to CD-ROM Box 2-3, you can see an example of phonetic transcription. We talk more about the speech samples themselves a little later.

English consonants are produced by altering the manner and place of articulation or by voicing. **Manner of articulation** refers to the different ways that speakers can block airflow through the oral cavity using different types of constrictions. For example, notice the difference between producing the sound /t/ as in *tea* and the sound /s/

Table 2-1   The Vowels of English

	Front	Central	Back
High	i *key*		u *loot*
	ɪ *lip*		ʊ *look*
Mid	e *made*	ʌ, ə *mud*	o *boat*
	ɛ been	ɝ, ɚ *curd*	
Low	æ *mad*		
	a *hot*		ɔ *bought*

Table 2-2   The Consonants of English

		Bilabial	Labiodental	Dental	Alveolar	Palatal	Velar	Glottal
Plosive	Voiceless	p *pea*			t *tea*		k *king*	
	Voiced	b *bee*			d *dig*		g *gap*	
Fricative	Voiceless		f *fig*	θ *thumb*	s *sea*	ʃ *shoe*		h *high*
	Voiced		v *vest*	ð *them*	z *zoo*	ʒ *garage*		
Affricate	Voiceless					tʃ *chew*		
	Voiced					dʒ *juice*		
Liquid	Central				r *rug*			
	Lateral				l *luck*			
Glide		w *wing*				j *you*		
Nasal		m *men*			n *nose*		ŋ *ring*	

as in *sea*. Different manners of blocking airflow lead to qualitatively different sounds. Another way of modifying speech sounds is to produce blockages at different places in the oral cavity. This is referred to as **place of articulation.** For example, the sound /p/ in *pea* is produced with the lips, and the sound /k/ in *key* is produced with the back of the tongue. Finally, consonants differ in **voicing**. They may be voiced or unvoiced. Voiced sounds are produced with vibration of the vocal folds (e.g., /v/) and voiceless sounds are produced with the vocal folds open (e.g., /f/).

Phonetic transcription of speech is useful when we study the speech production of young children or the speech of persons with phonological disorders. In both of these cases, speech patterns do not necessarily correspond directly to those of adult or mature speakers. By using the symbols from the International Phonetic Alphabet (Tables 2-1 and 2-2), clinicians and researchers can capture in writing precisely how children produce sounds in words. This is helpful for maintaining records of the child's speech development and to compare child production to standard adult production.

Syllables

Suppose that you are asked to read aloud an invented nonsense word such as "gigafibber." Try reading this nonword aloud to yourself right now. How did you go about deciding how this word is to be pronounced? You probably divided the words into shorter chunks or segments. Most likely, you tried to say the word syllable by syllable. **Syllables** are units of speech that consist of consonants and vowels. Vowels are the central component or the nucleus around which the rest of the syllable is constructed. A syllable may consist of a single vowel (e.g., the *a* in *alone*), although syllables usually contain combinations of consonants and vowels. The most common and easy to produce combination is a consonant and a vowel (e.g., *ba, si*), but syllabic complexity can be increased by adding consonants before the vowel (e.g., *ri, tri, stri*) or after it (i.e., *am, amp*).

Change in pitch, stress, intensity, and duration of sounds in connected speech production is called **prosody**. Falling pitch and intensity are associated with statements, whereas rising pitch is associated with question forms. Stress patterns distinguish between the multiple meanings of some words. For example, in the sentence *The <u>con</u>trast is startling,* the word *contrast* is a noun, but in the sentence *The red and blue flowers con<u>trast</u> with each other,* it is a verb. The difference in stress pattern helps distinguish the two meanings.

THE BUILDING BLOCKS OF LANGUAGE

Language is often characterized as having three interrelated components: content, form, and use (Bloom & Lahey, 1978). Content refers to the meaning of language, form refers to the structure of language, and use refers to the way speakers select different forms that best fit the communication context. Any sentence requires an interaction of all three components of language.

Language Content

Language content is the component of language that relates to meaning. Speakers express ideas about objects and actions, as well as ideas about relationships such as possession or cause and effect. Sometimes, these meanings can be expressed by a single word. Other times, these meanings are expressed through groups of words. The linguistic representation of objects, ideas, feelings, events, as well as the relations between these phenomena, is called **semantics**.

Children develop a **lexicon**, which is a mental dictionary of words. Word learning is a lifelong process primarily because there are so many words that make up a language, but also because new words are being added all the time (think about all the computer-related vocabulary that has become part of our daily language during the past 10 years). What makes word learning even harder is that most words have multiple meanings. For example, the word *bark* can refer to something that a dog does or the stuff on the outside of a tree trunk. Imagine how confusing the sentence *That tree has funny bark* might be to a young child who had only heard the word *bark* used with reference to the noise her dog made.

Language Form

Language form, or the structure of language, involves three linguistic systems: phonology, morphology, and syntax. We introduced the concept of phonology when we discussed writing about the sounds of speech. **Phonology** is the study of the sounds we use to make words. For example, /b/, /r/, and /l/ are English language sounds. In Spanish, there are different sounds, such as the trilled /r/ sound, that do not occur in English. Recall that we said a phoneme was the smallest meaningful unit of speech. Take the words /fæn/, /mæn/, and /kæn/ (fan, man, and can). We know that the sounds /f/, /m/, and /k/ are phonemes in English because putting these different sounds in front of the root /æn/ results in a change in meaning.

Morphology has to do with the internal organization of words. A morpheme is the smallest grammatical unit that has meaning. The word *bird* is a morpheme. It cannot be divided into parts that have any meaning in and of themselves (such as "b" and "ird"). *Bird* is an example of a **free morpheme** because it can stand alone as a word. There are also **bound morphemes**, which are grammatical tags or markers in English. An example of a bound morpheme is the final *-s* in *birds*, which adds grammatical meaning. In this case, *-s* marks plurality, meaning that there is more than one bird. Other examples of bound morphemes include *-ed* (which marks past tense as in the sentence "He jumped over the wall.") and *-ing* (which marks the present progressive tense as in the sentence "He is running."). In English, most bound morphemes are placed on the ends of words. However, some are placed on the beginning of words. An example is *un-*, meaning "not" as in *uninteresting*. Some readers may think information about linguistics is uninteresting. However, professionals who assess and treat individuals with communication disorders need to know this information.

Syntax refers to the linguistic conventions for organizing word order. Basically, syntax is the formal term for grammar. In English, we say *blue ball*; in French the proper order is *balon bleu*, or "ball blue." The meaning is the same, but the rules governing word order are different for the two languages. Sentences that are ungrammatical may still make sense. Imagine a young child who tells her mother, "Him holded baby doggie." The sentence is ungrammatical because an object pronoun is used in place of the subject (*he*), the regular past tense marker is applied to the word *hold* that has an irregular form (*held*) for the past tense, and the child omitted an article (*the* or *a*) before the object noun phrase (*a baby doggie*). Even though this sentence is ungrammatical, we know exactly what the child meant.

Language Use

Words are combined into sentences to express complex ideas. **Language use** concerns the goals of language and the means by which we choose between alternative combinations of words and sentences. There are sociolinguistic conventions, called **pragmatics**, that help us decide what to say to whom, how to say it, and when to say it. Imagine that you are telling your friend about a movie you saw recently. You might say, "That had to be the most uninteresting screenplay I've ever seen," or "That film was so dull I could hardly keep my eyes open," or even "Talk about a boring movie." We choose different sets of words that we believe will best communicate our meanings to the audience we are addressing.

Effective language requires an interaction of content (semantics), form (phonology, morphology, syntax), and use (pragmatics). Speakers think of something to say and the best words to say it (content) and put those words in sentences (form) that address their goal (use) given the nature of the speaking situation (use). Similarly, listeners interpret the words (content) and sentences (form) they hear with reference to what they already know about the language being spoken (content and form) and the situation they are in (use).

THE DEVELOPMENT OF SPEECH AND LANGUAGE

By the time most children are 3 or 4 years old, they can integrate language content, form, and use to understand and produce basic messages. By the time they reach the age of 9 years, most children are capable of understanding and expressing quite complex messages. Communication ability continues to change into adulthood, where it plateaus around age 50. Late in life, communication skills often decline as a result of hearing loss and the loss of mental functions. Some of the basic milestones of speech and language development are listed in Table 2-3.

We describe some of the important milestones in communication development from infancy to very old age in the next section of this chapter. We refer to the period from 0 to 24 months as "from crying to short phrases." We refer to the period from 2 to 5 years as "from early sentences to stories." The school-age years start at kindergarten (age 5) and go through high school (age 18). Finally, we discuss language change during adulthood. We discuss important language characteristics related to content (semantics), form (phonology, morphology, syntax), and use (pragmatics) in each of the four developmental stages.

Knowledge of speech and language development is important to speech-language pathologists, audiologists, and deaf educators. To identify atypical development, you must know what is typical. To assist children and adults with communication disorders, you must be able to determine what their communication abilities are. These skills require a solid grounding in speech and language development.

Individual Differences

It is important for you to understand that there is a fair amount of variation in the *rate* of communication development. That is, some children develop language faster than others do, and some adults' language skills decline faster than others' do. There is also some variation in the *way* language develops. Some children are risk-takers; they will try to say words that are difficult for them to produce even if the words are not pronounced correctly. Other children prefer not to produce words that may be difficult for them to say until they are sure they can say them correctly. Some children learn

Table 2-3 Basic Milestones of Speech and Language Development and the Typical Age Range at Which They First Appear

Speech and Language Milestones	Age Range of First Appearance
Understands simple words (*mommy, daddy, dog*)	6–8 months
Reduplicated babbling (*ba-ba*)	6–8 months
Variegated babbling (*ba-do-ke-ga-do*)	6–8 months
First word	10–14 months
Two-word utterances	16–20 months
First grammatical morphemes	1;10–2;2 years
Multiword sentences	2;2–2;6 years
Combinations of sentences that describe events	3;2–3;6 years
Understood by unfamiliar listeners (95% of consonants produced in adult-like manner)	3;10–4;2 years
Identifies beginning sounds in spoken words	5;0–5;8 years
Decodes words	6;0–6;6 years
Tells complex stories	8–10 years
Written stories are more complex than spoken stories	11–13 years
Combines information from multiple sources into research papers	14–15 years
Refines personal speaking and writing styles	15–20 years
Uses vocation-specific vocabulary	21–24 years
Consistent difficulty recalling names and content words	45–47 years

Footnote: Children's ages are represented by the convention years;months. So, 1;10 indicates the age, 1 year, 10 months.

lots of nouns (50 or more) before they start producing two-word utterances; other children learn and use social phrases (e.g., *thank you, see ya later, hi daddy*) some time before they have 50-word vocabularies. Finally, there is variation in communication style. Some children and adults are relatively reticent; they tend not to say a whole lot about anything. Other children and adults are quite gregarious; they tend to say too much about everything!

As a result it is difficult, if not impossible, to pinpoint what is "normal." Neither can we pinpoint what exactly happens in language development at a particular developmental age. Because there is so much individual variation, we talk about *typical* development instead of normal development, and we provide age ranges for the first appearance of the speech and language behaviors that we discuss. We celebrate diversity in language development and use, and we recognize that differences between speakers make communication more interesting. However, we also know that some children have developmental difficulties that place them at significant risk for social, educational, and vocational difficulties later in life. The well-informed speech-language pathologist knows how to tell when language development is so far outside the typical range that it can result in negative social, educational, or vocational consequences.

FROM CRYING TO SHORT PHRASES: AGES 0 TO 24 MONTHS

Content

Children do not seem to understand different words until they are around 6 months of age. Then, they begin to wave "bye-bye" when they are encouraged to do so by their parents, or they may hold up their arms when their sister says, "How big is baby? Soo big!" By the end of their first year of life, infants usually understand about 20 different words. They start to say words other than "mama" and "dada" between the ages of 10 and 14 months, and their vocabulary can expand to 200 or more words by the time they reach 2 years of age. It is interesting that children often learn words that contain sounds that they have difficulty saying (Storkel, 2006).

Once children have built an adequate lexicon (a personal mental dictionary), they begin to combine words into two- and three-word utterances. This happens a little before or a little after they are 18 months of age. The ability to produce two-word utterances marks the child's desire to express relationships between ideas, and it shows that children are learning about word order. For example, children will combine a modifier like "big" or "more" with nouns to create such utterances as "big dog" or "more cookie." Many of their utterances describe relationships between agents (someone or something that causes an action), actions (the activities), objects (things that are acted upon), and locations (places). These combinations of meanings result in utterances like the following:

Frog go	(Agent + Action)
Frog pond	(Agent + Location)
Go back	(Action + Location)
Daddy shoe	(Agent + Object)

Form (Phonology)

Even before they are born, young children are actively sorting out and grouping the sounds of the language they hear. In experiments, mothers have repeatedly read the same nursery rhyme aloud to their unborn children. At birth, these infants have been found to listen longer to the nursery rhyme read by their mothers than to a rhyme read by another woman (DeCasper, LeCanuet, Busnel, Granier-Deferre, & Maugeais, 1994; DeCasper & Spence, 1986). At birth, infants prefer to listen to speech than to other types of complex sounds (Vouloumanos & Werker, 2007). Also, newborns listen longer to the sound patterns of their own language than to those of another language (Jusczyk, 1997). Thus, from as early as children are exposed to speech, they are beginning to process information about the speech and language patterns of their native language.

BOX 2-2 Examples of Jargon and Early Words

CD-ROM segments Ch.02.02 and Ch.02.03 show a little boy, Ryan, playing with Meghan, who is a graduate student in speech-language pathology. Listen carefully to what Ryan says in segment Ch.02.02. Can you understand anything Ryan says? He sounds like he is talking, but he is not using any identifiable words in this segment. This is a good example of jargon. Sometimes Ryan uses sentence-ending intonation patterns. Toward the end of the segment, you'll hear Ryan say something that sounds a lot like a question. If you can figure out what the words are, you are a better transcriber than we are.

When you play segment Ch.02.03, you will hear Ryan say the word *cup* pretty clearly. The rest of his utterances are examples of babbling and jargon. Notice that his babbling sounds a lot like English. One longer utterance contains variegated babbling and ends with the word *cup*.

Speech is secondary to biological functions such as respiration and feeding. As infants gain control over these motor functions, speech begins to emerge. The earliest phase of speech development is called **babbling**, in which infants begin to produce a number of types of sounds such as growls, squeals, raspberries, and adult-like vowel sounds. As children gain greater independent control of the muscles that produce speech, they combine different consonants and vowels and string sets of different syllables together in a way that has a speech-like quality. Around the age of 7 months, infants start to use their voice to make syllable-like strings, a process called **canonical babbling**. In babbling they produce rhythmic syllables over and over (e.g., *bababa*), termed **reduplicated babbling**, as well as combining different syllables (e.g., *bawabedo*), termed **variegated babbling**. Later, their babbling starts to take on adult-like intonation patterns. This type of speech is known as **expressive jargon**, which sounds like statements and questions with the exception that none of the strings of syllables are recognizable words. Children exhibit expressive jargon interspersed with real words until they are 2 years old.

As children approach their first birthday, they begin to use words. Early words contain the same sounds observed in the later stages of babbling. Common first words, such as *mama*, *dada*, or *papa*, contain those sounds that the child regularly uses in babbled speech.

Form (Morphology and Syntax)

The ability to sequence actions is one of the critical foundations of language, which involves joining sequences of sounds to make words and sequences of words to make sentences. Therefore, sequenced organized behaviors such as combinations of symbolic play schemes (pretending to pour tea into a cup and then pretending to put the cup to a doll's mouth) are important prerequisites of morphology (sequences of morphemes) and syntax development (sequences of words that form sentences).

As most children near 2 years of age, they start to use two-word utterances such as *Billy go* or *go there*. These utterances are best characterized by semantic relations such as "agent + action" and "action + location." Utterances of this type are the building blocks of syntax because they usually reflect the word order of language.

Language Use (Pragmatics)

In mainstream American culture, we communicate with our children from the first minute we see them. Mothers and fathers hold their infants, look into their faces, and talk to them. When infants make gurgling noises, their parents are quick to say things like, "Yes, I know. You're all full now, aren't you?" We build conversations with our children by treating everything they say and do *as if* it was true intentional communication. It is important to remember, parents from some cultures do not treat their young children in quite the same way. Dr. Peña and Dr. Jackson discuss this in greater detail in Chapter 3.

Children communicate without words before they communicate with words. For example, when infants want something they cannot reach, they may point to it and vocalize loudly, "uh, uh, uh!" Even though they are not saying words, they are clearly communicating a form of a command, *Get that for me, Mom!* Other forms of early intentional communication include looking at a parent, and then looking at an object, and then looking back to the parent, and then back to the object, and so on until the parent gets what they want. This behavior is very important because it shows children that communication gives them some degree of control over their environment.

Once children start to produce words, they can communicate many different functions with just a few words. In a famous study of his son's early language development, Michael Halliday (1975) identified eight communication functions that Nigel used before he was 2 years old. These functions are listed in Table 2-4.

Table 2-4   Early Communication Functions Evident During the First 2 Years of Life

Label	Function	Words and Gestures
Instrumental	To satisfy needs	"want" + pointing
Regulatory	To control others	"go" (meaning, go away)
Interactional	To establish contact	"hi"
Personal	To express individuality	"mine"
Heuristic	To get information	"What that?"
Imaginative	To pretend	"you batman"
Informative	To explain	"Sara ball" (meaning, that ball belongs to Sara)

Source: Based on Halliday, M.A.K. (1975). *Learning how to mean.* London: Arnold.

FROM EARLY SENTENCES TO STORIES: AGES 2 TO 5 YEARS

Content

Children's vocabulary grows almost exponentially during the preschool years. Children *say* approximately 200 different words at 2 years of age, and this increases to approximately 1,800 different words by age 4, when they probably *understand* as many as 3,000 or 4,000 different words. During this period, children continue to expand their noun and verb vocabularies. They also learn prepositions (over, under, in front of, between), words that express time (before, after, until), words that express physical relationships (hard, soft, large, small), adjectives (blue, red, big, little), and pronouns (me, you, they, our, herself).

Children are also busy learning how to create sentences that express complex relationships between words. For example, children say sentences like, "Billy is riding his red bike in his backyard." This sentence expresses at least five different relationships. The basic relationships are agent (Billy) + action (is riding) + object (bike). The words, *red bike* tell about the state (color) of the bike. By adding the word *his* in front of *red bike*, the speaker specifies an ownership relationship. The pronoun makes it clear that it is the agent (Billy) who is the owner. The prepositional phrase *in his backyard* states two important relationships. We know where the event occurs (in the backyard), and we also know that the backyard belongs to Billy. This example shows how many relationships can be expressed in a relatively simple sentence.

Form (Phonology)

From age 2 years on, children begin to produce speech sounds with increasing accuracy. The earliest set of phonemes acquired by children is /m, b, n, w, d, p, h/; these sounds are often acquired by the time children are 3 years old. The next set of phonemes that children acquire, typically between 3 and 5 years of age, includes /t, ŋ, k, g, f, v, tʃ (ch), dʒ (j)/. The last set of phonemes to be acquired includes /ʃ (sh), θ (voiceless th), s, z, ð (voiced th), l, r, ʒ (ge as in garage)/. These sounds are sometimes referred to as the "late eight" sounds. Children may start to acquire these sounds as early as 4 years of age, but these may not be fully acquired until 7 or 8 years of age. It is important to remember that children will use these phonemes inconsistently for a long time before they are mastered. Thus, children might use a phoneme in places where it doesn't belong in a word, as when they substitute /t/ for /k/ resulting in /tæp/ *tap* for /kæp/ *cap* or distort a sound such as /s/ (e.g., young children may produce a "slushy" sound

BOX 2-3   Two-Word Utterances

Watch segment Ch.02.01. Brandi and her little sister Erin are looking at a book together. Listen to Erin's two-word utterances. How might we describe the utterances, "going night-night" and "getting out"?

in which the air comes out over the sides of the tongue instead of /s/ in which the air comes out over the tip of the tongue). Speech sound acquisition is a gradual process.

BOX 2-4   Examples of Jargon and Early Words

If you look at the transcriptions of the speech samples in parts 1, 2, and 3 of the CD-ROM segment Ch.02.01, you can see that each child uses increasingly more of the sounds that are expected for his or her age. You can also see that individual children differ from the norm. For example, /g/ was in the middle set of sounds acquired for 3 to 5 years, but Erin, who is 2, is already using it in her speech.

Part 1: Erin (Age 2) and Brandi

B: What is that?
E: A frog. /ə fag/
B: A frog!
B: And what are they in, Erin?
B: Look, what are they in?
E: A room. [ə bum]
B: A room, that's right.
B: And do you know what that is?
E: M-hum. [mhəm]
B: What is that?
B: Is that a window?
E: (nods head yes)
B: Yea. Now what is going on, what are they doing there?
E: Going night-night. [go naɪnaɪ]
B: They're going night-night.
B: What's the frog doing?
E: Get, getting out. [gɛ gɛɪ aʊ]
B: He's getting out!

Part 2: Older Erin (Age 4)

There was a little frog. [dɛ wa ə lɪdəl fag]
And then, he, the frog, that frog was mean and that frog was happy.
[æn dɛn hi də fag dæ fag wʌð min æn dæ fag wʌð hæpi]
And he would> [æn hi wʊð]
And there was a possible thing. [æn dɛr wʌð ə pasəbəl fɪŋ]
And the frog look like> [æn də fag lʊk laɪk]
And he was mean. [æn hi wʌð min]
And he, and he was sad. [æn hi æn hi wʌð sæd]
And he was mad. [æn hi wʌð mæd]
And they were mad. [æn deɪ wʌ mæd]
And he was mad and he was sad. [æn hi wʌð mæd æn hi wʌð sæd]

Form (Morphology and Syntax)

During this period, children progress from producing primarily one- and two-word utterances to producing sentences that may contain up to 10 words. As children begin to express more precise meanings with multiword utterances, the use of grammatical morphology and syntax becomes important.

Some of the earliest grammatical morphemes to emerge include forms such as the plural *-s* (*The boys ride*), the possessive *-s* (*The girl's bike*), and the progressive *-ing* (*The dog's barking*). Around 3 years of age, children begin to mark verb tense using the third person singular *-s* (e.g., *my sister swims*) or the past tense *-ed* (e.g., *The man jumped*). Later, children increase the complexity of their utterances using the copula and auxiliary form of "be" as in "Daddy *is* a clown" (a copula form) or "He *is* running" (an auxiliary form).

As children produce longer sentences, they must use appropriate word order (syntax) if they are to be understood. From the time that children use two-word combinations, changes in word order reflect differences in meaning. For example, a child may say "daddy shoe" to indicate the shoe belongs to daddy and "shoe daddy" to ask her daddy to put her shoes on. Ways that young children (between 2 and 3 years of age) add syntactic complexity include using modifiers (e.g., *want blue ball*) and using new forms such as questions (e.g., *see ball?* with a rising intonation). By age 3, children start to use prepositions (It's *on* my chair), they use *and* to conjoin elements (I want juice *and* cookie), and they use longer question forms (e.g., *Why you not here?*). By age 4, children are using passive sentences such as *The girl was bitten by the snake* and some complex forms like *I know how to cut with scissors*.

Use (Pragmatics)

Before children can produce short sentences, adults assume most of the responsibility for conversing with them. By age 3, children begin to play a much larger role in conversation. Look at the example of a conversation between Jennifer and her mother. Notice that Jennifer does not have control over all the morphology and syntax necessary to express her ideas grammatically. Nonetheless, she is assertive as she expresses new ideas and asks a question, and she is responsive when she answers her mother's question.

BOX 2-5 Morphosyntactic Development

Go back to the speech samples in CD-ROM segment Ch.02.01 again and notice how the children's sentences increase in morphosyntactic complexity. For example, when Erin uses a two-word utterance to describe an action, she uses the progressive *-ing* only (i.e., "going night-night"). The older Erin is able to express past tense forms such as *was* and *were*. However, she does not use the past *-ed* on the end of *look* as might be expected. Even after children have begun to use these forms, they may apply them inconsistently.

Jennifer: Sara be at school.
Mother: She'll be home pretty soon.
Jennifer: Can I go school, Mommy?
Mother: Some day. Right now, you get to go to Mother's Day Out. Don't you like Miss Sally?
Jennifer: Yea, that fun to go there.

One important development during the preschool years is the beginning of narration, the ability to express a chain of events in the form of a story. Children's first stories are personal narratives that consist of one or two sentences. For example, an early personal narrative might go as follows:

Look, I painted a picture. And it got on me. See my shirt? I washed it and it's not go away.

Toward the end of the preschool period, children start to tell stories that contain fictional elements. Many fictional stores follow a similar sequence called a **story grammar**. Stories usually contain **setting** information plus one or more **episodes**. To have a minimally complete episode, the narrator needs to say what motivated the main character to take an action (the **initiating event**), what actions the character took in response to the initiating event (**attempts**), and what the result of the action was (**consequence**). As children develop, they produce more complete and complex episodes that include the character's thoughts and feelings about the initiating events (**internal responses**), the character's ideas about the actions he can take (**plans**), his thoughts or feelings about the consequence of his actions (**reactions**), and the resolution or moral of the story (**ending**).

FROM ORAL LANGUAGE TO WRITTEN LANGUAGE: THE SCHOOL-AGE YEARS

Content (Semantics)

Children's vocabularies continue to expand dramatically during the school-age years. It has been estimated that children acquire as many as 3,000 different words annually during the school-age years. At that rate, high school seniors may know as many as 80,000 different words (Miller & Gildea, 1987).

School-age children have a greater understanding of relationships between concepts and increasing knowledge about the meanings of words. This is seen in their ability to comprehend and use figurative language such as metaphors and idioms. **Metaphors** are expressions in which words that usually designate one thing are used to designate another. For example, All the world is a stage. **Idioms** are expressions that have literal and figurative meanings. For example, the expression *reading between the lines* could mean looking for words in the white space between the lines of this book. However, you probably know that this idiom really means to comprehend meanings or to make inferences about meanings that go beyond the literal meanings of the individual words.

Form (Phonology)

Beyond the age of 5 years, children's speech continuously becomes more adult-like. As mentioned earlier, some of the latest sounds are not perfected until children are 7 or 8 years old. Children this age also become more adept at producing consonant clusters such as *str-* and *sl-*. They produce most words accurately, but some **phonological processes** are occasionally observed in the production of complex words or in the production of words containing sounds that are late to be acquired. For example, children may still have difficulty producing multisyllabic words such as *spaghetti* or *pharmacy*.

In the late preschool years and early school-age years, children become aware of and start to mentally manipulate the sound structure of the words they say and hear. This ability is known as **phonological awareness**, and it has been shown to be a skill that is critically important for learning to read. For example, children can tell that *fan* and *man* rhyme. Later, they realize that *hot* and *horse* begin with the same sounds. By the time they are in second grade, children should be able to segment words into all their constituent phonemes (*sun* is /s/ -/ʌ/ - /n/) and to delete phonemes (say *school* without the /s/).

Form (Morphology and Syntax)

Children use a greater variety of complex sentence forms during the school-age years. That is, they become adept at putting multiple clauses (subject–verb combinations) into single sentences. The earliest and most common complex sentences are formed with conjunctions such as *and* (He came to my party *and* brought me a present). Later, children learn to use adverbial clauses that express time (*After we went to the movie*, we got an ice cream cone) or causality (I want you to come over *because* I don't like to play alone). By the time they are 8 years old, children routinely form sentences that have multiple clauses such as, *We wanted Steve to help us study for our science test, but he wouldn't because he thought he was so much smarter than everyone else.*

An important part of language development during the school-age years is learning literate (more formal) language structures. As they read and write with greater frequency, children's language sometimes takes on a "literate" sound. For example, the sentence *Readers might be pleased to discover that we will not require memorization of the cranial nerves* sounds more like written language than "I'll bet you will be glad to hear this. We are not going to make you memorize the cranial nerves." Near the end of the elementary school years and into the middle school years, children experiment with the kinds of syntactic devices that are required for literate language, and they discover when and how to use these structures.

Use (Pragmatics)

A number of important changes in language use occur during the school-age years. School-age children engage in longer conversations. They also become more adept at shifting topics and at shifting the style of their speech to match the nature of the speaking context and their relationship with the person they are talking to. Similarly, their narratives become longer and more complex. School-age children can weave multiple

BOX 2-6 A Fictional Story

CD-ROM segment Ch.02.01 shows six children who were filmed as they told the story, *Frog Where Are You?* (Mayer, 1973). We spliced sections of their narratives together to create the entire story, starting with Erin (age 2) and ending with her sister Brandi, who is an eighth-grader. Note that as children get older, the length of children's language increases and their descriptions become more complete and complex. Notice that, beginning at age 8, the children's language sounds more literary. The story propositions are named in parentheses following the children's utterances.

Frog Where Are You?

Part 1: Erin (Age 2) and Brandi

> **B:** What is that?
> **E:** A frog.
> **B:** A frog!
> **B:** And what are they in, Erin?
> **B:** Look, what are they in?
> **E:** A room. **(Setting)**
> **B:** A room, that's right.
> **B:** And do you know what that is?
> **E:** M-hum.
> **B:** What is that?
> **B:** Is that a window?
> **E:** (nods head yes)
> **B:** Yea. Now what is going on, what are they doing there?
> **E:** Going night-night. **(Setting)**
> **B:** They're going night-night.
> **B:** What's the frog doing?
> **E:** Get, getting out. **(Initiating Event)**
> **B:** He's getting out!

Part 2: Older Erin (Age 4)

> There was a little frog.
> And then, he, the frog, that frog was mean and that frog was happy.
> And he would>
> And there was a possible thing.
> And the frog look like>
> And he was mean.
> And he, and he was sad.
> And he was mad.
> And they were mad.
> And he was mad and he was sad. **(Setting)**

Part 3: Trey (Kindergartner)

Trey: Well, he escaped while they were sleeping. **(Initiating Event)**

Trey: And then they woke up. And and it was morning, and he was gone.

Adult: Oh no.

Trey: He looked in the book and the puppy looked in the jar a little bit more closer. **(Attempt)**

Trey: He stuck his head in there.

Adult: M-hum.

Trey: And then the little boy, and Tom and Spot looked out the window. **(Attempt)**

Adult: Yes, they did.

Trey: And Spot fell out.

Adult: And then, then what?

Adult: Well, what's happening here?

Trey: Then the glass broke.

Adult: It sure did.

Trey: And then they were yelling with, and and see if the frog would come out. **(Attempt)**

Part 4: Ashley (Grade 3)

Jimmy went outside in the woods with Spot calling, "Mr. Frog, Mr. Frog, where are you?" **(Attempt)**

Jimmy looked in a mole hole and called, "Mr. Frog." **(Attempt)**

And the mole shot up, scolding Jimmy. **(Consequence)**

While Spot was near a beehive shaking a tree, and it fell.

Jimmy was looking in an owl hole calling, "Mr. Frog, Mr. Frog." **(Attempt)**

The owl came out and Jimmy fell. **(Consequence)**

Part 5: Jorge (Grade 6)

The boy was surprised to find the owl in the hole and fell to the ground, **(Reaction)** while the bees were still chasing the dog.

The owl chases the boy around the rock.

When the owl leaves, he climbs the rock.

And the owl said the frog's name. **(Attempt)**

And then, then a deers, a deer lifted his head, and the boy was on top of the deer's head. **(Setting)**

Part 6: Jennifer (Grade 6)

And the moose took off! **(Initiating Event)**

The dog was barking at the moose. **(Attempt)**

Then the moose stopped at a cliff, and the dog and the boy flew over the cliff into a marshy area.

The boy fell in the water. **(Consequence)**

Then the boy heard a sound. **(Initiating Event)**
The dog crawled on top of the boy's head.
Ribbit, ribbit.
Shhhhh, the boy said to the dog.

Part 7: Brandi (Grade 8)

The little boy told the dog to be very quiet.
He was going to peek over to see what was there. **(Plan)**
So the boy and the dog looked over the wall. **(Attempt)**
They found two frogs, a mother and a father. **(Consequence)**
Then they climbed over and noticed a whole bunch of little babies were hopping through some grass.
And the little boy said, "There's our frog!" **(Reaction)**
So the little boy scooped up their frog, and the dog and him started going back home. **(Reaction)**
And they said, "Goodbye" to the little frog family, saying they would come back to see them soon. **(Ending)**
The end.

episodes into their stories, and they can tell and write in different **genres** (personal accounts, mysteries, science fiction, horror stories, etc.).

Children also improve at persuasion and negotiation during the school-age years. To be persuasive, speakers need to be able to adjust their language to the characteristics of their listeners and state why the listener should do something that is needed or wanted. Politeness and bargaining are often helpful as well. The first grader's use of persuasion may be limited to getting a friend to share a new toy. However, by high school, students need to use persuasion and negotiation quite well to gain privileges such as use of their parent's car for the evening.

ADULTHOOD

By the end of the school-age years, development in language form, content, and use has reached a very high level of complexity. As young persons transition from high school to higher education or the workplace, their language continues to change in ways that reflect their vocational choices and interests. Later in life, language begins to decline as a result of cognitive, motor, and environmental changes.

Content (Semantics)

Vocabulary continues to expand throughout the adult years. This is especially true for vocation-specific words. Biologists have different vocabularies from pharmacists, engineers, or speech-language pathologists because members of these professions tend to talk about different things. Shared vocabulary is often used to create social and economic bonds between members of a vocation or people with shared interests.

Late in life, neurological changes may lead to declines in some semantic functions. The ability to comprehend words does not decline much with age. However, the number of different words that are used decreases, as does the speed with which words can be recalled (Benjamin, 1988). There appears to be a "use it or lose it" quality to the mental lexicon. Older adults who have remained mentally active (those who still work, have busy social lives, and read and write frequently) and have better memory have fewer declines in semantic abilities than do older adults who watch more television.

Form (Phonology)

As part of the aging process, muscles atrophy and cartilage stiffens. Physiological changes lead to some changes in the voice. For example, older male speakers may use a somewhat higher pitch and their voice may sound hoarse compared to younger male speakers. In addition, respiratory support for speech diminishes so that it may be necessary for some speakers to pause more frequently. Specifically in regard to articulation, it has been observed that older speakers produce consonants less precisely than do younger speakers. Speaking rate may also slow. Generally speaking, articulatory changes in speech production of older adults are not considered problematic.

Form (Morphology and Syntax)

Older speakers demonstrate some changes in their use and understanding of morphology and syntax. Older speakers tend to use a diminishing variety of verb tenses and grammatical forms. Older speakers also may produce grammatical errors somewhat more frequently than younger speakers do. Some changes observed in the area of syntax are more closely related to changes in the lexicon and pragmatics. For example, older speakers may rely more on pronouns than on specific nouns when telling a story. Errors may be observed in the production of complex structures such as passive sentences or embedded structures that place demands on memory. It may also be more difficult for older speakers to understand syntactically complex utterances such as "I saw the lady who had a rose in her hair that the little girl picked from a garden on her way to school." This difficulty relates to declines in memory, processing ability, and vocabulary (Waters & Caplan, 2005).

Use (Pragmatics)

Throughout their adult lives, individuals continually refine their discourse to match the needs of the situation. They use persuasion, argument, narration, and explanation in different ways depending on their communication goals, their understanding of the formality of the situation, and assumptions they make about what their listeners already know or think about the topic. Communication style is also related to social and cultural expectations. Manners of expressing oneself are used to create bonds among members of subgroups of society. For example, compare the way newscasters explain a story on National Public Radio's "All Things Considered" to the way the same story might be reported by the newscaster on your local rock-and-roll station.

With aging come shifts in income levels, employment, social status, and leisure time. Many times, older adults relocate to settings like retirement communities or nursing homes where there are few younger individuals. A recent study on perceptions of older persons' communication noted changes in discourse style that included dominance of conversations, unwillingness to select topics of interest to listeners, increased verbosity, failure to take the listener's perspective, and more of a rambling style (Shadden, 1988). Discourse changes like the ones just mentioned could be related to memory loss, a desire for prolonged contact, and decreases in opportunities for socialization with a wide range of people. Once again, it is worth mentioning that there are large individual differences in the degree of discourse change and the ages at which these changes occur.

SUMMARY

People communicate by exchanging meanings with one another. This can be done nonverbally, through gestures and facial expression, but meanings are usually exchanged through spoken, signed, or written language. Languages are symbolic systems that require the integration of form (phonology, morphology, and syntax), content (semantics), and use (pragmatics). Nearly all children begin to develop language during the first year of life, but there is a great deal of individual variation in the rate of development.

During infancy, children explore the world around themselves with their sensory and motor systems, begin to communicate a variety of meanings nonverbally, and learn their first words. Children begin to produce two-word utterances around age 18 months, and they create their first short sentences around age 2. Language development literally explodes during the preschool years. By the time children are 5 years old, they know more than 4,000 different words, produce nearly all the sounds of speech correctly, use complex sentences, and tell short stories. The development of reading and writing creates many more opportunities for language development during the school-age years. By the time students graduate from high school, they know as many as 80,000 different words; they can create complex stories with multiple episodes; and they know how to weave sentences together to explain, persuade, and negotiate effectively. Language becomes more specialized during the adult years to match career and social choices. There is a gradual reduction in language skills in older adults. Just as there was individual variation in the rate of language growth, there is also a great deal of individual variation in language decline. The most common aspects of language decline involve word retrieval difficulties, difficulty comprehending nuances of meaning, and a tendency toward a more rambling verbal style.

BOX 2-7 Personal Story by Ron Gillam

One day, when my daughter Jennifer was nearly 3 years old, she and her older sister, Sara, were playing with some toys together. Jennifer had some zoo animals in a small train, and she was pretending to drive the train to another part of their make-believe zoo. She said to Sara, "Move over. I'm going over there." Sara responded, "You sure are bossy." Jenn replied, "I amn't either!" Sara moved, Jenn managed to get her train where she wanted it, and they resumed playing without further incident.

I found Jenn's use of "amn't" to be particularly interesting. I was relatively certain that she had never heard anyone say "amn't" before. Her utterance was ungrammatical, but it showed a great deal of grammatical knowledge about copula verbs and negative contractions. I suspect that she realized that people often used *isn't*, *aren't*, *wasn't*, and *weren't*. If it was all right for people to add the negative contraction to the copula verbs *is*, *are*, *was*, and *were*, why couldn't she add the negative contraction to the copula *am*? Her error was consistent with a number of grammatical morphology rules, but it was not consistent with some phonological rules related to connecting nasals in English. The important point is that Jennifer, like nearly all children, was actively re-creating the rules of language that she was exposed to. Her creativity within the learning process resulted in an interesting and amusing error.

STUDY QUESTIONS

1. What is the difference between language production and comprehension?

2. What is the critical difference between these terms: *phonemes*, *syllables*, and *morphemes*?

3. What linguistic systems are involved in language form, language content, and language use?

4. Why can't we pinpoint the language abilities a child should have at 3 years and 9 months of age?

5. Name one important development that occurs in each area of language (content, form, and use) during each of the four major developmental periods (infancy, the preschool years, the school-age years, and adulthood).

6. What are some examples of sounds that may be difficult for children to produce at the time they enter kindergarten?

KEY TERMS

Allophone
American Sign Language
Attempt
Babbling
Bound morpheme
Canonical babbling
Communication
Consequence
Ending
Episode
Expressive jargon
Free morpheme
Genre
Idiom

Initiating event
Internal response
Language
Language content
Language form
Language use
Lexicon
Manner of articulation
Metaphor
Morphology
Phoneme
Phonological awareness
Phonological processes
Phonology

Place of articulation
Plan
Pragmatics
Prosody
Reaction
Reduplicated babbling
Semantics
Setting
Story grammar
Syllable
Syntax
Variegated babbling
Voicing

REFERENCES

Benjamin, B. J. (1988). Changes in speech production and linguistic behaviors with aging. In B. B. Shadden (Ed.), *Communication behavior and aging: A sourcebook for clinicians*. Baltimore, MD: Williams & Wilkins.

Bloom, L., & Lahey, M. (1978). *Language development and language disorders*. New York: John Wiley & Sons.

DeCasper, A., LeCanuet, J.-P., Busnel, M.-C., Granier-Deferre, C., & Maugeais, R. (1994). Fetal reactions to recurrent maternal speech. *Infant Behavior and Development, 9*, 133–150.

DeCasper, A., & Spence, M. (1986). Prenatal maternal speech influences newborn's perception of speech sounds. *Infant Behavior and Development, 17*, 133–150.

Halliday, M. A. K. (1975). *Learning how to mean*. London: Arnold.

Jusczyk, P. W. (1997). *The discovery of spoken language*. Cambridge, MA: MIT Press.

Mayer, M. (1973). *Frog where are you?* New York: Dial Press.

Miller, G. A., & Gildea, P. M. (1987). How children learn words. *Scientific American, 257*, 94–99.

Shadden, B. B. (Ed.). (1988). *Communication behavior and aging: A sourcebook for clinicians*. Baltimore, MD: Williams & Wilkins.

Storkel, H. L. (2006). Do children still pick and choose? The relationship between phonological knowledge and lexical acquisition beyond 50 words. *Clinical Linguistics & Phonetics, 20*, 523–529.

Vouloumanos, A., & Werker, J. F. (2007). Listening to language at birth: Evidence for a bias for speech in neonates. *Developmental Science, 10*, 159–164.

Waters, G., & Caplan, D. (2005). The relationship between age, processing speed, working memory capacity, and language comprehension. *Memory, 13*, 403–413.

SUGGESTED READINGS

Aitchison, J. (1994). *Words in the mind: An introduction to the mental lexicon*. Cambridge, MA: Blackwell.

Hoff, E., & Shatz, M. (Eds.). (2007). *Blackwell handbook of language development*. Boston: Blackwell.

Pinker, S. (2007). *The language instinct: How the mind creates language*. New York: William Morrow.

Tomasello, M. (2003). *Constructing a language: A usage-based theory of language acquisition*. Cambridge, MA: Harvard University Press.

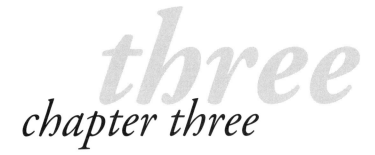

chapter three

The Social and Cultural Bases of Communication

ELIZABETH D. PEÑA AND JANICE E. JACKSON

LEARNING OBJECTIVES

1. To learn how individuals learn to use, speak, and understand the language of their community.

2. To understand how culture and communication are related.

3. To compare and contrast the processes of socialization and acculturation.

4. To understand the implications of a mismatch between the culture of the home and the culture of the school.

5. To understand how dialects are formed.

Children learn to use language in a remarkably short span of time. In childhood and as adults, we use language to communicate, problem solve, cooperate, teach, learn, and plan. These tasks take place within social contexts, and they follow conventions that are understood by the particular linguistic community that uses the language. Whether we learn English, Spanish, Farsi, Tagalog, or multiple languages depends on the language that is spoken at home and in the greater community. Languages differ structurally (e.g., their grammar and phonology) and socially. In this chapter, we consider the social and cultural bases of language and their implications for working with people from different cultural and linguistic backgrounds than our own.

THE SOCIAL CONTEXT OF COMMUNICATION

Children learn rules of communication through everyday interactions with their family. In addition to learning the specific language that the family speaks, children learn how, when, why, and with whom to use their language. Different families have different customs, including ways of talking and interacting. For example, some families may interact in a quiet manner while others use a loud tone of voice. Some families expect children to perform certain kinds of communicative behavior for others. They may tell their children things like, "Show me your head" or "Tell Aunt Sally what happened to us yesterday." Other families may expect children to "speak when spoken to" and not perform or "show off" in front of others. These differing beliefs are related to a number of variables such as ethnic background, religious beliefs, **socioeconomic status**, familial education, family makeup (nuclear/extended), neighborhood, country of origin, and gender.

A helpful framework for understanding differing worldviews is the collectivism–individualism continuum (Hofstede, 1986). In this framework, there are two ends in a continuum. Collectivism is one end of the continuum. A collectivistic worldview focuses on group harmony. As such, cultural values include understanding others'

BOX 3-1 CD-ROM Summary

The CD-ROM that accompanies this chapter contains eight short video segments of children from diverse cultural and linguistic backgrounds. In addition, there is an audio segment of adults who are from different parts of the United States or who learned English as a second language. The first segment (Ch.03.01) demonstrates how a young child might learn to point in response to an adult request that later leads to school-like activities and testing behavior. The second segment (Ch.03.02) shows a typical, English-as-a-second-language error that may lead to misdiagnosis. The third segment (Ch.03.03) demonstrates different varieties of English. The following four segments (Ch.03.04, Ch.03.05, Ch.03.06, and Ch.03.07) highlight features of African American English. Finally, the last two segments (Ch.03.08 and Ch.03.09) demonstrate code switching between languages and between dialects.

perspectives and moods. Sharing is another important value from a collectivistic perspective. At the individualistic end, the focus is on achievement. Self-expression and opinion are valued from this worldview. These two general perspectives influence what people communicate about and how they interact. We need to have an understanding of the variation in these beliefs to understand how they can influence how people talk and how they interact. These beliefs influence parent–child communication, peer interaction, and school talk.

In early childhood, for example, if you are a person who believes that communication begins early, you might interact with babies in a way that assigns meaning to things that babies do. When a baby cries, you might say things like, "Oh, you're hungry?" or "Do you want to be held?" On the other hand, if you don't believe that these early signals have intentional meaning, you might try to meet the baby's needs, but you might not say anything to him. You may not think your child is communicating with you. Rather, you may think of yourself as being "in tune" with your baby's needs.

What constitutes "first words" for parents also varies according to what they believe about communication. In mainstream American society, we focus on first words as demonstrating an important early milestone in development. However, other cultures may not view this as an important time. Some cultures think of complete sentences or phrases as an indication of "talking." An example that comes to mind is a referral for a speech-language evaluation where a Spanish-speaking mother had stated that her son had not started talking until age 2. At first, we were concerned that this child spoke so "late." However, in discussion with the mother, we found out that her son began *combining words* at age 2. For this mother, "talking" meant the use of phrases and sentences—single words did not count as talking. To understand this mother's concerns with respect to her child's development, we needed to better understand what she was reporting from *her* point of view and what her expectations were.

We have seen that individual families may have different beliefs and customs that relate to communication. Families function within a society and culture that guide and influence their beliefs and customs. But each individual within the family has slightly different experiences. Culture is constantly changing and adapting. Consequently, **culture** can be defined as a set of beliefs and assumptions shared by a group of people that guide how individuals in that group think, act, and interact on a daily basis. The members of the cultural group implicitly understand these beliefs. The way language is used is a reflection of the cultural group to which that person belongs.

SOCIALIZATION: LEARNING THE RULES OF FAMILY AND SOCIETY

Socialization and **acculturation** are two terms used to describe how people learn about culture. In our discussion, we refer to socialization as the process by which an individual learns his or her own culture, and we refer to acculturation as the process by which the individual learns or adapts to another culture.

The process of socialization includes learning how to interact with others. This interaction is reflected in how we use language to communicate. Language learning is an important step in becoming a fully integrated member of a cultural group. When we learn a mutual language, and the syntactic and pragmatic rules that govern that language, we can communicate. In learning English, for example, we learn that word order dictates meaning. For example, "She kissed him," tells who did what and who received what; on the other hand, "He kissed her" has the opposite meaning. In addition, we learn the social or pragmatic rules for using the language that we've learned. In learning language rules, we learn whom to talk to and when. We learn formal or polite ways of interaction as well as informal ways of communicating. One example is what we call people. The first author's son knows her as "Mom," but knows who others are referring to when they call her "Liz," "Elizabeth," or "Dr. Peña."

Specific customs and conventions govern how language is used. Anyone who has tried to learn another language knows that the grammar is different. For example, in some languages, such as Spanish and French, nouns have gender, and the article is used to mark gender and number. This is different from the English articles *a* and *the* that are neutral to gender. English speakers can use *a* and *the* in front of masculine or feminine nouns as in *a girl* or *a boy*.

Also, different conventions govern language use (pragmatics). How close should you stand when talking to someone? How much time is given to order in a restaurant? How long must a customer wait before receiving a bill? There is a whole ritual of behavior and communication in restaurants. For example, in many restaurants in the United States it is not unusual to receive the bill toward the end of the meal, even while eating dessert. However, in other countries, the customer must *ask* for the bill because the bill signals that the customer is getting ready to leave. Bringing the bill before the customer finishes a meal might be interpreted as hurrying them along, which would be considered rude.

There are regional differences within countries as well. For example, in the United States, the amount of information that is given when asking questions is indicative of different social interaction rules. On the East Coast, it has been our experience that you get an answer to the question you ask, and nothing more. The respondent may not want to assume lack of knowledge and embarrass you by telling you something you didn't ask about. On the other hand, West Coast respondents may give additional information "just to be friendly." When visiting the East Coast, someone from the West Coast may ask a general question expecting information beyond that which was specifically requested and be disappointed that his or her "real" question was not answered.

The rules of your community may determine whether you "get right to the point" or "beat around the bush." These are values consistent with individualism and collectivism perspectives, respectively. In some communities, it is considered appropriate for people to carry on a conversation for a while, asking about family and friends, discussing the weather, and then sitting a spell before they even begin to broach the "true" nature of their visit (e.g., to ask for someone's assistance or to negotiate the price of a car). If someone like a teacher or an outsider introduced him- or herself and then began to ask a series of straightforward questions, he or she might be considered rude and highly suspect.

Variation in Socialization Practices

We tend to interpret behavior based on our own expectations and experiences. Someone who has a different set of expectations may misinterpret a behavior that seems perfectly reasonable for someone else. This is especially true for communicating across cultures. It is important for speech-language pathologists and audiologists to remember that parents may teach ways of interacting that reflect their own culture and their own values. Parents teach children both directly and indirectly by providing them with examples and models of appropriate communication. Through these interactions, children learn to be active participants in their own culture. Parents universally want their children to be contributing adult members of society. What differs is the path that learning takes. Parents, based on their own culture and experiences, teach the behaviors that are important to them (Rogoff, 1991).

Potential for Home and School Mismatch

Because parents do not universally socialize children in the same way, there is a potential for **mismatch** when two cultures come into contact with each other. This is seen particularly when children from nonmainstream cultures enter the public school system. In most mainstream public schools, educators have selected the curriculum content, the way that it is delivered, how children are taught, and the language in which children are taught (English). Educators in the public schools have a shared knowledge of child development and the skills that children have when they begin school. This shared knowledge is based on mainstream culture and experiences that focus on individual achievement. Greenfield and colleagues (Greenfield, 1997; Greenfield, Donaldson, Berger, & Pezdek, 2006; Greenfield, Trumbull, Keller, Rothstein-Fisch, Suzuki, & Quiroz, 2006) propose two general pathways of development based on the collectivism–individualism framework. Schools in the United States tend to focus on an individualistic perspective, centering on child independence and self-fulfillment. Many children from immigrant groups, however, are socialized from a collectivistic perspective that focuses on group membership and social responsibility. When children who are not from the American mainstream culture enter the school system, their experiences may not match educators' expectations about what they should know or how to display that knowledge. Children may enter the mainstream school system with little knowledge of the language that is spoken in the school.

BOX 3-2   "Show Me"

CD-ROM segment Ch.03.01 shows an 18-month-old child pointing to body parts in response to the parent's requests. Because the parent is an educator, she knows the types of question demands that will occur later in school and uses questioning that matches that of schools. By the time this child begins school, he will have had many opportunities to practice this type of question–answer routine.

WHAT SHOULD WE DO IF THERE IS A MISMATCH?

Speech-language pathologists, audiologists, and other educators can potentially reach inappropriate conclusions about the abilities of children from diverse backgrounds if they do not understand issues related to normal cultural and linguistic variation.

We need to understand how first and second languages are learned, how languages and dialects vary, and how socialization goals might affect school performance. It is important that those who work with individuals from different cultural and linguistic backgrounds keep these issues in mind so as not to interpret a mismatch as a disorder. Learning about different developmental and socialization pathways may help to develop an understanding of why home and school mismatches may occur.

Learning a Second Language

Second language learners take from 1 to 3 years to learn face-to-face communication—what Cummins (1984) calls **basic interpersonal communication skills (BICS)**. These children make take as long as 5 to 7 years to learn higher-level, **decontextualized language**, which Cummins terms **cognitive academic language proficiency (CALP)**. Sometimes children who are assessed in their second language may appear to be fluent in English because they have good BICS. However, they may score poorly on educational and language tests because they have yet to master the nuances of CALP. Thus, it is important that educators take both languages into account when making educational decisions about children who are second language learners and those who are from bilingual environments.

Differences in Language Form and Acquisition

A second issue with respect to children from different cultural and linguistic backgrounds has to do with the ways that languages are structured and the order of acquisition of these structures. For example, earlier in this chapter we said that gender agreement was important in Spanish and French. Gender agreement is not learned in English because it does not exist in English. Examining performance in only one

BOX 3-3   Learning English as a Second Language

CD-ROM segment Ch.03.02 shows a 4-year-old Spanish-speaking girl speaking in English. In response to a statement by the English-speaking adult, "She's a boy," Magali says, "No, her a girl." This grammatical error is typical for a child in the process of learning English but could be mistaken for an indication of language impairment. Additionally, notice that this young language learner is relatively fluent in English even though she has been speaking it for less than a year. Because of her limited exposure and experience with English, it would not be appropriate to assess her only in English.

language of a bilingual child may exclude important information that is not specific to that language.

There may be differences in the order of acquisition across languages. We have the expectation that children learn certain things at a given age: generally easier things are learned early and harder things are learned later in development. Children's performance is often judged either informally or formally by comparison to what is known about this developmental progression. However, some language tasks may be more complex in one language in comparison to another language. One example is the acquisition of prepositions that convey directionality or location. In English, these occur relatively early in development (about age 1–2). In Spanish, directionality is often expressed in a verb phrase and is learned relatively later in comparison to English. So, we need to have an understanding of the development of both languages to make appropriate judgments about language competencies.

The Effect of Experience on School Performance

The school situation has **communicative demands** and unwritten rules about how children and adults interact. In American mainstream schools, children are expected to be able to tell stories, relate known events, ask and respond to direct questions, respond to "known-answer" questions (names of objects, attributes), and respond behaviorally to indirect requests. A typical question format that is seen in classrooms is responding to known-answer questions. Here, we may see teachers asking children questions that adults know the answer to. The purpose of this type of question is to elicit a display of knowledge consistent with the individualistic pathway of development. This allows the teacher to assess whether children know a certain concept, whether they understood a lesson, or whether they have certain background knowledge.

Children who have had experience with adult–child interaction in which the adult asks the child to respond to known-answer questions are likely to respond in a way that is consistent with those expectations. We see a lot of this kind of questioning in American mainstream parent–child interaction. Mothers and fathers may ask known-answer questions that require pointing (such as looking at books and responding to "Where's the cat, dog, shoe, ball, etc.?"), or choices ("Do you want up or down?"), or naming ("What's this"). However, some children may have little experience with this style of questioning. They may be more familiar with responding to questions that require them to provide information that is not known to the adult, so they may see this type of question as a request for relating an event or story. Thus, care must be taken to ensure that children's classroom interaction differences are not misinterpreted as low performance or low ability.

These three issues (the nature of second language learning, differences in language form, and different socialization experiences) together may lead to mismatch between communication expectations and experiences. This mismatch potentially leads to miscommunication, lowered expectations, stereotypes, and inappropriate referrals and classification. Understanding how culture and language can affect these decisions can help to lessen the negative impact that mismatches may have.

DIALECTS AND BILINGUALISM

There are different languages and different dialects in the world. What makes a dialect a dialect and what makes a language a language? A **dialect** is typically defined as a variation of a language that is understood by all speakers of the language. One language may have several different variations. For instance, in the case of English, there are British variations, North American variations, Australian and New Zealand variations to name a few. And within those countries there are even more variations or dialects of English. Everyone speaks a dialect—some variety of the "mother" language that we learned as a child. Often it is the "sound" of a particular dialect that we notice first. In the United States, we notice that people in New York sound different from people in the South, yet they are both understandable to a speaker of English. On the other hand, different languages have different phonology, lexicon, and syntax (sound system, vocabulary, grammar) and are not understood by people who don't speak those languages.

At what point does a dialect become a language? According to Pinker (1994), the linguist Max Weinrich maintained that "A language is a dialect with an army and a navy." That is to say, the primary determination of what is called a dialect and what is called a language is one of power—not of linguistics. Dialects are as linguistically legitimate as any language, but without the power to "promote" themselves to the level of language. Therefore, you can be sure that whatever the standard language is in any given community, it belongs to those with the most power.

How Are Dialects Formed?

Historically, dialects have evolved as the result of social transitions such as large-scale geographical patterns of movement by people, the development of transportation routes, or the establishment of education systems and government. Languages change over time. When a group of people are separated by geographical barriers such as oceans, rivers, or mountain ridges, the language that was once spoken in similar ways by everyone will change within each of the two groups. The two resulting varieties are

BOX 3-4 "Mary Had a Little Lamb"

Watch CD-ROM segment Ch.03.03, "Accents." You will hear people with different accents and dialects recite this familiar poem. Listen to the rhythm and intonation patterns of each of the different samples. Listen to how they produce the vowels and consonants. Speech patterns typically affect rhythm, intonation, and individual sounds. Can you guess where each person is from? Do you really notice certain patterns? Typically, people notice a speech pattern that is different from their own or from what they have heard often. Are there some that sound more pleasing to you than others? Know that both positive and negative attributes can be assigned to the same speech pattern. It is important to note that these attributes are assigned based on individual experiences and not on some objective value of the language.

usually understandable to both groups. A perfect example is the English spoken in the United States and the English spoken in England. When the first settlers arrived in the Americas, they sounded the same as their fellow countrymen left behind in England. Over time, the lack of contact among those in the Colonies and those in England resulted in two distinctly different forms of English. In this way American English and British English are both dialects of the language of English. Within the United States there are dialect varieties of English as well. Most of these varieties are related to geographical regions. There are Northern dialects, Southern dialects, and Midwestern dialects. As many as several thousand people or as little as a few hundred people may speak a dialect. A hallmark of dialect variation is intonation, prosody, and phonology. We often refer to these sound differences as **accents.**

Because language is dynamic, dialects change and evolve as communities change and evolve. The more isolated a speech community is, the more preserved the speech style will be. For example, on some small coastal islands (such as Tangier Island off the coast of Virginia and the Gullah Islands off the coast of southern Georgia), speech patterns have remained relatively unchanged for generations. To outsiders, groups of people like these might have speech that sounds quite old-fashioned or unusual.

The Social Context of Dialects and Languages

Although language scientists have no difficulty in defining dialect in a neutral manner, society seems to have much more difficulty with this. Because language occurs in a social context, it is subject to certain societal judgments. Individuals attribute, often unfairly, certain characteristics to people with certain dialects. Certain dialects may be seen as exotic or romantic, whereas others may be viewed as problematic and "difficult to understand." To know more than one language can be seen as a positive or a negative depending on which languages the individual speaks. In any given society, the ways of a "favored" group become favored as well. The customs themselves have no inherent value but become valued or favored simply as a result of their use by a favored group. Most people would not consider cucumber sandwiches or snails inherently desirable. Yet because they are consumed in favored "upper-class" circles, they become desirable to many.

In much the same way, the dialect of any favored group will become the favored dialect in a community. It is crucial to understand that this favored status has no basis in linguistic reality, just as cucumbers and snails are not in any real sense better than any other food. Because a particular dialect is considered to be the standard to be achieved, the language itself is not necessarily better or more sophisticated than the other varieties of the language. Conversely, the speech patterns of a stigmatized group often become as stigmatized as the group. In truth, the dialect of a socially stigmatized group may not be linguistically impoverished or more unsophisticated than the standard variety.

Historically, the dialects of American English evolved as immigrants came to the United States. Immigrants from different parts of England had different varieties of English, as was the case with immigrants coming from Poland, Ireland, and Italy. In the areas of the Northeast United States where these people immigrated, the different varieties of English are quite distinct—New Yorkers sound different from Bostonians who sound different from those living in Maine and so on. As settlers moved west, the different varieties of English began to blend more as groups interacted more. That is why dialect differences in the western United States are not quite as distinct.

Dialects can also be indicative of close contact with other languages. As we noted before, the languages that many immigrants spoke when they initially came to this country had an impact on English. This phenomenon is seen today with our newest immigrant populations. Again, in individuals learning a second language, the home language and the language of the larger community influence each other. These issues are seen in both African American English (AAE) and in bilingualism. In the next two sections, we examine issues regarding AAE and bilingualism within this social context.

The Case of African American English

The speech variety used by the African American population in the United States illustrates most of the dialect issues discussed so far, as well as the bilingual issues discussed in the next section. Linguists and language specialists most often refer to this variety of speech as African American English, or AAE. In the past, it has also been called Black English, Negro dialect, Non-Standard Negro dialect, and Ebonics. AAE may be viewed as a dialect of English because English words are used and there is much overlap with English grammar. However, when viewed from historical and political perspectives, AAE can be considered as a unique language.

AAE has been the subject of great debate over the past several decades. Early debates centered on the legitimacy of AAE as a language variety and the true linguistic competence of those who spoke AAE. Debates in the late 1990s centered on the legitimacy of using AAE as an educational tool to improve classroom performance in schools where children speak primarily AAE. Although the latter is too in-depth a topic for this discussion, we can provide some insight on what linguists and other language specialists do know about AAE.

When groups are socially stigmatized, their language will likely be stigmatized as well. This is certainly true of AAE, which is used by a large segment of the African American community. Frequent misconceptions and myths have long surrounded its use. Indeed, AAE is commonly incorrectly presumed to refer to the use of slang or urban vernacular terms used either by impoverished individuals with less education, or the language of the "street" (i.e., "jive" or "hip"). Consequently, it is pertinent to first briefly note what AAE is not. AAE is not "bad English," "broken English," or slang. AAE is not an impoverished form of General American English (GAE), African Americans are not the only speakers of the variety, and neither do all African Americans use AAE. Moreover, the use of AAE is a linguistic phenomenon, not an ethnic one. So, members of other ethnic groups who are familiar with AAE features and who find value in their usage use features of AAE.

So, what then is AAE? AAE is a language variety used by a large segment of the African American population. The variety has ties to the West African linguistic roots of the African American community's African slave ancestors (Baugh, 1999). That is to say, AAE has pronunciation, grammatical rules, and semantic rules in common with a variety of West African languages (Howe & Walker, 2000; Smitherman, 1977). The variety's unique evolutionary history in the United States allowed for the preservation of many forms across generations.

Although there is debate about the scale and nature of English and African linguistic influences in the development of AAE (Wolfram & Thomas, 2002), it is agreed that the beginnings of AAE start with the African slaves that were brought to America as captives in the transatlantic slave trade. Most African slaves were taken from the west coast of Africa. Languages spoken in this part of Africa are part of the Niger-Congo family of languages, one of the world's major language families and the largest group of languages in Africa, consisting of more than 600 different languages (Bendor-Samuel & Hartell, 1989). These languages, although not mutually intelligible, have similar grammars. For example, members of the West African family of languages tend to follow the same sound rules (e.g., not clustering consonants at the ends of words); conjugate verbs using regularized agreement patterns where the verb remains constant for person and number; and have similar tense and aspect patterns such as habitual aspect and past, present, future, near past, and remote past tenses. In short, Niger-Congo languages have shared **grammatical patterns** among one another, as well as some distinct grammatical differences from the Indo-European family of languages of which English is a member. Some distinctions remain in the AAE used today, in particular, regularized agreement (e.g., *I go, you go, we go, everybody go*), and some tense and aspect patterns.

To illustrate how patterns could be developed and retained over generations, consider the following. Upon arrival in America, Africans initially retained their African linguistic patterns. The majority of slaves working as field laborers had limited direct contact with English, which reinforced the retention of the African-turned-slave's primary linguistic patterns (including rules governing grammar, sound, and meaning). Conversely, slaves working in plantation homes or on small plantations had more direct contact and interaction with English. It is hypothesized that the slaves did what all learners of second languages do—first, they learned the names of things (nouns); then, verbs; and later, adjectives and other forms. As with all learners of second languages, what remained most constant in their English use were the grammatical patterns of their first language(s). For example, word classes such as nouns and verbs were frequently organized according to the slave's African linguistic patterns. This is similar to the way English speakers initially say *blanca casa* (*white house*) when learning Spanish, instead of using Spanish grammar where the adjective follows the noun (e.g., *casa blanca*).

It is crucial to understand that slaves were never taught English directly. Neither were they taught to read. The common penalty for literacy during the time of slavery was death. This is an important distinction in understanding how African Americans are unlike other immigrant groups. Historically, immigrants to America have had access to programs designed to teach English and encourage assimilation. Furthermore, immigrants typically have a favored view of their new country and strong intrinsic motivation to become a part of their new country's society by learning the language and ways of their new land as well as access to formalized means to "learn" the new language. Africans, on the other hand, were not welcome to assimilate into American society and had no access to formalized instruction. English, therefore, was not "learned" in the formal sense, but rather parsed into the slaves' existing linguistic repertoire with its grammatical, sound, and meaning rules. Further, social and legal isolation of the group and its language served to reinforce the language patterns of the African-turned-slave. This is described as the *Creole Hypothesis* of AAE (Dillard, 1972; Wolfram & Thomas, 2002).

So, why would language forms from so long ago still exist? Well, following the end of slavery (around 1865), **Jim Crow segregation** began. Blacks were legally denied access to social and political interactions with mainstream society. Legal segregation dictated that blacks could not live where whites lived, go to school where whites went to school, eat where whites ate, attend church where whites worshipped, swim where whites swam, or even drink from a fountain where whites drank, and so on. Linguistically, this social stratification served to preserve speech patterns of the African American community. As we noted earlier, when speech communities are isolated, their patterns are likely to be preserved. The social isolation of legalized segregation continued from the late 1800s until the dismantling of Jim Crow segregation in the mid- to late 1960s—less than 50 years ago. Furthermore, despite the official desegregation of the African American community, many sociologists contend that the socioeconomic stratification that continues has sustained the isolation of a large segment of the African American population from the mainstream population.

Let's consider some specific features. Table 3-1 highlights some of the features found in AAE, many of which are considered to be reflective of West African language rules, especially the tense and aspect patterns, which are notably different from GAE; in particular, the use of the aspectual marker *be*, which does not exist in GAE (e.g., she *be* running). Although this *be* appears to be used like a GAE auxiliary (e.g., she *is* running), it is an aspect marker that denotes an activity or state of being (mad, sad, happy, etc.) that occurs habitually over time, but may or may not be happening now.

AAE includes features that are identical to those in GAE, as well as additional features not found in GAE, called contrastive features. There two types of contrastive features: (1) those that have no counterpart in GAE, such as the aspectual *be* described previously that denotes habitual aspect, and (2) features that are used obligatorily in GAE, but used variably in AAE. The latter are most often morphological endings such as past tense *-ed*, possessive *'s*, and plural *-s*. In AAE, these forms can be "zero-marked" or omitted as in the sentence *Yesterday my mom bake a cake*, or *That my brother hat.* Additionally, where GAE requires irregular agreement on all third-person cases, AAE calls for a regularized agreement pattern (e.g., *I go, you go, we go, everybody go*). The fact that AAE utilizes agreement patterns different from GAE is not a reflection of an error of GAE, rather a different agreement pattern. The collapsing of groups of consonants at the ends of English words (e.g., *tesses* instead of *tests*) is not an error of GAE pronunciation rules, but an adherence to pronunciation patterns found in some West African languages (see Table 3-1 for commonly used features).

Table 3-1 African American English Grammatical Features

Grammatical Feature	Examples
Copula/auxiliary deletion	He running to the store He a doctor
Verb regularization (same verb form for all subject cases)	"I play, you play, he play, we play, they play."
Zero possessive marker	That my brother car I go to my auntie house
Zero past tense *-ed* marker	Yesterday we play ball
Zero plural marker	Fifty cent Four chair
Reflexive pronouns	He did it hisself She gonna hurt herself, itself, theirselves
Expletive "it" (*it* used for *there's*)	It's a girl in my class named Amber It's a dog in your yard (vs. there's a dog…)
Tense and Aspect Features	
Habitual "be"	She be sewing (She sews habitually on specific occasions over time)
Completive past tense	He done gone (He already left)
Remote past tense	He been gone (He left a long time ago)
AAE Sound Rules	**Example**
No consonant pairs on word endings	"jus" (for *just*) "men" (for *mend*)
No /th/ sound: /d/ or /f/ used in its place	"dis" (for *this*) "birfday" (for *birthday*)

BOX 3-5   AAE Features

CD-ROM segments Ch.03.04, Ch.03.05, and Ch.03.06 show children using specific features of African American English. Segment Ch.03.04 is an example of nonuse of past tense *-ed* marker. Notice here that the past tense context is indicated by the use of the irregular past tense verb *went*, which precedes the nonmarked *graduate*, "*When* she, um *graduate*, everyone was there for her party."

Segment Ch.03.05 shows third-person /s/ regularization in the form of using *eat* instead of *eats*, copula deletion in the form of substituting *they* for *they're*, and the phonological pattern of using /d/ for /th/ in the sentence: "But the real principal *eat* lunch with *dem*, because *they* bad."

Another example of third-person regularization is included in segment Ch.03.06. In this clip, the feature is not as easily identified because of the phonetic context. Listen and see what you hear. Is Danny saying, "*he teach us college stuff like . . .*" or "*he teaches college stuff like . . .*"?

Today, AAE is used on a continuum by its speakers, some of whom use many features frequently, whereas others use a few features infrequently. Some speakers move up and down the continuum depending on the particular communicative context. In formal work settings, some speakers may use only GAE patterns. Then, in a casual home and family environment, these same individuals may use more AAE features. This ability to use AAE in some settings and not in others, or to vary its usage throughout one event, is known as **code switching**. For many in the African American community, the use of AAE features has become a social identity marker that is embraced. That is, some speakers willingly move between GAE and AAE and have no desire to abandon AAE in favor of GAE. They feel this way because AAE is part of their cultural identity and their connection to the African American community. Still others wish to use only the more socially esteemed variety of GAE that is most accepted in mainstream American society.

We have discussed the difference between languages and dialects as relating primarily to power and influence as opposed to any linguistic reality. The major difference between AAE and other dialects of English is the base language. Typically, dialects emerge as the speakers of one language diverge and experience differences in that language. AAE differs from this model in that, at its core, it appears to embody grammatical forms from at least two languages (or language families): Indo-European English and Niger-Congo West African languages. Further, whereas dialects tend to be bound by geographical location (e.g., southern dialect speakers tend to be found in the South, not in New England), AAE has no such boundaries. Speakers of AAE can be found all over the country. Despite this difference, though, most linguists typically consider AAE to be a dialect of English because it uses English words and has more similarities than differences to GAE. But its differences have been significant enough, historically, to cause debate about its legitimacy and origin, as well as the misdiagnosis of children's

---

BOX 3-6   Code Switching: AAE and GAE

CD-ROM segment Ch.03.07 shows Danny performing intonational code switching when imitating a GAE-speaking classmate. He uses intonation and pitch indicative of GAE that differs from his typical use of pitch and intonation, "Stop, stop, get off, I'm telling Mr. Naughlin."

Segment Ch.03.08 shows Danny performing grammatical code switching to GAE in the presence of a non-AAE-speaking visitor. He starts to use aspectual "be," which has no GAE equivalent word, and then changes to a GAE translation, "He *be putting* big words *he puts* big words." Note that although *he puts big words* is similar in meaning to *he be putting big words* . . . it does not highlight the same habitual aspect that *be* refers to in AAE. He also switches from a regularized third-person /s/ production to the GAE irregular third-person /s/, "He *don't* He *doesn't* need to . . ." These types of switches were not observed in Danny's speech before the visitor arrived and appeared to be a result of accommodating a non-AAE speaker.

linguistic competence. Similar issues of misdiagnosis also occur with children who are bilingual, as discussed in the next section.

Bilingualism

Most of us would probably agree that a **bilingual** individual is someone who speaks and understands two languages. When we start to look at the nature of bilingualism and at people who are bilingual, we see enormous variation. There are varying definitions of bilinguals and different implications for the practice of speech, language, and hearing sciences.

It used to be that bilingualism was defined as a "balanced" use of two languages by a person. However, studies on these so-called balanced bilinguals demonstrated that they had different strengths in each of their languages and that the two languages did not, in fact, mirror each other. Grosjean (1989) points out that the way we define bilingualism influences how we interpret bilingual behavior. He suggests that the "balanced" definition of bilingualism (meaning, two monolinguals in one) reflects the idea that a bilingual individual must have equal fluency in both languages, and that anything short of that is therefore inadequate. But even bilinguals who are highly fluent in two languages have different strengths depending on the situations in which they use each of the languages. Over time, bilinguals move in and out of relative fluency in the two languages based on the social and educational demands that affect their lives.

At any given point in time, it is much more likely that a bilingual individual will present an "unbalanced" profile. This is why Grosjean (1989) suggests that we think of bilinguals as bilinguals, and not as two monolinguals. Because there are different types of bilinguals, it is important to take into account the dynamic nature of language and how two languages might be learned.

It is important to understand how an individual becomes bilingual. Some people who have studied a foreign language in school may then travel, live, or work in a country where that language is spoken. This type of bilingual is usually referred to as an **elective bilingual**. Other people learn a second language because they have immigrated to another country, very likely because of economic reasons, and must learn a second language to interact in the community. This person is likely not to have formal education learning the second language. This person is referred to as a **circumstantial bilingual**.

The nature of bilingualism also relates to when the person learned the first and second languages. Some individuals are exposed to two languages from birth. Perhaps their families know and use two languages at home. These bilinguals are considered to be **simultaneous bilinguals**. Some individuals learn a second language when they go to school (often kindergarten or preschool) or learn a second language as an adult. These individuals are considered **sequential bilinguals**.

It's important to examine the status of each language and understand that different types of bilinguals will have different profiles. A kindergarten child who was exposed to two languages from birth will perform differently from a child whose first exposure to English is in kindergarten, even though both of these children may be classified as bilingual. Young children present a special case because they are still learning language.

They may still be learning their primary language when they begin to learn a second language, or they may be learning two languages at once. Thus, their bilingualism is not fully established.

We consider bilingualism to be a continuum of relative proficiency in a speaker's first language (L1) and their second language (L2). Proficiency in any language is task dependent. So, individuals who are bilingual may be highly proficient in their first language (L1) for certain tasks, while they may be more proficient in their second language (L2) for a completely different set of tasks. For example, it is not uncommon for young children to know "home" vocabulary (e.g., functions, body parts, names of relatives, social routines) in the home language and "school" vocabulary (e.g., colors and numbers) in English. Finally, bilinguals in interaction with other bilinguals may mix, switch, or borrow words across languages in a rule-governed way. Additionally, they may code switch in response to the situation or to their listeners.

These descriptions are important so that speech-language pathologists and audiologists can understand how and when bilinguals came to know two languages. Understanding bilinguals' language learning circumstances and timing may help us make more appropriate clinical judgments about their language learning abilities and may help us to respond to their needs in a culturally sensitive manner. Also, it is important to assess in both or all the languages of an individual to gain a complete understanding of the person's speech and language functioning. Finally, because bilingual status is constantly changing as a result of social and academic interactions, language testing should be viewed as having only short-term stability.

When two languages come into contact with each other, they typically influence each other mutually. One common occurrence is that the grammar of the home language may influence word order in the second language. For example, in Spanish, articles and nouns must agree in number and gender (masculine/feminine), but in English gender is not marked, and the article *a* is singular, whereas *the* can be singular or plural, with plurality marked on the noun. An English speaker learning Spanish may make article–noun agreement errors: *el casa* (the [masculine, singular] house [feminine, singular]) instead of the correct *las casas*.

There is also evidence that the second language may influence the first language. In several studies of bilinguals across several languages, Bates and colleagues (Bates,

---

BOX 3-7   Code Switching: Spanish and English

Watch CD-ROM segment Ch.03.09. At first, Magali interacts with an adult who speaks only Spanish to her, and that is her stronger language. Together, Magali and the adult make up a story about a frog's birthday party. They also draw a frog, adding water, a table, and a birthday cake. Magali turns to the other adult once the drawing is complete and says to her, "There we go," while picking up the puppet. The Spanish speaker continues to address Magali in Spanish only, telling her to explain to the other adult what is happening in the picture. Once again, Magali turns to the second adult and explains in English, "That is the happy birthday." You can see that Magali is aware of her audience and switches between the two languages appropriately and effortlessly.

Devescovi, & D'Amico, 1999; Bates & MacWhinney, 1981; Hernandez, Bates, & Avila, 1994; Liu, Bates, & Li, 1992) have found that, in comparison to monolinguals, bilinguals employ the grammatical cues of both their languages at the same time. For example, Spanish speakers rely heavily on noun–verb agreement as an important grammatical cue, whereas English speakers rely on word order as a primary cue. Spanish-English bilinguals used both word order and noun–verb agreement in Spanish and English.

A final issue that is important to consider when working with individuals who come from a different language background is that of culture. In the earlier part of this chapter, we discussed the process of socialization—or coming to know one's own culture and language. We also need to consider the process of acculturation. We said that this was the process by which a second culture was acquired. It is important to realize that several processes are in action in the acculturation process. Just as with learning a second language, the reasons for acculturation may vary. On one hand, an individual or family may want to maintain the home culture but may have to make some adaptations to succeed in school or work. On the other hand, some families feel that their culture may be stigmatizing, and they may want to adapt to the new culture as fast as possible. Still other families may blend aspects of the home and host cultures. It is important to understand that there are many ways that families acculturate.

SUMMARY

This chapter introduced you to some of the issues related to examination of culture and language. Culture and language change over time, and culture is reflected in the language that we use every day. It is important to understand the process of learning a first and second language and of learning a first and (possibly) second culture. We

---

BOX 3-8   Personal Story

A recent graduate relates a story of how he remembers first becoming aware that people raised in different cultural communities differed linguistically. During high school, he worked at a pizza parlor on the weekends, and sometimes the manager would allow him to break away from cleaning out the dough vats (an oftentimes dangerous and messy job) to operate the cash register. While he stood proudly at the cash register, a young African American female approached him holding two dimes and a nickel and she said, "Do you have a case quarter?" He stood there dumbly thinking, "What is a case quarter? Why is she asking me for a quarter when she is holding 25 cents in her hand?"

After several ridiculous queries on his part, the young lady patiently explained to him that a case quarter was simply a quarter, that her two dimes and nickel also equaled a quarter but would not activate the jukebox—a case quarter was necessary to do that. "Well," he thought to himself, "That makes perfect sense, why didn't I know that?" He didn't know that because he was not an integrated member of her cultural group and thus did not have access to some of the vocabulary used by that group. It was his first real experience with linguistic diversity.

know that lack of understanding of cultural and linguistic diversity can lead to erroneous assumptions about someone's ability. Furthermore, this lack of understanding can lead to misdiagnosis in speech-language pathology and audiology. Ultimately, we need to have an understanding of culture and language to better assess and treat individuals from diverse backgrounds.

STUDY QUESTIONS

1. Compare and contrast the processes of socialization and acculturation.

   a. How might differences in socialization practices affect school performance?

   b. What are reasons for acculturation?

2. Define and describe BICS and CALP.

3. How can language and culture affect test taking?

   a. Explain some potential problems with translating tests from one language to another.

   b. How might differences in test-taking experiences affect test performance?

4. Describe how dialects are formed.

5. List both positive and negative assumptions that might be made about dialects. What are some potential impacts of these assumptions?

6. What are some examples of different types of bilinguals?

7. Why would understanding how individuals become bilingual matter to a speech-language pathologist or audiologist?

8. Describe the origins of African American English (AAE).

   a. Explain how AAE might be considered a language.

   b. Explain how AAE might be considered a dialect.

KEY TERMS

Accent
Acculturation
Basic interpersonal communication skills (BICS)
Bilingual
Circumstantial bilingual
Code switching

Cognitive academic language proficiency (CALP)
Communicative demand
Culture
Decontextualized language
Dialect
Elective bilingual

Grammatical patterns
Jim Crow segregation
Mismatch
Sequential bilingual
Simultaneous bilingual
Socialization
Socioeconomic status

REFERENCES

Bates, E., Devescovi, A., & D'Amico, S. (1999). Processing complex sentences: A cross-linguistic study. *Language & Cognitive Processes, 14*(1), 69–123.

Bates, E., & MacWhinney, B. (1981). Second-language acquisition from a functionalist perspective: Pragmatic, semantic, and perceptual strategies. *Annals of the New York Academy of Sciences, 379,* 190.

Baugh, J. (1999). *Out of the mouths of slaves.* Austin: University of Texas Press.

Bendor-Samuel, J., & Hartell, R. L. (Eds.). (1989). *The Niger-Congo Languages—A classification and description of Africa's largest language family.* Lanham, MD: University Press of America.

Cummins, J. (1984). *Bilingualism and special education: Issues in assessment and pedagogy.* Austin, TX: Pro-Ed.

Dillard, J. L. (1972). *Black English: Its history and usage in the United States.* New York: Vintage.

Greenfield, P. M. (1997). You can't take it with you: Why ability assessments don't cross cultures. *American Psychologist, 52*(10), 1115–1124.

Greenfield, P. M., Donaldson, S. I., Berger, D. E., & Pezdek, K. (2006). Applying developmental psychology to bridge cultures in the classroom. In S. I. Donaldson, D. E. Berger, & K. Pezdek (Eds.), *Applied psychology: New frontiers and rewarding careers* (pp. 135–152). Mahwah, NJ: Erlbaum.

Greenfield, P. M., Trumbull, E., Keller, H., Rothstein-Fisch, C., Suzuki, L., & Quiroz, B. (2006). Cultural conceptions of learning and development. In P. A. Alexander, P. R. Pintrich, & P. H. Winne (Eds.), *Handbook of educational psychology* (2nd ed.). Mahwah, NJ: Erlbaum.

Grosjean, F. (1989). Neurolinguists, beware! The bilingual is not two monolinguals in one. *Brain and Language, 36,* 3–16.

Hernandez, A., Bates, E., & Avila, L. (1994). On-line sentence interpretation in Spanish-English bilinguals: What does it mean to be "in between"? *Applied Psycholinguistics, 15,* 417–446.

Hofstede, G. (1986). Cultural differences in teaching and learning. *International Journal of Intercultural Relations, 10*(3), 301–320.

Howe, D. M., & Walker, J. A. (2000). Negation and the Creole-Origins Hypothesis: Evidence from early African American English. In S. Poplack (Ed.), *The English history of African American English* (pp. 109–139). New York: Wiley-Blackwell.

Liu, H., Bates, E., & Li, P. (1992). Sentence interpretation in bilingual speakers of English and Chinese. *Applied Psycholinguistics, 13,* 451–484.

Pinker, S. (1994). *The language instinct: How the mind creates language.* New York: William Morrow.

Rogoff, B. (1991). *Apprenticeship in thinking: Cognitive development in social context.* New York: Oxford University Press.

Smitherman, G. (1977). *Talkin and testifyin: The language of Black America.* Boston: Houghton Mifflin.

Wolfram, W., & Thomas, E. R. (2002). *The development of African American English.* Malden, MA: Blackwell.

SUGGESTED READINGS

Baker, C. (2001). *Foundations of bilingual education and bilingualism* (3rd ed.). Bristol, PA: Multilingual Matters.

Goldstein, B. (2004). *Bilingual language development and disorders in Spanish-English speakers.* Baltimore, MD: Brookes.

Green, L. (2002). *African-American English: A linguistic introduction.* New York: Cambridge University Press.

Gumperz, J. (1982). *Discourse strategies.* New York: Cambridge University Press.

McCardle, P., & Hoff, E. (Eds.). (2006). *Childhood bilingualism: Research on infancy through school age.* Tonawanda, NY: Multilingual Matters.

Trumbull, E., Rothstein-Fisch, C., Greenfield, P. M., & Quiroz, B. (2001). *Bridging cultures between home and school: A guide for teachers: With a special focus on immigrant Latino families.* Mahwah, NJ: Erlbaum.

section II

Individuals with Speech Disorders

four

Speech Science

THOMAS P. MARQUARDT AND CHRISTINE L. MATYEAR

LEARNING OBJECTIVES

1. To learn the major structures and functions of the central and peripheral nervous systems.

2. To learn the localization of speech and language functions of the cerebrum.

3. To understand the basic processes of respiration, phonation, resonation, and articulation for speech production.

4. To learn the acoustic properties of the speech sounds of English.

5. To learn how speech sounds are categorized based on voicing, place, and manner of production.

Speech production for most individuals requires little effort. We can speak for long periods of time without undue fatigue. The reason is that the physiological effort for speech production is minimally taxing. Biting to open a difficult candy wrapper or blowing up a balloon may be more physically demanding.

Speaking involves the interaction of respiratory, laryngeal, and articulatory structures, all governed by the nervous system. We consider each of these components in turn but with the understanding that they do not function independently but rather as a whole during speech production.

We first review terms helpful to understanding the relationship among structures of the body (Table 4-1). These terms provide an orientation to the structures of the nervous system as well as respiratory, laryngeal, and articulatory systems. Take a moment to review them before we continue.

NERVOUS SYSTEM

The nervous system is composed of a series of complex, densely connected structures that make speech and language possible. The vital building blocks of the systems are neurons supported by an infrastructure of other cells essential to their operation. The nervous system is divided into the central nervous system (CNS), which consists of the brain and spinal cord, and the peripheral nervous system, made up of neurons that carry information to and from the CNS.

The Neuron

The nervous system contains as many as 10 billion neurons and perhaps many more. The neurons differ in size and shape, depending on their location and function. Most often we think of these cells as being microscopic and densely packed. In some cases, however, neurons are very long. If we considered the unusual example of the giraffe, there are neurons that extend from the surface of the brain to the tail end of the spinal cord, a total distance of perhaps 14 feet.

Regardless of the size, shape, or function of neurons, they have common architectural features. If you examine the neuron shown in Figure 4-1, you can identify a cell body, a nucleus and nucleolus, dendrites, and an axon. Neurons may have many dendrites, but only one axon. They also may or may not have **myelin**, a fatty insulator

Table 4-1 Orientations in Anatomic Descriptions

Superior: toward the top	**Inferior:** toward the bottom
Posterior: toward the back	**Anterior:** toward the front
Medial: toward the middle	**Lateral:** toward the side
Ventral: toward the belly	**Caudal:** toward the back
Superficial: near the surface	**Deep:** away from the surface
Proximal: toward the middle	**Distal:** away from the middle

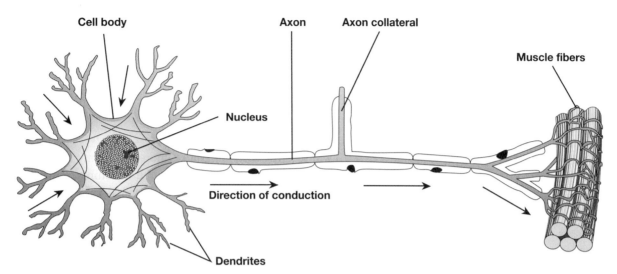

Figure 4-1 The neuron. *Source:* Rothenberg, M. A., & Elling, M. K. (2003). *Paramedic: Anatomy and physiology* (p. 31). Sudbury, MA: Jones and Bartett.

covering the axon that speeds transmission of impulses, and *neurilemma*, a covering of the axon that allows it to regain function after being damaged. Only nerves of the PNS have neurilemma, so they are the only neurons that can effectively reestablish function after damage to the axon.

Neurons can be described by their function. A neuron is termed an **efferent** if it conveys impulses from higher to lower structures. In most cases, efferent neurons are *motor neurons* and make up the nerves that carry impulses to muscles and glands from the brain and spinal cord. Neurons that bring information to a higher structure of the nervous system are termed **afferent**. Afferent neurons are *sensory* and bring information, for example, from the ear, eye, and nose to the brain. *Interneurons* make up the neural tissue of the brain and spinal cord. They are far more numerous than the sensory and motor neurons are combined.

Neurons communicate with one another by means of synapses, functional gaps between the axon of one neuron and the dendrites and cell bodies of surrounding neurons. When a neuron is excited, a wave of electrical activity (depolarization) sweeps down the axon to end branches where **neurotransmitters** are released to excite or inhibit the response of surrounding neurons. Neurotransmitters are the chemical messengers of the nervous system. A large number of different types of neurotransmitters facilitate or inhibit responses and make a complex functional networking of groups of neurons possible. Networks of neurons work together in a group, but a single neuron may be involved in more than a single network. In fact, neurons may be influenced by hundreds of other neurons as a result of varied synaptic relationships.

There is also another important group of cells in the nervous system, **glial cells**. Glial cells perform a number of functions: (1) they form the fatty myelin covering of axons that affect the speed of transmission of an impulse down the axon; (2) they serve as a blood–brain barrier for nutrients delivered to neurons; and (3) they remove dead cells from the nervous system.

The brain has characteristic areas of gray and white matter. The gray matter is composed primarily of neuron cell bodies. White matter is given its appearance by the myelin covering on axons that make up the projections or transmission lines between different parts of the brain.

CENTRAL NERVOUS SYSTEM

The CNS includes the cerebrum, brainstem, cerebellum, and spinal cord (Figure 4-2). It is encased within the skull and spinal column, covered by tissue layers (**meninges)** and surrounded by circulating cerebrospinal fluid. The *cerebrum* has two **cerebral hemispheres** that are similar but not identical in appearance. There are differences in the size of the areas of the two hemispheres, but we do not yet fully understand the functional importance of the differences.

Cerebrum

Each hemisphere has four lobes: frontal, parietal, temporal, and occipital (Figure 4-3). The lobes of the hemispheres have unique but not exclusive functional roles. The frontal lobe is responsible for motor planning and execution, the temporal lobe is important

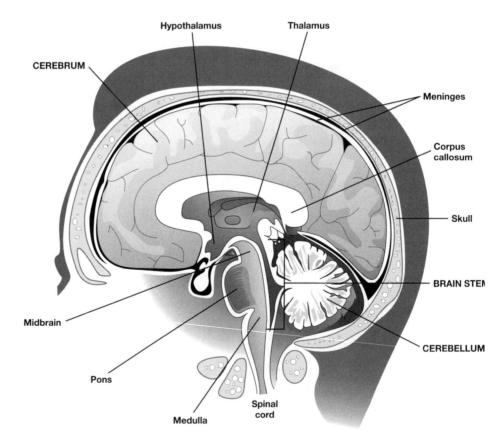

Figure 4-2 Structures of the central nervous system. *Source:* Rothenberg, M. A., & Elling, M. K. (2003). *Paramedic: Anatomy and physiology* (p. 169). Sudbury, MA: Jones and Bartett.

for auditory processing, the occipital lobe for visual processing, and the parietal lobe for sensory association and spatial processing.

The surface of the cerebrum is folded with prominences (**gyri**) and depressions (**sulci**). The gyri and sulci are identified most typically by brain lobe and position. For example, three gyri of the frontal lobe are the superior, middle, and inferior frontal gyri (Figure 4-3).

The two hemispheres are separated by a deep longitudinal fissure, but are joined by a series of connecting pathways that form the **corpus callosum.** The frontal lobe is demarcated by the lateral **(Sylvian) fissure** and by the central (**Rolandic) fissure**. The Sylvian and Rolandic fissures serve also as landmarks for the anterior border of the parietal lobe and the top of the temporal lobe. The occipital lobes lie at the back of each hemisphere.

The surface of the cerebrum is gray matter, that is, neuron cell bodies. Deep under this mantle of gray matter is white matter, given its appearance by the presence of myelin on the neuron axons. Lying within each hemisphere are groups of cell bodies (nuclei) important for sensory and motor processing: the **basal ganglia** and **thalamus**. The basal ganglia are important for the control of movement. Damage to these structures results in involuntary movements such as tremors that you might observe in an older adult with Parkinson's disease or writhing arm movements in a child with cerebral palsy. Sensory information is projected to the cortical surface through the

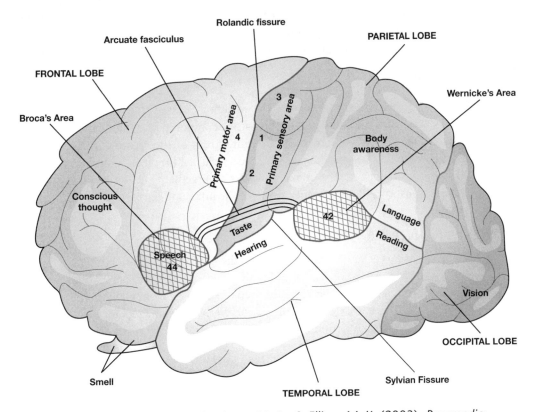

Figure 4-3 The cerebral cortex. *Source:* Rothenberg, M. A., & Elling, M. K. (2003). *Paramedic: Anatomy and physiology* (p. 169). Sudbury, MA: Jones and Bartett.

thalamus. What this means is that all the information from our senses, with the exception of our sense of smell, is routed through the thalamus on its way to the surface of the cerebrum. An example of a nucleus of the thalamus is the medial geniculate, a structure within the auditory pathways described in Chapter 13.

Brainstem

The **brainstem** lies at the base of the brain in front of the cerebellum and includes in descending order the *midbrain*, *pons*, and *medulla*. The brainstem is a conduit for sensory information coming from the receptors of the body for touch, temperature, pain, and pressure as well as vision, hearing, balance, and movement, and for motor pathways to the muscles of the body. The strategic position of the brainstem is clearly evident in Figure 4-2. Many of the nerves that bring sensory information from the head and neck and that project to the muscles of this region are located in the brainstem, so these structures are important to speech production.

Cerebellum

The *cerebellum* lies in back and on top of the brainstem and includes two hemispheres. The cerebellar cortex is highly convoluted such that its surface area is large. It is connected to the brainstem by three pathways that allow for the (1) input of sensory information from the body, (2) output of signals for motor execution to the body musculature, and (3) input from the cerebrum for control of cerebellar function. The cerebellum is important for balance and for ensuring coordination of various body movements; specifically, the timing, amount, and speed of movement.

Spinal Cord

The *spinal cord* lies within the vertebral column. In contrast to the cerebrum and cerebellum, the outer part of the cord is composed of white matter with a butterfly-shaped area of gray matter in the interior. Areas of the spinal cord are identified by the surrounding vertebrae. There are 7 cervical, 12 thoracic, 5 lumbar, and 5 sacral vertebrae, plus a coccyx. The spinal cord has enlargements at the cervical and lumbar levels for sensory and motor innervation of the arms and legs.

PERIPHERAL NERVOUS SYSTEM

Groups of nerves extending from the CNS make up the *peripheral nervous system*. The nerves can be divided into highly specialized cranial nerves that extend from the cerebrum and brainstem, and the spinal nerves that extend from the spinal cord.

There are 12 pairs of *cranial nerves* specialized for sensory, motor, or sensory and motor functions (Table 4-2). The cranial nerves most important for speech production include the trigeminal, facial, glossopharyngeal, vagus, accessory, and hypoglossal that innervate the musculature of the head and neck. It would be helpful at this point to review each of the nerves to learn their names and function, as shown in Table 4-2.

Table 4-2 Cranial Nerves

Number	Name	Function
I	Olfactory	Sensory for smell
II	Optic	Sensory for vision
III	Oculomotor	Motor for eye movement
IV	Trochlear	Motor for eye movement
V	Trigeminal	Motor for mastication (chewing) Sensory for face, maxillary teeth, and eyes
VI	Abducents	Motor for eye movements
VII	Facial	Motor for facial movements Sensory for taste for front of tongue
VIII	Vestibulocochlear	Sensory for hearing and balance
IX	Glossopharyngeal	Motor for pharyngeal movements Sensory for taste at back of tongue
X	Vagus	Motor for intrinsic laryngeal and pharyngeal movements Sensory for motor for thoracic and abdominal viscera
XI	Accessory	Motor for shoulder movements
XII	Hypoglossal	Motor for tongue movements

There are 31 pairs of *spinal nerves* that arise from the spinal cord and innervate sensory and motor functions of the body below the level of the neck. In contrast to the cranial nerves, the spinal nerves are not specialized for sensory or motor functions but innervate specific areas of the body. They carry general sensory information from specific areas of the body, such as the side of the leg or bottom of the arm, and serve as a final common pathway for motor impulses from the CNS to the muscles. In general, input from the cervical level is to the hands and arms, from the thoracic level to the trunk of the body, and from the lumbar, sacral, and coccygeal levels to the front and back of the legs and the feet.

HEMISPHERIC SPECIALIZATION/LOCALIZATION OF FUNCTION

The two cerebral hemispheres are specialized in terms of the types of information they are most adept at processing. The left hemisphere is specialized for sequential functioning; the right hemisphere for holistic processing. Because speech and language are processed over time, the left hemisphere has a dominant role in this aspect of communicative functioning. The right hemisphere's holistic processing makes it more adept at face recognition, comprehending and expressing emotion, and music. This functional asymmetry is true, in most cases, whether the person is right or left handed.

Although the two hemispheres are specialized for the types of information they are best able to handle, it is clear that they work together during communication. When talking with a friend, for example, you listen not only to what he says, but how he says it and the intonation of the phrases, and you observe his facial appearance and the gestures he uses. What your friend communicates is more meaningful than simply the words he uses.

Earlier, we mentioned that the lobes of the cerebral hemispheres have different functional responsibilities. For example, we mentioned that the temporal lobe is responsible for auditory processing and the occipital lobe for visual processing. More specific functional roles can be assigned to cortical areas of the left hemisphere, not like a mosaic, but more like an increased role of one area compared to another in carrying out a particular processing task.

Localization of function for the left hemisphere based on the Brodmann numbering system is shown in Figure 4-4. We do not discuss the functional specialization in detail in this chapter, but rather focus on sensory and motor behaviors and speech and language representation. Both anatomic and functional descriptions may be employed for this purpose. Anatomically, particular gyri are identified; in functional terms, Brodmann's areas are described. Brodmann's numbers demarcate areas where specific types of processing take place. An example may be helpful: The area responsible for

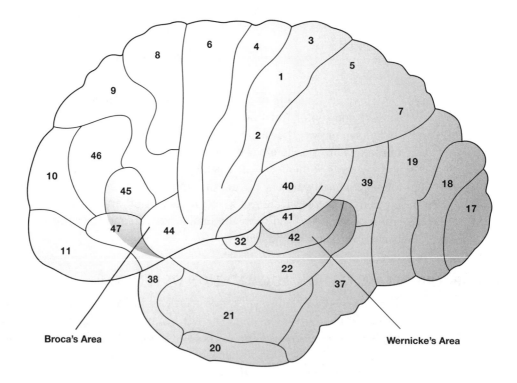

Figure 4-4 Cortical speech centers. *Source:* Chiras, D. D. (2008. *Human biology* (6th ed., p. 200). Sudbury, MA: Jones and Bartlett.

programming speech movements is Brodmann's area 44; it also could be described as the posterior part of the third (inferior) frontal gyrus.

The frontal lobe has important representation of motor functions for the opposite side of the body on the precentral gyrus (Brodmann's area 4), which lies just in front of the frontal fissure. More than 50 years ago, researchers studied this area while doing brain surgery. They found they could cause movements of various parts of the left side of the body by stimulating this "motor strip" on the right side of the brain. Stimulating the gyrus near the top of the brain caused movements of the lower limb; stimulating the gyrus at a lower point caused arm and tongue movements. They also observed that a larger area could be stimulated to obtain tongue or thumb movements than for arm movements. They demonstrated that the representation for body movements is in the form of an inverted and distorted body image with the feet and legs located on the medial aspect of the hemisphere and the body, neck and head, and then hand represented laterally. The body scheme is distorted because there are a larger number of neurons that project to areas with highly developed motor skill such as the tongue and thumb. This motor strip is the primary origin for direct motor pathways to the muscles of the body.

Just behind the lateral fissure is the postcentral gyrus of the parietal lobe (Brodmann's areas 1, 2, 3). Here there is a sensory representation of the body in a form similar to that of the motor strip. That is, the feet and legs are represented near the top of the gyrus, with the trunk, face, and hands along the side. Broad areas of the frontal and parietal lobes, like the other lobes of the brain, contain association cortex. These areas do not have highly specialized functioning but are involved in processing various types of information.

Several areas of the left side of the brain are important to speech and language. **Broca's area** (area 44) and surrounding tissue of the posterior part of the inferior frontal gyrus are important for the programming of movements for speech production. Damage in this location causes problems in the planning and carrying out of speech movements.

The temporal lobe includes an area critical for understanding auditory information (**Wernicke's area**). This area (Brodmann's area 42) is located on the back part of the first temporal gyrus. It is linked to the supramarginal and angular gyri that are important to language interpretation. Damage to Wernicke's area results in a marked deficit in understanding what is heard. Also, other areas of the temporal lobe are important for reading.

The cerebrum could not function unless there were pathways that carry information from one place to another within and between the hemispheres of the brain. Particularly important to speech and language is the *arcuate fasciculus* that connects Wernicke's area to Broca's area. Damage to this connecting pathway causes difficulty in repeating what is heard because the information cannot be conveyed efficiently between Wernicke's and Broca's areas. The Broca's area-arcuate fasciculus-Wernicke's area complex is critical to speech and language functioning. Damage to this area produces classifiable types of language disorders in adults, which are the focus of the chapter on aphasia (see Chapter 12).

MOTOR PATHWAYS

Motor activity is controlled by two major tracts of the nervous system—pyramidal and extrapyramidal. The **pyramidal tract** is a direct pathway from the cortical surface to the peripheral nerves (Figure 4-5). Pyramidal tract neurons frequently are referred to as upper motor neurons, and peripheral nerve neurons as lower motor neurons. The lower motor neurons that innervate muscles are a final common pathway because all input to the body by necessity must be channeled through these nerves. The origin of the pyramidal tract is centered on the motor strip (Brodmann's area 4), approximately the area of the precentral gyrus. Representation of motor function, as we have discussed, is inverted, with the feet and trunk of the body represented on the superior aspects of the frontal lobe and the face and hands represented on the lateral aspect of the hemisphere. The neurons of the pyramidal tract form pathways that travel through the interior of

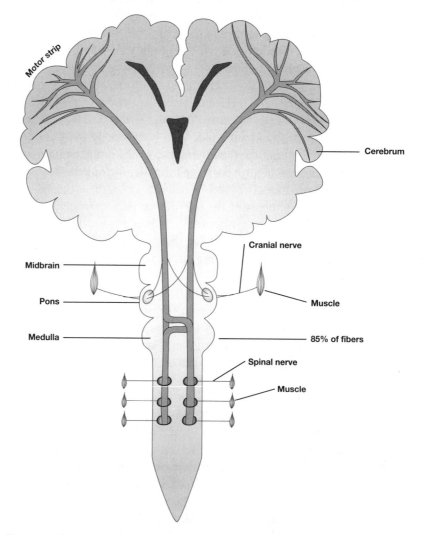

Figure 4-5 Schematic diagram of pyramidal tract. *Source:* Rothenberg, M. A., & Elling, M. K. (2003). *Paramedic: Anatomy and physiology* (p. 176). Sudbury, MA: Jones and Bartett.

BOX 4-1 Neuroimages of the Brain

On CD-ROM segment Ch.4.01, compare the neuroimages from computerized tomography and magnetic resonance imaging in terms of how the brain structures are revealed.

---

each hemisphere to either the cranial nerves of the brainstem or to the spinal nerves. Approximately 85% of the fibers traveling to the spinal nerves cross to the opposite side of the body at the medulla. Therefore, the left side of the body receives innervation from the right side of the brain and vice versa.

For the cranial nerves, the innervation is somewhat different. Axons from both the left and right hemispheres innervate the motor cranial nerves with the exception of part of the facial nerve. When an individual has a stroke in the frontal lobe of the left hemisphere, most of the motor functions of the head and neck are spared because innervation from the right side of the brain to these nerves has not been interrupted.

The **extrapyramidal tract** is a complex system important for control of movements. It originates in an area just in front of the motor strip (Brodmann's area 6) but overlaps with the pyramidal tract on the frontal lobes. This tract is indirect to the extent that input is from the cerebral cortex to basal ganglia deep within the cerebrum, with internal loops that project back to the cerebrum and downward to influence lower motor neurons. The extrapyramidal tract's role is to modulate the complex motor activity of the nervous system. Damage to the system results in problems with the level of background electrical activity within muscles and the development of involuntary movements such as tremors.

There are a number of modern methods for studying brain anatomy and function including, among others, computerized tomography (CT) and magnetic resonance imaging (MRI). CT scans are based on computer-processed X-rays; MRI relies on intense magnetic fields that affect the spin axis of electrons. Other modern techniques such as functional magnetic resonance imaging and positron emission tomography are important new developments because they allow brain activity to be investigated during the performance of speech and language tasks.

The nervous system governs speech production by providing input to the more than 100 pairs of muscles of the respiratory, laryngeal, and articulatory structures with continual on-line sensory monitoring of the process. We examine each subsystem of speech production and then consider the dynamic process by which these components are used to produce articulate speech.

RESPIRATION

Respiration is the power source for speech production. The primary components of the respiratory system are the lungs, rib cage, the air passageways, and diaphragm. The lungs lie within the bony framework of the rib cage. They have access to the upper airway by means of the bronchioles, bronchi, and trachea, which are a series of air-filled tubes of varying diameters. The lungs fill a large portion of the thorax (chest cavity), which is separated from the abdominal cavity by a large muscle called the diaphragm (Figure 4-6).

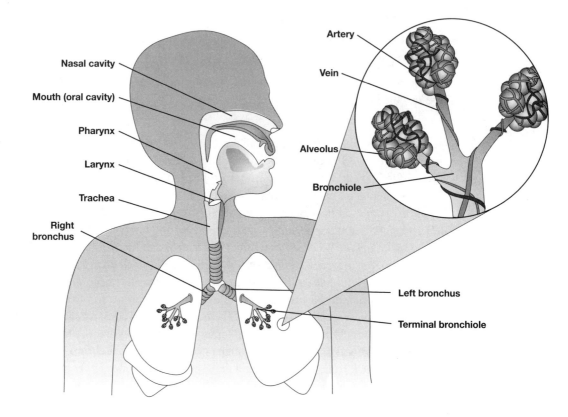

Artery
Vein
Alveolus
Bronchiole

Nasal cavity
Mouth (oral cavity)
Pharynx
Larynx
Trachea
Right bronchus

Left bronchus
Terminal bronchiole

Figure 4-6   The lungs with an enlargement of the alveolar sacs. *Source:* Rothenberg, M. A., & Elling, M. K. (2003). *Paramedic: Anatomy and physiology.* Sudbury, MA: Jones and Bartett.

The internal structure of the lungs is analogous to the branching structure of an inverted tree (Kent, 1997) composed of a trunk (trachea) and a series of branches (bronchi and bronchioles) that end in air-filled sacs (alveoli). The alveoli are the end organs where the exchange of oxygen and carbon dioxide takes place. In their natural state, the lungs are spongy and elastic.

The lungs are surrounded by 12 pairs of ribs that extend from the thoracic vertebrae at the spinal column to the front of the body (Figure 4-7). Seven pairs of "true" ribs attach to the sternum and three additional pairs of "false" ribs attach to the base of the lowest true rib. The lowest two pairs of ribs do not attach to the sternum anteriorly and are termed "floating ribs." At the top of the thorax are additional bones that protect the lungs and serve as attachment points for our upper limbs, the two scapulas (shoulder blades) and the two clavicles (collar bones).

The movement of air during breathing results from changes in lung volume and the resulting changes in air pressure within the lungs (alveolar pressure). In the body at rest, the lungs are slightly inflated and would collapse if punctured. The thorax, in contrast, is compressed and would expand if unlinked from the lungs. Membranes called pleura link the lungs and thorax. These include the visceral pleura that surround each lung and the parietal pleura that lines the interior surface of the rib cage and the upper surface of the diaphragm. The pleura of the lungs and thorax are bonded together by

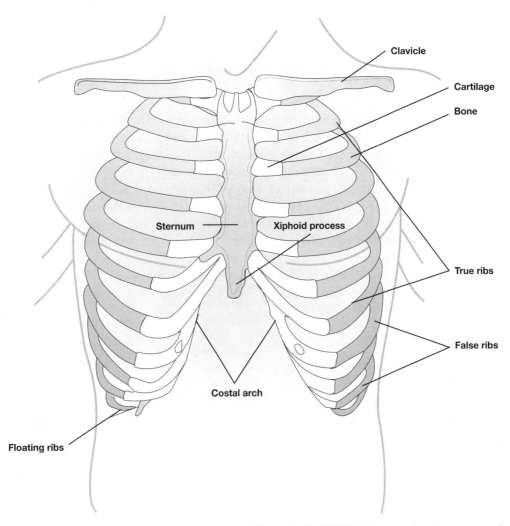

Figure 4-7 The rib cage. *Source:* Rothenberg, M. A., & Elling, M. K. (2003). *Paramedic: Anatomy and physiology* (p. 63). Sudbury, MA: Jones and Bartett.

negative pressure so that as the shape of the thoracic cavity changes, the lungs, which are linked to its surface by the pleurae, have to conform to the change. At a mechanically neutral point in the respiratory cycle (**resting expiratory level**), the opposing forces of the lungs (collapse) and thorax (expand) are in balance and air pressure in the lungs (alveolar pressure) is equal to the air pressure outside the body (atmospheric pressure). This assumes, of course, that the airway from the lungs is open.

Respiration is the process of moving air in and out of the lungs. We know from elementary laws of physics that for an enclosed gas such as air, pressure is inversely related to volume (Boyle's law) and that air flows from areas of high pressure to areas of low pressure (Law of Gases). An increase in lung volume causes a reduction in the air pressure within the lungs, resulting in an inward flow of air (inspiration); a reduction in lung volume causes an increase in air pressure in the lungs and an outward flow of air (expiration).

Changes in lung volume are caused by the application of active muscle forces to the respiratory system. The respiratory system is elastic; it is subject to being stretched and is capable of rebounding from the distortion. Some muscles increase the size of the lungs (inspiratory muscles) by pulling them to a larger volume; other muscles decrease the size by compressing the lungs (expiratory muscles). After the lungs are stretched to a larger volume or compressed to a smaller volume by contraction of the respiratory muscles, the relaxation of those muscles causes the lungs to return to their rest position (resting expiratory level). This is much like a coiled spring that can be stretched or compressed, but that returns to its original shape when released. Recoil (relaxation) forces of this type in the respiratory system are described as passive.

Primary inspiratory muscles that expand the size of the lungs are the *diaphragm* (Figure 4-8), a bowl-shaped partition between the lungs and abdominal contents, and the *external intercostals*, a sheet of 11 muscles that lie between the ribs. These muscles act to increase the front to back, side to side, and top to bottom volume of the lungs. In effect, they cause an increase in the size of the lungs by pulling them to a larger volume. They are supplemented by other muscles that help to raise the rib cage, sternum, and clavicle during more demanding inspiratory activity, such as taking a deep breath.

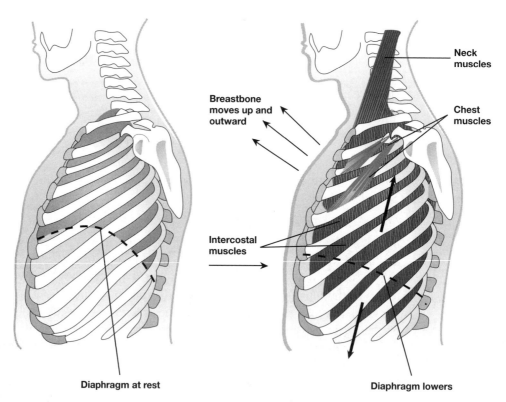

Figure 4-8 The diaphragm. Source: Chiras, D. D. (2008). *Human biology* (6th ed., p. 160). Sudbury, MA: Jones and Bartlett.

Expiratory muscles work to reduce the volume of the lungs by narrowing the rib cage and by compressing the abdominal contents so that they press upward on the diaphragm. You probably have noticed during a demanding singing activity that the muscles of your abdomen were fatigued after a particularly long passage. That is because you were using muscles such as the *rectus abdominis* to push inward on the abdominal contents, which forced the diaphragm upward to reduce lung volume. At the same time, the *internal intercostals*, another series of muscles lying between the ribs, pulled down on the rib cage and expiratory muscles of the back pulled down on the back of the ribs to reduce the volume of the lungs.

As you probably have deduced by this point, changes in lung volume are accomplished by application of muscle forces to the respiratory apparatus. With the application of these forces, there is a storing up of recoil (relaxation) forces in the lungs, rib cage, and abdomen that have the potential, when released, of increasing or decreasing the pressure within the lungs. When the volume of the lungs is increased from a mechanically neutral point (resting expiratory level), relaxation results in a decrease in lung volume, an increase in lung pressure, and an outward flow of air. Compressing the lungs to a smaller volume than at rest stores up recoil (relaxation) forces that will cause the lungs to expand to a larger volume with an inward flow of air when respiratory muscles are relaxed.

During quiet breathing (breathing while sitting quietly), the diaphragm and external intercostals actively increase lung volume to develop an inward flow of air. When the pressure within the lungs is equal to atmospheric pressure, the flow of air stops. The process of inspiration results in the storing of recoil forces primarily in the lungs and abdomen. When released, these forces produce a reduction of lung volume and expiration. Note that during this quiet breathing cycle, inspiration is active and expiration is passive. That is, muscles are active in expanding the lungs, but are not active as the lungs collapse back to their original size because the relaxation forces make the lungs smaller without help from expiratory muscles.

During speech, the respiratory system provides a stable air pressure within the lungs. This activity is accomplished by the balancing of active (muscle) and passive (recoil) forces to maintain a constant pressure while lung volume is decreasing with the loss of air. This maneuver includes the active use of inspiratory and expiratory muscles during the expiratory phase of speech production to act like brakes and accelerators to maintain a constant pressure.

Speech breathing is different in two important respects from quiet breathing—the lungs are increased to a larger volume and the expiratory phase is extended. More air is taken into the lungs while talking. The amount of air inspired is determined by the length and intensity of what the speaker intends to say. Obviously, if you want to shout or to read a paragraph aloud without stopping to take a breath, you take in more air and use a greater portion of the total volume of air in your lungs.

During quiet breathing, inspiration and expiration take about the same amount of time. However, this pattern is altered during speech with an extended expiratory phase in the respiratory cycle. The effect of respiratory activity for speech, then, is to provide an extended stable air pressure to the larynx and upper airway.

PHONATION

The larynx is a small hollow structure lying in the anterior neck. Part of the air passageway, it is located between the top of the trachea (or windpipe) and the bottom of the pharynx (throat cavity). It is composed of cartilages, muscles, membranes, and other connective tissue. The function of the larynx in speech production is to convert respiratory energy, the energy of air put into motion by movement of respiratory muscles, to sound energy (phonation, or voicing).

Lying horizontally across the hollow, tube-like center of the larynx is a valve that we can close to block the flow of air. This valve is formed by a pair of complex structures called the vocal folds. In speech science, we are interested in the vocal folds because their vibration creates the sound of human voicing, but it is also important to note that they serve two vital functions: They help protect the lungs from accidentally aspirating (inhaling) foreign matter, and they permit us to perform muscular actions such as "bearing down."

When we swallow, the vocal folds close tightly and a leaf-shaped cartilage called the epiglottis, which is located at the top of the larynx, folds down to cover the vocal folds. Together these structures help ensure that food and liquid travel as they should around the inside of the larynx and down into the esophagus (food passageway) into the stomach rather than down center to trachea and into the lungs. If foreign matter (e.g., excessive mucus or food) should become lodged in the trachea or the lungs, the air pressure from the lungs can force the vocal folds open explosively (coughing) to help expel the material back into the oral cavity. When we need to hold our breath to perform effortful muscular tasks such as weight lifting or bearing down (e.g., during childbirth), the vocal folds also close tightly, trapping air in the lungs and providing greater downward force to assist the abdominal muscles.

To understand the role of the vocal folds in speech production, however, we must first understand how they fit into the overall structure of the larynx. The skeletal structure of the larynx consists of three large unmatched and three pairs of matched cartilages. Of these, the following four are most important for speech production: the cricoid, the thyroid, and the paired arytenoids cartilages (Figure 4-9). All of these cartilages can move with respect to one another and as a consequence are able to affect the vocal folds, either stretching or shortening them and either tensing or relaxing them. These changes in the vocal folds lead to changes in the quality of the human voice.

The laryngeal cartilages move with respect to one another through the action of various intrinsic muscles (muscles that connect one laryngeal cartilage to another). The entire larynx moves with respect to the rest of the body by the action of various extrinsic muscles (muscles that attach the larynx to structures outside of the larynx). In addition, the various cartilages and muscles are attached to one another by connective tissues (ligaments and tendons) and are lined by mucous membranes. Altogether, the larynx is a specialized, airtight portion of the respiratory passageway.

The four laryngeal cartilages that affect the vocal folds, the cricoid, the thyroid, and the two arytenoids, have distinctive shapes and ranges of motion. The large cricoid cartilage is roughly circular, being shaped something like a signet ring (narrow in its

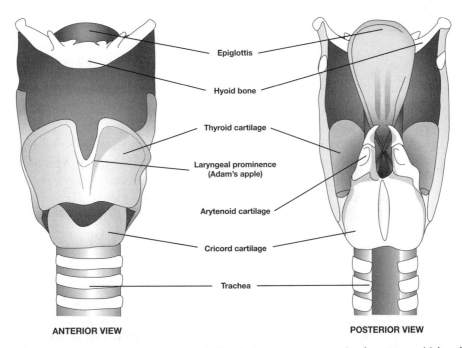

Epiglottis

Hyoid bone

Thyroid cartilage

Laryngeal prominence
(Adam's apple)

Arytenoid cartilage

Cricord cartilage

Trachea

ANTERIOR VIEW

POSTERIOR VIEW

Figure 4-9 Layrngeal cartilages. *Source:* Caroline, N. (2007). Emergency care in the streets (6th ed., p. II.8). Sudbury, MA: Jones and Bartlett.

anterior aspects and wide in its posterior aspect). It is seated horizontally at the very top of the trachea and is in fact a modified tracheal ring. Compared to the other laryngeal cartilages, it is relatively stationary; however, it provides a base for the others to move against.

The large thyroid cartilage, roughly prow-shaped (like the front of a boat), is formed by two large flat plates called lamina that come together in front to form the thyroid angle (the outside edge of this angle is what we can perceive as the "Adam's apple" in men). The posterior edges of the thyroid lamina sport two protrusions each. Extending upward are two large cornua (horns), and extending downward are two small cornua. The large cornua attach the thyroid cartilage to a small horseshoe-shaped bone called the hyoid bone that lies at the base of the tongue. The small cornua attach the thyroid to the cricoids, forming two small ball-and-socket joints on the lateral aspects (the sides) of the wide portion of the cricoid. The thyroid can rock up and down and can glide forward and backward at these joints.

The two small arytenoid cartilages (a matched pair) are roughly shaped like four-sided, triangle-based pyramids. They are seated on top of the wide portion of the cricoid, one on the left and one on the right, each in its own small ball-and-socket joint. In this position, the arytenoid cartilages can rotate their front peaks toward or away from one another, and they can glide forward and backward.

Several intrinsic muscles of the larynx create the movements of the cartilages. The ones we are most interested in are the internal thyroarytenoid muscles, also known as the thyrovocalis or simply the vocalis muscles. Coursing horizontally from the inside of the thyroid angle to the anterior points of the arytenoids cartilages, these muscles form the body of the vocal folds (Figure 4-10).

The connective tissues of the larynx include tendons, which attach muscles to cartilages, and ligaments, which connect cartilages to cartilages. Of great importance to us are the vocal ligaments, which also course horizontally between the inside of the thyroid angle and the arytenoids cartilages. These ligaments lie parallel to the thyroarytenoid muscles and form the edges of the vocal folds.

The mucous membrane that lines the inside of the larynx is contiguous with the membrane that lines the trachea and the throat cavity. As it courses down the laryngeal pathway, the left and right sides of the mucous membrane fold over on themselves twice, creating four flaps of soft tissue. Two such folds cover and surround the edges of the vocal ligaments and the thyroarytenoid muscles and are called the "true vocal folds" (or simply the vocal folds). The other two folds, lying parallel to and slightly above the true vocal folds, are called the "false vocal folds."

The vocal folds thus course horizontally from the inside of the thyroid angle, each attaching to one of the small arytenoids cartilages. Each vocal fold consists of muscle (thyroarytenoid muscle), connective tissue (vocal ligament), and a surface cover (mucous membrane). Lying as they do, the vocal folds are subject to being moved in various ways. They can be spread apart (abducted) or pulled together to the point of touching (adducted) by the action of the muscles that move the arytenoids cartilages. They can be tensed by the **adduction** of the vocalis muscles. They can be stretched by

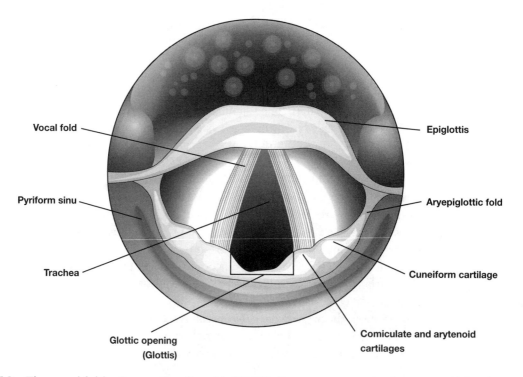

Figure 4-10 The vocal folds. *Source:* Caroline, N. (2007). Emergency care in the streets (6th ed., p. II.9). Sudbury, MA: Jones and Bartlett.

the action of the muscles that move the thyroid cartilage. Tension in the folds can also be affected by action of the extrinsic muscles that move the entire larynx up or down in the neck. What are the consequences of these movements for speech?

When the vocal folds are abducted (spread apart), the gap between them (called the **glottis**) is part of the open passageway that lets air flow into and out of the lungs. The sound of such air movement is either very soft and quiet (when the glottis is very wide) or harsh and noisy (when the glottis is somewhat constricted). However, when the vocal folds are adducted (brought together to touch), the airway is blocked. Under this condition, air being exhaled from the lungs builds up pressure (subglottal pressure) below the closed vocal folds. When subglottal pressure becomes intense enough to cause the vocal folds to bulge upward, they are eventually blown open and release a minute puff of air. The folds then fall back and are sucked back together by a combination of elastic recoil and aerodynamic forces. Elastic recoil, or myoelasticity, refers to the tendency of soft tissue, when deformed by some force (in this case subglottal pressure) to rebound to its original shape when that force is removed. The aerodynamic force in this case is called the **Bernoulli effect**. When the speed of airflow along a surface increases, the air pressure against that surface decreases. As air rushes out between the vocal folds when they are blown apart, the pressure against their surfaces reduces, and they are sucked back together by the partial vacuum that is created. The entire cycle can then repeat.

As long as subglottal pressure is maintained, the vocal folds will continue to move in this fashion at a very rapid and fairly regular rate (e.g., 200 times per second). This motion is called vocal fold vibration, and the series of small puffs of air emerging from between the adducted vocal folds sounds like a low hum (called phonation or voicing). The more slowly the vocal folds vibrate, the lower pitched the hum, and the faster they vibrate, the higher pitched the hum. This process is termed the aerodynamic myoelastic theory of vocal fold vibration.

The perceptual quality of the sound of vocal fold vibration (pitch, timbre, loudness) is affected by the size, shape, and amount of tension in the vocal folds and by the rate and volume of airflow from the lungs. Heavier, more massive, vocal folds naturally vibrate more slowly than lighter, less massive ones. We understand this instinctively: Men tend to have deeper-pitched voices than women because they have more massive vocal folds that vibrate slowly. Infants and children have even less massive vocal folds than women and correspondingly higher-pitched voices because their vocal folds vibrate rapidly. But no matter what a speaker's intrinsic pitch is, that person can change it by using the muscles of the larynx to stretch, contract, tense, or relax the vocal folds. And these changes in the physical properties of the vocal folds require corresponding adjustments in the flow of air from the lungs to maintain steady vibration and to control loudness. In short, the interaction between the respiratory and the laryngeal systems permits speakers to modulate their voices to an amazing degree. The result is the capacity to sing a wide range of melodies, loudly or softly with great emotion, and to speak from a shout to a whisper to convey emotions from ecstasy to rage and to communicate in statements of fact to interrogatives by adjusting laryngeal airflow.

The humming sound of vocal fold vibration (also called voicing or phonation), however, is only part of the story. The sound produced in the larynx must pass through the upper airways before it can emerge as speech. To understand how the upper airways modulate the sound of vocal fold vibration, we first need to understand something about the nature of that sound. The sound produced as the vocal folds vibrate is complex and periodic.

As discussed in Chapter 14, complex periodic sound is composed of a series of simple periodic sounds (pure tones) called **harmonics.** Each harmonic tone has a unique frequency and amplitude. Frequency is measured in cycles per second or Hertz (Hz). The lowest of these harmonic frequencies is called the **fundamental frequency (F0)** and represents the rate of vocal fold vibration (what we perceive as the pitch of the voice). Each subsequent harmonic has a frequency that is an integer multiple of the FO (e.g., if F0 = 120 Hz, subsequent harmonics will have frequencies of 240, 360, 480, 600, 720, . . . Hz).

Amplitude is represented in decibels (dB) of sound pressure level or intensity level. The amplitudes of the harmonics in human phonation vary in a predictable fashion. F0 has the highest amplitude, and the subsequent harmonics have increasingly lower amplitudes. For typical human voicing that is neither overly loud nor overly soft, the amplitudes of the harmonics drop off at a rate of about 12 dB per octave (an octave being a doubling of the frequency). That means that the amplitudes of the harmonics drop off by about 12 dB in the interval between F0 and the second harmonic, another 12 dB between the second and the fourth harmonics, another 12 between the fourth and the eighth, and so forth. A graph called an amplitude spectrum shows the amplitude and frequency of each of the harmonics in a sample of human voicing (Figure 4-11).

When the sound of phonation travels up from the larynx and through the upper airways (also called the supralaryngeal tract or simply the vocal tract), the sound is modulated by the size and shape of the vocal tract. Some of the harmonics are amplified and some are reduced in amplitude (damped) with the result that the humming sound of phonation acquires perceptual overtones called resonant or formant frequencies. As

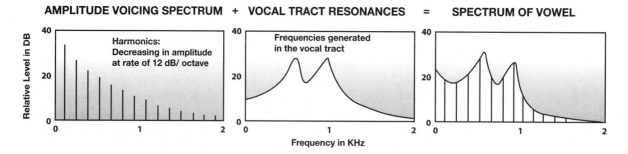

Figure 4-11 Voicing and vocal tract resonances together produce a vowel sound. Source: Fant, G. (1960). *Acoustic theory of speech production*. Hague: Mouton & Co.

BOX 4-2   Endoscopy of the Larynx

CD-ROM segment Ch.4.02 shows the larynx as revealed by endoscopy. The speed of the vocal folds has been slowed so that each cycle of vibration can be observed. Stroboscopy is a method used to slow down the apparent speed of vibration of the vocal folds. A pulsing light exposes the folds and gives sequential views of a series of vibrations that, when seen together, make the folds appear as if they are moving 100 times slower. The man is producing vocal fold vibration at several frequencies with different pitches. What is the relationship between increasing pitch and the mass and tension of the vocal folds?

---

the size and shape of the vocal tract changes, the resonances or formants of the voice change frequency correspondingly, creating the distinctively different sounds that are the consonants and vowels of speech. The process by which the different speech sounds are produced by changes in the vocal tract is called articulation.

Articulation

Articulation is the process of forming speech sounds by movement of the articulators (structures used to produce speech sounds). The articulatory system creates sound sources and shapes the resonance of the vocal tract to produce the recognizable speech sounds of the language. This is the primary focus of our discussion in this section.

The *vocal tract* is made up of a series of interconnected tubes from the larynx to the opening of the mouth and nose. (See Figure 4-12.) The *oral cavity* extends from the lips to the back of the throat. The *nasal cavity* extends from the opening at the nares to the *velopharynx*, the opening between the nose and mouth where the oral and nasal cavities are joined. The shape and size of the oral cavity are highly malleable and constantly changing during the course of speech production as a result of movements of the tongue, lips, jaw, and velum. The configuration of the nasal cavity, in contrast, is fixed. The *pharyngeal cavity* is the portion of the vocal tract that extends from the vocal folds to the nasal cavity and is subdivided into the laryngopharynx, oropharynx, and nasopharynx.

Articulation requires the coordinated movement of moveable structures for the production of speech sounds. The articulators can be considered as fixed or mobile. Fixed structures include the teeth, the alveolar ridge, and the hard palate. Mobile articulators are the jaw, tongue, face, and structures of the velopharynx.

The teeth are embedded in the alveolar ridge of the *maxilla* (upper jaw) and *mandible* (lower jaw). The chisel-like incisors are important to the production of sounds in English such as the voiceless and voiced /th/ sounds and sounds produced between the lower lip and upper incisors such as /f/ and /v/ in which contact is made between a mobile structure, such as the tongue and lips, and the teeth. The alveolar ridge, the bony semicircular shelf of the upper jaw, is important to the production of sounds such as /t/, /d/, /s/, and /z/. Extending from the alveolar ridge is an inverted bowl-shaped

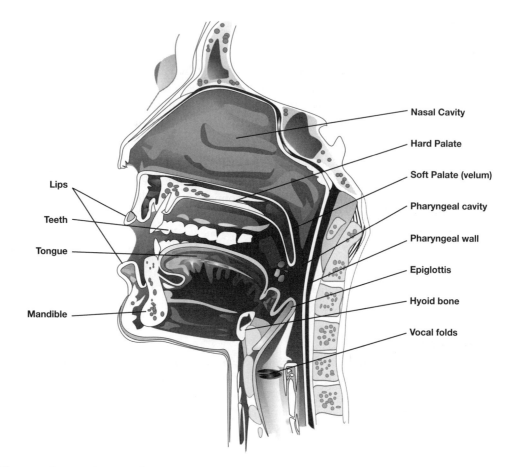

Labels on figure: Nasal Cavity, Hard Palate, Soft Palate (velum), Pharyngeal cavity, Pharyngeal wall, Epiglottis, Hyoid bone, Vocal folds, Lips, Teeth, Tongue, Mandible

Figure 4-12　The vocal tract. *Source:* Chiras, D. D. (2008). *Human biology* (6th ed., p. 154). Sudbury, MA: Jones and Bartlett.

hard palate formed by the palatine processes of the maxilla and the horizontal plates of the palatine bones. The hard palate is important as a contact point for multiple sound productions that involve the tongue such as articulatory contacts for the formation of the /sh/ at the midpalate and /j/ at the back of the hard palate.

The face is important to communication beyond the production of individual speech sounds. Expressions of anger, happiness, surprise, and fear are difficult to envision without the facial posturing that accompanies the emotion. The facial muscles are similar in function to a purse string used to gather the opening for closure. The primary rounding and closing muscle is the *obicularis oris*, a tear-shaped muscle that forms the interior of the upper and lower lip in circular fashion. Other facial muscles work in opposition to the obicularis oris to retract and open the lips. Primary movements of the face during speech production provide a point of closure for the stops /p/ and /b/ as well as the fricatives /f/ and /v/.

Another mobile articulator is the mandible. The mandible has the largest mass of any of the articulators and functions as a platform for the tongue. The mandible lowers or raises the tongue depending on the height of the vowel produced. For example, if you produce the vowels "eee" and "ahh," you will notice that the jaw is raised for the first vowel and lowered for the second. The jaw also is raised to make it easier for the tongue to make articulatory contacts.

The upward and downward movements of the jaw are different during chewing and speech production. While chewing food, the jaw moves asymmetrically as food is ground between the teeth; during speech production the mandible moves up and down symmetrically.

Mandible movements are accomplished by muscles that extend between the sides of the jaw and the skull and between the mandible and the hyoid bone at the base of the tongue. Some muscles connect to a midline connective tissue structure extending back from the mandible to form the floor of the mouth. You can identify two muscles responsible for jaw closure quite easily. If you bite down and place your fingers at the angle of the jaw approximately an inch below the outer ear, you can feel the *masseter* muscle flex. Now repeat this action, but place your fingers on the lateral aspect of the forehead to palpate a muscle, the *temporalis*, that extends from an attachment on the mandible to insert broadly on the temporal area of the skull.

The tongue is perhaps the most important articulator. It is composed of intrinsic muscles that allow it to change shape. It can be shortened, lengthened, widened, narrowed, flattened, and made thicker. The extrinsic muscles of the tongue anchor it to the hyoid bone, mandible, temporal bone, and pharynx and position the tongue in the mouth. The tongue may be protruded, retracted, raised, or lowered depending on the speech sound being produced. The tongue has several identifiable parts including the root, body, dorsum, blade, and tip (from back to front), which are important in the description of the production of speech sounds. Because many speech sounds are produced by constriction (narrowing) of the vocal tract, the tongue has a strategic role in their formation within the oral cavity.

The speech sounds of English, with several exceptions, are oral, meaning they are produced with the opening between the oral and nasal cavities (velopharyngeal port) closed. Raising the velum and inward movement of the sides of the pharynx closes the opening. During speech production, movements of the velum are actively utilized to open and close the velopharyngeal port for nasal (e.g., /m/) and oral (e.g., /b/) speech sounds.

To this point, we have viewed the fixed and mobile articulators independently and considered their actions in isolation. It is important to remember that respiratory, phonatory, and articulatory movements are overlapping and conjoined in a complex series of actions during the production of speech. We consider this topic after a discussion of sound sources for speech.

Speech Production

So far, we have studied the three systems of speech production, respiration, phonation, and articulation, one by one. To fully understand the production of speech, however, we must now consider how all three systems function together to produce not only the segmental elements of speech called consonants and vowels, but also the suprasegmental elements (also called *prosodic* elements, or **prosody**) called stress and intonation.

Speech is produced during the expiratory phase of respiration (exhalation) when we control the release of air from the lungs by a gradual relaxation of the inspiratory muscles using what is called a "checking action." The resulting airflow is sufficient to make the vocal folds vibrate if they are adducted and there is sufficient tension in the vocalis muscles. Greater airflow produces sounds with higher amplitude (what we perceive as greater loudness). More tense vocal folds also require greater airflow to vibrate, but the vibration is at a higher frequency (what we perceive as higher pitch). So, respiration and phonation are interdependent and together permit us to modulate both pitch and loudness across a wide range of values.

Articulation can operate much more independently, however. Changes in phonation neither cause nor require changes in articulation, and articulation can change without significantly affecting phonation. For example, we can articulate the vowel [a] and allow phonation to change from a low pitch to a high pitch and back down again: We call that singing a scale. Conversely, we could articulate all the vowels at the same pitch. Most of the time, of course, we capitalize on our ability to control phonation and articulation to produce an enormous variety of perceptually distinct sounds: thousands of combinations of consonants and vowels with variations in rhythm. In this section, we explore the acoustic nature of these simultaneous productions.

The **source-filter theory** (Fant, 1960) of speech production explains how respiration, phonation, and articulation operate together. The respiratory system is the source of power for speech: Without the controlled flow of air from the lungs, there would be no sound. The phonatory system is the primary sound source for speech: The complex periodic sound we call voicing is present in the majority of speech sounds. Another source of sound exists too and must be taken into account in any full description of speech production: It is the complex, aperiodic sound (also called frication or noise) that is produced when airflow is forced through a narrow opening. Such narrow openings can occur between various articulators such as the tongue and the alveolar ridge, for example, when we make the sound [s]. Noise is also produced when air pressure is built up and released in the production of sounds such as /p/ and /t/. The articulatory system is the sound filter for speech, which means that the sound sources are modulated into distinctly different speech sounds in the vocal tract. We look next in more detail at this process of sound filtering.

The vocal tract, as we have mentioned, is an air-filled hollow tube, the size and shape of which can be changed by movements of the articulators. One of the properties of air-filled cavities is their ability to resonate, to produce a series of sound waves at particular frequencies as air flows through them. Think about the tones that can emerge from a simple musical instrument like an Australian didgeridoo when the musician blows into the hollow tube. Those tones are the resonances, or reverberations, that occur as the motion of air molecules within the tube become regular and organized; that is, they settle into a frequency of reverberation. Long instruments have low-frequency resonances and shorter instruments have higher-frequency resonances.

Most woodwind instruments with which we are familiar are more complex; they have a sound source in addition to a resonating cavity. Think of the sound of a vibrating reed in a clarinet. In a clarinet, just as in a didgeridoo, resonances or reverberations build up inside the air-filled cavity of the instrument and those tones, or frequencies, emerge. But in a clarinet, the sound of the vibrating reed (a complex, periodic sound with an FO and a whole series of mathematically related harmonics) is also emerging at the same time. The combined effect of the resonances of the tube and the harmonics of the sound emerging at the same time are what makes the sound of the clarinet distinctive. In effect, the energy of the resonances combines with the energy of those harmonics that are closest to the resonances in frequency, with the result that the frequencies of those harmonics are amplified (made more intense, made to sound louder) and the same harmonics in the complex, periodic sound are damped (made less intense, made less audible). This amplitude modulation of the harmonics by the resonances in an air-filled cavity is what we are calling *filtering*.

The air-filled cavity that is the human vocal tract behaves very much like the air-filled cavity of the clarinet, although the human vocal tract is more complex than the clarinet and can produce a wider range of different sounds. How are they alike? The human vocal tract, like the didgeridoo and the clarinet, produces resonances when air is forced through it. The human vocal folds, when they are vibrating, produce complex periodic sound, like the reed of a clarinet. That sound source then interacts with the resonances produced in the vocal tract: Those harmonics with frequencies closest to the frequencies of the vocal tract resonances are amplified and stand out auditorily compared to the frequencies of the other harmonics, while the rest of the harmonics are damped.

How is the human vocal tract different from an instrument like the clarinet? There are three main ways: (1) the vocal tract can change size and shape in ways that a clarinet cannot; (2) the human vocal folds can change frequency in a way that the clarinet's reed cannot; and (3) humans can generate both complex, periodic (voicing) and complex, aperiodic (fricative sound) sound sources.

First, the vocal tract can change size and shape through movements of the articulators. For example, it can be shaped as one very long tube that produces low-frequency resonances or a shorter tube that produces higher-frequency resonances. The vocal tract can also be shaped as two tubes. For example, if the mandible is moderately elevated and the tongue is thrust forward in the mouth, the vocal tract is divided into two cavities. In this example, the oral cavity forms one tube, shorter and narrower, while the pharyngeal cavity forms a second one, longer and wider. Each tube produces its own distinctive set of resonances. Each different shape into which we form the vocal tract by movements of the articulators changes the filtering effect of the air-filled cavities.

Second, we can change the rate at which the vocal folds vibrate. By changing the tension in the folds and adjusting airflow appropriately, we can modulate the pitch of our voice and change the F0 and the frequencies of all of the harmonics. Remember that voicing is the primary sound source for speech. If the vocal folds are vibrating, the amplitudes of the harmonics of the voiced sound source are filtered by the resonances of the two tubes, creating a complex set of frequencies that characterize that particular shape of vocal tract. In speech, these resonances combined with the energy of the harmonics closest to them in frequency are called **formants**.

Third, remember that we can also produce another kind of sound source with our vocal tract. If the vocal folds are not vibrating, but frication noise is being produced as a sound source, formants are still produced in the vocal tract, although they will not be as distinct as they are when voicing is the sound source. Listen to yourself saying the two sound [s], the initial sound in the word *sue*, alternating with [sh], the initial sound in *shoe*. You should hear that [sh] has lower tones; those are the resonances of formant frequencies of the two sounds. Listen to yourself speak in a whisper: You can distinguish all the consonants and vowels even without the presence of voicing, although the whisper is not as distinct as voiced speech. But even greater complexity occurs when both voicing and frication are being produced as dual sound sources. Compare the sound of /s/ with the sound of /z/. The first has only frication as the sound source, but the second has both voicing and frication as dual sound sources. It is an amazing instrument, the human vocal system.

Phonetics

Phonetics is the study of speech sounds. The sounds of speech are sometimes called *segments*. They are the consonants and vowels that we produce in sequence to make words. Words in turn are produced in sequence to make phrases. At the level of the word or the phrase, we create different emphases such as stress or intonation (e.g., "I am going," "**I** am going," "I **am** going," "I am **going**," "I am going?"). These effects are sometimes called the *suprasegmental* or *prosodic* characteristics of speech. The International Phonetic Association has developed a classification system for all the sounds of human language using these criteria. They have also created a system of symbols called the International Phonetic Alphabet that can be used to represent the segmental and suprasegmental characteristics of speech. Let's take a brief look at this notation system.

All sound segments are classified according to their production characteristics. To define consonants fully, four and sometimes five descriptors typically are used:

- *Voicing:* Are the vocal folds vibrating?
- *Nasality:* Are the nasal cavities contributing to the resonance of the sound?
- *Manner of articulation:* How high is the mandible; how closed is the oral cavity?
- *Place of articulation:* Where is the narrowest point of constriction in the oral cavity?
- *Secondary articulations:* Is the tongue shaped in a particular way that affects the perceptual quality of the sound (e.g., tip curled up or sides curled down)?

For example, a consonant produced with the vocal folds vibrating, the nasal cavities connected to the oral and pharyngeal cavities, the mandible completely elevated, and the tongue tip touching the alveolar ridge would sound like [n] and would be called a voiced, alveolar, nasal (stop). In comparison, a consonant produced with the vocal folds not vibrating, the opening from the pharyngeal cavity to the nasal cavities blocked off, the jaw somewhat less elevated, and the lower lip touching the upper incisors would sound like /f/ and would be called an unvoiced, labiodental fricative.

Vowels are described in a similar fashion, using three primary criteria:

- *Height:* How high, mid, or low within the oral cavity is the tongue?
- *Frontness/backness:* Is the tongue positioned front, central, or back within the oral cavity?
- *Lip shape:* Are the lips spread, normal, or rounded?

Voicing is not a criterion because all vowels are considered voiced. For example, a vowel produced with the tongue low in a very wide open mouth and thrust slightly forward in the mouth and the lips in a spread position (like a smile) sounds like the vowel in "sap" and is called the low, front, unrounded vowel. In contrast, a vowel produced with the tongue very high in the mouth and retracted backward with the lips in a rounded position (like a kiss) sounds like the vowel in "soup" and is called the high, back, rounded vowel.

The suprasegmental characteristics of speech are produced by modulating three qualities of sound:

- *Loudness:* How are the volume and rate of airflow changing?
- *Pitch:* How is the rate of vocal fold vibration changing?
- *Duration:* How long is a sound being sustained?

For example, the difference between two otherwise very similar sounding words such as **sub**ject (noun) and sub**ject** (verb) is created by placing greater emphasis on either the first or second syllable of the word. Such emphasis is called *stress*. We give the percept of stress by making the vowel in the stressed syllable longer, louder, or higher pitched (sometimes all three). Another example is the way we differentiate between a statement of fact, "It's a good thing," and a question, "It's a good thing?" To make the distinction with our voice instead of with the order of the words, we contrast the intonation of the two phrases by changing the pitch of the voice during the production. The statement has an overall falling pitch, while the question has an overall rising pitch.

Before we finish this section of the chapter, we must mention two other topics: **coarticulation** and *motor equivalence*. Coarticulation is the simultaneous production of two sequential sounds. The words and phrases that we form using the vocal organs are not just simple sequences of individual speech sounds. The segments of speech in a phrase do not behave like individual beads on a string. The production of these sounds is a fluid process in which the articulators move smoothly from one position to another and the respiratory/laryngeal system creates a dynamic range of sound qualities in a continuous stream. In many cases, production of one segment actually overlaps with the production of a following sound, creating an auditory blend of the two at the boundary or transition between them. For example, if you make the sound /s/ in isolation, you will typically produce it with the lips spread as you force air through a narrow gap between the tongue and the alveolar ridge. And when you produce the sound /w/, you will have your lips rounded and your tongue in a relatively high and backed position within the oral cavity while the vocal folds are vibrating. But when you form the word *swing*, you will probably find yourself rounding the lips in anticipation of the /w/ while still producing the initial /s/ sound. To the listener, the two sounds are quite understandable despite this overlap. Examples of similar coarticulation or overlapping productions of adjacent sounds are common in speech.

We have learned that a change in the shape of the vocal tract changes the acoustic signature of the sound being uttered and that there are characteristic patterns of formants for each segment of speech. Therefore, it might seem that coarticulation and other variations in the way segments are produced might be thought to interfere with their intelligibility. Fortunately, speakers learn through years of experience listening to and producing speech that there is more than one way to produce sounds with similar acoustic signatures. For example, say the following vowels of English: "a, e, i, o, u." During vowel production, the mandible is usually quite depressed, creating a fairly open oral cavity, and the tongue moves up and down with the movements of the mandible. Now try saying the same vowels with your teeth clenched together as though your jaw were wired shut. Notice that the tongue and the lips can make the necessary movements without the mandible and that the vowels sound correct. Technically the vocal tract is not the same during the two sets of utterances, but acoustically the sounds are enough alike to permit the segments to be perceived as such. These are the motor equivalences of the sounds that allow us to identify sounds despite differences in their mode of production.

SUMMARY

Speech production is a complex behavior that requires the coordination of respiratory, laryngeal, and articulatory systems. The speech output of this coordinated activity is programmed by the nervous system based on our experience with the complex

---

BOX 4-3 Personal Story

Did you ever wonder how an infant can lie back in its mother's arms and suckle without having to stop and take a breath? Like many mammals, the newborn human infant has the ability to breathe and swallow at the same time. This capability is a result of the configuration of the infant vocal tract and its relationship to the larynx. Unlike adult humans, infant humans have hardly any pharyngeal cavity. The infant vocal tract is composed largely of the nasal cavities and the oral cavity. The larynx is so high in the neck that the epiglottis actually articulates with the velum, or soft palate. The consequence of this arrangement is that the infant's airstream can flow from the nose through the larynx into the trachea at the same time that milk is able to flow from the mouth down the esophagus. Interestingly, most other species of mammals, in both their infantile and adult forms, have the same configuration: Like human infants, they are "obligate nose breathers."

At around 2 years of age, the shape of the human vocal tract begins to change: The larynx descends lower into the neck, creating a separation between the velum and the epiglottis. The dorsum, or back of the body, of the tongue also lowers to create the anterior wall of a third cavity in the vocal tract: the pharynx. This transformation is effectively complete by about age 6. The reshaped vocal tract with its three resonating areas, the nasal cavities, the oral cavity, and the pharyngeal cavity, is one of the crucial elements in the human ability to produce the wide range of speech sounds used for language.

movement of our articulators and the variable quality of the sound we produce. The speech sounds of our language can be described in terms of how we produce them segmentally in terms of phonation and articulator position and suprasegmentally in terms of prosodic variations at the level of the syllable and the phrase.

STUDY QUESTIONS

1. Describe three sound sources for speech production.

2. How are consonants different from vowels?

3. What are the parts of the vocal tract?

4. Why does increasing the length of the vocal folds increase their frequency of vibration?

5. What is the difference between static and mobile articulators?

6. What change in respiratory activity would be needed to talk louder?

7. Why is the vocal fold frequency of vibration higher for women than for men?

8. What are some functions of the larynx in addition to its role as a sound source for speech?

9. What is a formant?

10. What are the major structures of the central nervous system?

11. Describe the representation of speech and language in the nervous system.

12. How do neurons differ from glial cells?

13. Which cranial nerves are most important to speech production?

14. Compare the functions of the pyramidal and extrapyramidal tracts.

15. Describe three places for consonant production.

KEY TERMS

Adduction
Afferent
Basal ganglia
Bernoulli effect
Brainstem
Broca's area
Cerebral hemispheres
Coarticulation
Corpus callosum
Efferent

Extrapyramidal tract
Formant
Fundamental frequency (F0)
Glial cells
Glottis
Gyri
Harmonic
Meninges
Myelin
Neurotransmitters

Prosody
Pyramidal tract
Resting expiratory level
Rolandic fissure
Source-filter theory
Sulci
Sylvian fissure
Thalamus
Wernicke's area

REFERENCES

Fant, G. (1960). *Acoustic theory of speech production.* Hague: Mouton & Co.

Kent, R. (1997). *The speech sciences.* San Diego, CA: Singular.

SUGGESTED READINGS

Andrews, M. (2006). *Manual of voice treatment* (3rd ed.). Clifton Park, NY: Thomson.

Awan, S. (2001). *The voice diagnostic protocol.* Gaithersburg, MD: Aspen.

Behrman, A. (2007). *Speech and voice science.* San Diego, CA: Plural.

Boone, D., McFarlane, S., & Von Berg, S. (2005). *The voice and voice therapy* (7th ed.). Boston: Pearson.

Clopper, C., Pisoni, D., & de Jong, K. (2005). Acoustic characteristics of the vowel systems of six regional varieties of American English. *Journal of the Acoustical Society of America, 118,* 1661–1676.

Minifie, F., Hixon, T., & Williams, F. (Eds.). (1973). *Normal aspects of speech, language and hearing.* Englewood Cliffs, NJ: Prentice Hall.

Smith, A., & Robb, M. (2006). The influence of utterance position on children's production of lexical stress. *Folia Phoniatrica et Logopedica, 58,* 199–206.

Webster, D. B. (1999). *Neuroscience of communication* (2nd ed.). San Diego, CA: Singular.

chapter five

Developmental Speech Disorders

BARBARA L. DAVIS AND LISA M. BEDORE

LEARNING OBJECTIVES

1. To understand the distinction between an articulation disorder and a phonological disorder.

2. To understand the causes of articulation and phonological disorders in children and adults.

3. To learn what factors are important in describing the severity of articulation and phonological disorders.

4. To understand how articulation and phonological disorders are related to language disorders in children.

5. To differentiate between organic and functional articulation and phonological disorders.

6. To learn how articulation and phonological disorders are identified and treated.

We are all capable of making many different types of sounds by changing the configuration of the articulators (the lips, tongue, teeth, jaw, and velum). When we communicate our ideas about the world around us, we produce specific kinds of sounds, called phonemes (e.g., /b/ or /a/), that we sequence together in a variety of ways to form words. Recall from Chapter 2 that phonology is the term for the language conventions (or rules) that govern how phonemes are combined to make words. The ability to *produce* sounds in sequence by moving the articulators is referred to as **articulation**. Articulation is somewhat different from other motor activities such as skiing, where Olympic athletes are always better than the rest of us at performance. With respect to speech production, nearly all normal adult speakers of a language are proficient at producing strings of speech sounds that are correct and easily understood by others.

Children with developmental speech disorders produce words that sound different from the words that are produced by most other speakers of a language. Because language is most often expressed through speech, severe difficulties with articulation can negatively affect the way linguistic knowledge (phonology, morphology, semantics, syntax, and pragmatics) is expressed. As you might expect, this has a negative effect on communication. That is why speech-language pathologists (SLPs) are interested in describing, assessing, and treating children with developmental speech disorders.

Developmental speech disorders are among the most common types of communication disorders treated by SLPs. As a result, this clinical disorder category is considered a core aspect of the scope of practice of certified SLPs. Few of these professionals will deliver assessment and intervention services to children without a portion of the caseload being composed of clients with some component of their communication disorder characterized as articulation or phonological impairment.

Our primary interest in this chapter is children. First, we describe the population of interest. Next, we discuss the developmental tools for describing speech disorders, including a framework for understanding what is normal in speech acquisition. Last, we provide an overview of assessment and treatment procedures for individuals with speech disorders.

BOX 5-1   Overview of CD-ROM Segments

In the CD-ROM segments for this chapter, you can view examples of children with articulation and/or phonological disorders:

Ch.5.01. A child with an expressive language disorder that co-occurs with a speech disorder.

Ch.5.02. A child with a mild speech sound production disorder.

Ch.5.03. A child with a severe speech disorder.

Ch.5.04. Use of gestures by a child with a severe speech disorder.

Ch.5.05. A young child with delayed speech development.

DEFINITION AND INCIDENCE

It is important to distinguish between an articulation disorder and a phonological disorder because this distinction is critical for the way speech production problems are assessed, described, and treated. Children or adults may have difficulty producing the sounds and sound sequences of their language (an **articulation disorder**) or with understanding and implementing the underlying rules for producing sounds and sequences (a **phonological disorder**). An individual with an articulation disorder may have difficulty with the movements of the vocal folds, lips, tongue, teeth, and jaw that are necessary for the production of understandable speech. An example of a simple articulation disorder is the substitution of a /w/ where /r/ is expected (e.g., *wed* for *red*). An example of a more complex articulation disorder is a girl with cerebral palsy who has difficulty coordinating and controlling respiration, phonation, and articulation. This person may know exactly what she wants to say. Nevertheless, she may not have adequate control over the movements of her articulators, causing most sounds to be produced in an unusual manner. She may also have breath support for only one or two words at a time. As a result, listeners may have a difficult time understanding what this individual is saying. These types of disorders are discussed in greater detail in Chapter 8.

A phonological disorder, in contrast, is considered to be a deficiency in the abstract system of knowledge that forms the rule system for sounds and sequences needed to convey a message in a given language. That is, a person may not have developed adequate mental representations of the sound system of the language that surrounds him or her. An example of a simple phonological disorder is the English-speaking child who thinks that the affricate /*ch*/ and the fricative /*sh*/ are completely interchangeable. (These sounds are interchangeable in some languages, but not in English.) The child can produce both sounds correctly but mistakenly uses one for the other, saying *shair* for *chair* or *choe* for *shoe*. An example of a more complex phonological disorder would be the child who represents the fricative sounds /*sh*/, /*th*/, /s/, /z/, /f/, and /v/) with the stop /t/, but uses fricatives like /*sh*/ to represent the affricates /D/ (*j*) and /*ch*/. The child might say the word *ship* as *tip*, but he would say the word *chip* as *ship*. We know this is a phonological problem and not necessarily an articulation problem because the child demonstrates the ability to produce fricatives. Yet, he or she produces fricatives for stops when producing words.

Some children have difficulty with both articulation and phonology simultaneously. For example, a child with a history of chronic otitis media accompanied by a mild hearing loss may not have been able to hear speech clearly. Such a child may not develop the same mental representation of speech sounds as a child with normal hearing. At the same time, this child will not have been able to monitor his or her productions and thus may not know if he or she is producing sounds or sound sequences correctly. Other children with both articulation and phonological disorders are those with severe limitations in the number of sounds they can produce. We have seen 5-year-old children whose inventory of speech sounds include only the nasals /m/ and /n/, the stops /p/, /b/, /t/, and /d/, and a few vowels. As a result of producing so few sounds, these children have developed unusual representations of the phonology of the language.

It can be quite difficult to determine whether a child has difficulty with articulation alone or with both articulation and phonology. However, as we discuss later, many assessment and intervention approaches are specifically designed to evaluate or treat either articulation problems or phonological problems. We use the term *articulation disorder* when we are referring to difficulties producing speech sounds and the term *phonological disorder* when we are referring to difficulties with phonological rules.

A FRAMEWORK FOR UNDERSTANDING ARTICULATION AND PHONOLOGY

Two scientific perspectives have been used for understanding individuals who have difficulty with speech production, speech perception, or phonological knowledge. Physiological systems for producing and perceiving speech have been the focus of phonetic science. Speaker knowledge of speech sounds in a language has been studied as an aspect of phonological science. The most salient difference between these perspectives is that phonetic science emphasizes the physical ability to produce speech, and phonological science emphasizes the acquisition of the rules for combining sounds to produce words in a specific language such as English or French. Both perspectives on understanding of speech have been employed by SLPs in assessment and treatment of clients with speech production deficits.

Phonetic Science

The discipline of phonetic science studies the three major subsystems of the body that are involved in producing speech: the respiratory system, the phonatory system, and the articulatory system. Chapter 4 provides an in-depth look at speech production processes. In addition, speech is served by perceptual processes of audition (hearing sounds) and discrimination (sorting sounds into recognizable categories). Perception is crucially important for acquisition of speech production skills as well as for ongoing speaker self-monitoring of his or her own speech production. Individuals with difficulty in the physiological processes involved in producing and perceiving speech are usually considered to have an articulation disorder.

Phonological Science

Speech is a system that is used to relate meaning with sounds. For meaning to be conveyed in a message, the speaker and listener must share a common understanding of how specific sounds and sound sequences are combined to form words. Recall from Chapter 2 that the individual sounds in a language are called phonemes. A phoneme is the smallest unit in a language that conveys meaning (i.e., /p/ and /b/ are phonemes used to convey the difference between *pig* and *big*). Two different types of phonemes, consonants and vowels, are discussed in Chapter 2. Recall that consonants are described by where they are produced (place of articulation) and how they are produced (manner of articulation), in addition to whether they are voiced or not (i.e., are the vocal folds vibrating?). Vowels (e.g., /a/, /i/, /o/, etc.) are made with a relatively open vocal tract and alternate with consonants to create syllables (Tables 2-1 and 2-2).

A variety of systems of analysis have been employed to describe difficulties in using the sounds and sound sequences of language. **Distinctive features** (Chomsky & Halle, 1968) reflect the underlying units of knowledge that are used to construct sounds in words. There are 15 binary (+/–) features in Chomsky and Halle's system, and each phoneme has its own "distinctive" set of features. For example, the sound /n/ is termed a nasal sound because air moves through the nose. In distinctive feature terminology, /n/ is +nasal, meaning that it is stored mentally as a +nasal sound. The other features of /n/ include +sonorant (spontaneous voicing is possible), +consonantal (there is obstruction in the oral cavity), +anterior (the obstruction is at the alveolar ridge), +coronal (the front part of the tongue is raised), and +voiced (the vocal folds are vibrating). The phoneme /n/ also has a minus (–) value for some features. For example, it is –syllabic (it's not a vowel), –strident (the airstream does not produce a high-frequency noise), and –lateral (it is not produced by lowering the sides of the tongue). From a distinctive feature perspective, an individual with a phonological disorder or delay may have difficulty retrieving and using the mentally stored units that specify sounds. In addition, the individual may not have figured out one or more of the important features of the language he or she speaks.

Another system for describing mental representations of sound is called phonological processes. Phonological processes are variations in the way phonemes are combined. When two sounds are produced in rapid sequence, they become more like each other. This is the process of assimilation. For example, vowels that are followed by nasals tend to become nasalized. This happens because the velum lowers for the nasal consonant while the vowel is still being produced. Say the words *fan* and *fad*. Can you hear how the vowel in *fan* is more nasalized? Another common phonological process is called deletion. In English, the last phoneme in a consonant cluster like /st/ is deleted when the cluster appears at the end of a word that is followed immediately by a word that begins with a voiceless consonant. For example, the final /t/ in the word *most* and the initial /t/ in the word *teams* are rarely produced separately in the phrase *most teams*. Unlike distinctive features that describe differences between the individual phonemes in a language, phonological processes are ways to describe phonological rules that operate above the level of the individual phoneme.

ARTICULATION AND PHONOLOGICAL DISORDERS

There are a number of important factors to consider in understanding and treating articulation and phonological disorders. In this section, we consider the concepts of disorder versus delay, the severity of disorders and delays, issues related to dialects, the etiology of articulation and phonological disorders, and the co-occurrence of articulation and phonological disorders with other types of communication disorders.

Delay versus Disorder

Description of articulation and phonological development as disordered or delayed is based on comparison of the child's speech to the articulation and phonological patterns of children of a comparable age who are developing normally (Davis & Bedore,

2008). Recall the discussion of early, middle, and late developing sounds in Chapter 2. Children who are considered to have delayed articulation development have speech production patterns that typically occur in children who are younger. For example, a 5-year-old child may produce all the sounds of English but may have difficulty using them at the ends of words, resulting in a pattern where *top*, *cat*, and *kiss* are produced as "to_", "ca_," and "ki_." Normally developing children between the ages of 24 and 36 months often leave off the ends of words. An older child who presents this pattern would be considered delayed because he or she is producing speech like a child who is chronologically 24–36 months old. A 38-month-old child who produces only one-syllable words beginning with /b/ and /d/ (i.e., "ba" for *ball* and "da" for *doll*) and no consonants at the end also would be considered delayed. She would be described as speaking like a child 12–15 months old who uses few different consonants and produces mainly one-syllable words.

In contrast to children with a **speech delay**, children with a **speech disorder** do not produce speech that is like children who are developing normally. A 10-year-old child who produces speech that is whispered and contains mostly vowels with only a few consonants shows skills that are not like a normally developing child of any age. He would be described as disordered.

Severity of Involvement

The severity of a speech delay or disorder is related to several important aspects of speech production:

- The number of sounds produced correctly (e.g., if the child is saying the word *watermelons*, how many of the sounds does she say correctly?)
- The accuracy of production (e.g., saying "*d*all" for "*b*all")
- The ability to produce sounds in different word positions (saying "l" in both *l*ike and in ki*ll*)
- The ability to produce sound sequences (saying *blu* instead of the simpler *bu*)
- The ability to produce various types of words (saying *top* as well as *marginal*)

Each of these factors is related to speech intelligibility. **Intelligibility** is the understandability of spontaneous speech and is a crucial factor for determining the need for and the effectiveness of therapy (Bernthal & Bankson, 2004).

BOX 5-2 Andrew 7

In CD-ROM segment Ch.5.01, notice that Andrew, age 7, is speaking in incomplete sentences. Instead of including all the sentence elements when he expresses himself, his sentences include only the main words. Andrew is telling his therapist about his dog who swims in the river. What sounds are missing?

Three adjectives are often used to indicate the degree of impairment: *mild, moderate,* and *severe.* Table 5-1 provides examples of how hypothetical children with mild, moderate, and severe speech impairments would produce a list of words of varying complexity. Mildly involved children have problems producing only a few sounds. They are able to produce most of the sounds of their language and can use these sounds in sequences both within words and in varied types of words. Children whose only speech errors are the substitution of /T/ for /s/ ("thee" for *see*) or the substitution of /w/ for /r/ ("wabbit" for *rabbit*) are considered to be mildly speech delayed. Individuals with mild delays are generally intelligible to most listeners, but their speech errors call attention to the way they speak. Frequently, the sounds that are produced incorrectly by these individuals are those identified in Chapter 2 as in the "late eight" group. Individuals with mild delays or disorders usually have excellent treatment outcomes.

The child with *moderate* impairment has more difficulty producing speech sounds correctly than the mildly involved child does. A 4-year-old child with a moderate speech disorder may have difficulty producing all velar sounds where the back of the tongue approximates the top of the mouth (i.e., /k/, /g/, and /˜/ as in *k*ite, *g*o, and ki*ng*). Moderately involved children may use sounds incorrectly in different word positions such as /d/ in place of /t/ at the ends of words (i.e., "po*d*" for "po*t*"). These children often have difficulty producing all the syllables in multisyllabic words (i.e., [pamus] for *hippopotamus*), leave sounds off the ends of words (i.e., "do-" instead of *dog*), and simplify some

Table 5-1 Examples of How Hypothetical 4-Year-Old Children with Mild, Moderate, or Severe Speech Disorders Might Produce Selected Words

Target Word	Mild	Moderate	Severe
Soup	/sup/	/tup/	/tu/
Rabbit	/wæblt/	/wæbl/	/æ³l/
Yellow	/jɛwo/	/wɛwo/	/ɛo/
Crayon	/kwelən/	/kelən/	/elə/
Butterfly	/bʌdəfwal/	/bʌfal/	/ʌal/
Refrigerator	/wifwldəweldə/	/fldəwelə/	/wl/

BOX 5-3 Alex, Age 3

In CD-ROM segment Ch.5.02, Alex, age 3, exhibits a mild speech delay for his chronological age. His speech is intelligible, but calls attention to the way he speaks because some of the sounds are missing or incorrect. Here he is looking at a book with the clinician and he says, "A dwaf, a pinwin, teddy beo" to describe a giraffe, a penguin, and a teddy bear. How would you describe his errors?

consonant clusters (two consonants "clustered" together without an intervening vowel) as in "bu" for *blue*. Children with moderate speech disorders are mostly intelligible to familiar listeners such as parents or family members, but they may not be understood by unfamiliar listeners, especially when the listener is not sure what the individual is talking about. Moderately involved children have a good prognosis for improvement, although the course of therapy may be longer than for children with mild difficulties.

Severe level of clinical involvement is found in individuals who are unintelligible to most listeners or who may not be able to use speech consistently to communicate. These individuals usually produce more than six sounds in error. They do not sequence sounds consistently to produce intelligible words. As a consequence, their ability to use sounds to communicate effectively is limited. Children with severe speech disorders may resort to using gestures to get their message across. For example, a 6-year-old child who produces only four different consonants, uses vowels inconsistently, and primarily gestures for communication would be considered to have a severe speech disorder. A 12-year-old child with cerebral palsy who does not have adequate control over breathing to support speech production would also be considered to have a severe disorder.

In very severe cases, an SLP may decide to use augmentative communication systems (i.e., systems in which the client pushes a button or points to a picture) as an alternative method for communication. Severe developmental speech disorders interfere with a child's ability to communicate in the long term.

Language and Dialect

There are an increasing number of speakers of languages whose rules for producing the sounds and sequences of sounds do not match English. The result is widely differing types of pronunciation found among nonnative speakers of English. Recall from

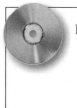

BOX 5-4   Andrew

In CD-ROM segment Ch.5.03, Andrew, age 7, is talking to the clinician about his dog. He notes that he has a new dog, and his big dog knows how to swim. He is very difficult to understand in this segment. These types of errors in a child age 7 connote a severe speech impairment. What types of errors do you hear?

BOX 5-5   Andrew

In CD-ROM segment Ch.5.04, Andrew is using gestures to supplement his comments about where he is going. The use of gesture is typical for Andrew and for individuals with severe problems with intelligibility because it helps to convey the message to the listener. In this instance, Andrew's gestures are not sufficient to help Jena understand exactly what he is trying to say.

Chapter 3 that speakers who have some competence in English, but who have a different primary language, are termed bilinguals (Gildersleeve-Neuman, Stubbe-Kester, Davis, & Pena, 2008). These speakers have the same ability to produce speech sounds and sequences; they simply have different rules for how to produce them based on the requirements of their primary language. If you have tried to learn a second or third language, you might have noticed that you do not produce words, phrases, and sentences in the same manner as native speakers of the language you are learning. One reason is that you are not proficient at producing the specific sound types and sequences of sounds of the new language. For example, there are no /b/, /d/, or /g/ sounds at the ends of German words. English speakers learning German may use these sounds at the ends of German words because they are present in English (e.g., *mob*). When speaking English, you will not spend time thinking about how to produce sounds or how to order them when you ask your roommate, "Where are your car keys?" In contrast, you may labor consciously in German to produce sounds correctly and to put them in order in ways that are different from your English pronunciation patterns.

It is important to discern dialectal differences from speech disorders. If a child's speech errors are related to learning a second language (i.e., the Latino child who says "shiken" for *chicken* because the /sh/ is a variation of the /ch/ sound in Spanish), the patterns are considered to be sound differences rather than delay or disorder. Children whose phonological production patterns are different because they are applying the phonological patterns of their first language to their second or third language are not usually placed in speech therapy. Children who have adequate speech production abilities and good language-learning capabilities often develop production patterns that are consistent with the phonological rules of the second language they are learning.

Etiology

Finding a cause of a developmental speech disorder in children is often quite difficult. Many children with articulation or phonological impairment are termed as having functional speech impairment. A functional impairment indicates that the cause of differences from normally developing children in speech development simply cannot be determined. With these individuals, the SLP describes articulation and phonological skills carefully and works to change deviant articulatory patterns to speech patterns that are appropriate for the child's chronological age. Behavioral description takes precedence over a search for etiological cause. The clinician does not utilize information about possible causes to plan therapy or to predict the child's prognosis for improvement.

Most developmental speech disorders are considered to be "functional." We do not know why a child has difficulty representing the phonology of the language that surrounds him. Phonological knowledge is based on descriptions of knowledge about language. No information is available to pinpoint possible etiologies for differences in the ways in which children learn the phonology of their language. Phonological perspectives provide rich descriptions of a child's pattern of differences from normal development; they do not provide explanations of *why* these children are different in their development.

Articulation disorder or delay is more likely to have a known etiology or to be associated with a risk factor for developmental delay. In general, SLPs use the term *articulation disorder* or *delay* when the peripheral organs of speech are involved (i.e., the input system of perceptual organs that receive sensation and discriminate sounds and/or the output system of jaw, tongue, lips, and so forth that produce sounds and sequences). Etiologies for articulation delay or disorder fall into three major categories: perceptual or input-related etiology, structural etiology, and motor or output-related etiology. Table 5-2 lists examples from each of these major etiological categories for articulation delay or disorder.

Co-Occurrence With Other Types of Disorder

Developmental speech disorders can co-occur with other types of speech and language problems. For example, children with expressive or receptive language problems and voice and fluency disorders often present with articulation or phonological impairment as well. For example, a second-grader may have a problem producing speech sounds at the ends of words. This same child would probably omit many grammatical morphemes in English that happen to occur at the end of words, which would affect his ability to express his ideas in complete sentences (an expressive language disorder).

Another example of co-occurring speech and language disorders is a 32-month-old child who may be using just four or five words to communicate, all of which contain only a consonant and a vowel put together (e.g., "da" for *doll*). This child may also have difficulty with understanding directions from her mother at home (language comprehension), with grammatical morphemes (e.g., plural *-s*, past tense *-ed*), and with combining words to form sentences. In these cases, the SLP must decide whether to work on both deficits at once or whether to work on each deficit separately. With some careful planning, it is usually possible to work on all of a child's problems at once.

ASSESSMENT AND TREATMENT

Infants, children, and adults form a dramatically diverse population of individuals who need assessment and remediation for developmental speech disorders. The goal of

BOX 5-6   Brian

In CD-ROM segment Ch.5.05, Brian, age 5, demonstrates delayed speech production abilities for his age. In talking with his clinician about the "good guy and the bad guy cars," he is difficult to understand. His most obvious error is the use of a /t/ sound where he should use a /k/ sound. View segment Ch.5.05 again and see if you can understand Brian now that you know which sound is substituted. His delay is considered moderate because he is talking in long sentences and is somewhat difficult for an unfamiliar listener to understand.

assessment is to determine the specific nature and severity of the disorder or delay. Specific assessment procedures and materials are needed relative to the suspected etiology and the chronological and developmental age and the primary language spoken. Using

Table 5-2 Examples of Common Etiologies That Are Representative of Major Classes of Organic Etiologies

Disorder Type	Definition	Speech Characteristics
Perceptual Etiology		
Otitis media	Middle ear fluid secondary to ear infection. Hearing loss is mild to moderate, and duration of loss is variable.	Fluctuating losses as are observed in children with otitis media are thought to put children at risk for delays in speech development. There is not a distinctive pattern of errors that is associated with this risk factor.
Sensorineural loss	Genetic or postnatal disease processes that result in moderate or severe hearing loss.	Children with moderate to severe hearing loss do not hear speech sounds adequately. Thus, it is difficult to impossible for children to learn to produce them without prolonged remediation. These children typically demonstrate *severe* difficulties. You can learn more about the impact of sensorineural hearing loss on speech and language in Chapter 14.
Structural Etiology		
Cleft lip and palate	Oral-facial malformations resulting from interruption of development during the prenatal period.	Children's speech may be very nasal even after closure of the palate. Children may have difficulty producing speech sounds that require high pressure such as /s/ or /ch/. You can learn more about cleft lip and palate in Chapter 6.
Motor Etiology		
Dysarthria	Neuromuscular impairment resulting in speech disorder.	Speakers with dysarthria have difficulties with respiration, phonation, articulation, resonance, and prosody. Speech involvement is usually *moderate* to *severe*. You can learn more about dysarthria in Chapter 8 in the section on cerebral palsy.
Apraxia	Neurological damage resulting in inconsistent speech production abilities.	The difficulties observed in the speaker with apraxia are a result of the inability to plan or program speech. Apraxia affects speech intelligibility and prosody. Errors are typically inconsistent and more likely to occur as length increases.

the information gathered, SLPs employ specific analysis procedures to understand the patterns of difference between the individual's productions and the relevant comparison population. Decisions about treatment will be based on results of the assessment and analysis.

Collecting Information

Speech Samples

Suspected developmental speech impairment requires analysis of a **spontaneous speech and language sample** to evaluate the use and integrity of speech production skills in communication. Clinicians collect a speech sample by talking and playing with the child. The spontaneous sample is analyzed to determine the child's ability to produce consonants, vowels, and sequences characteristic of the language community. Children with very severe impairment may not use vocalization consistently to communicate. In these cases, the use of gestures or other ways the person has to communicate and the intentionality of vocalizations needs to be evaluated.

Articulation Tests

If the child is capable of naming pictures or objects, a **single-word articulation test** may be administered to assess the child's ability to produce consonants in varied word positions. The *Goldman-Fristoe Test of Articulation* (Goldman & Fristoe, 1986; Hodson, 2004), for example, samples the consonants of English in all word positions. Vowels in English are not consistently tested by single-word tests, however. Very young and/or very impaired children may not be able to participate in a structured single-word test of articulation. In addition, individuals who are bilingual may not be tested validly on tests developed for English speakers. In these cases, the spontaneous sample is the only source of information for analyzing oral communication skills. Regardless of whether we obtain samples of single-word production from an articulation test or from spontaneous speech, we are interested in several measures of phonological development. We evaluate the number of speech sounds that are correctly produced or determine if children could use complex phonological structures such as consonant clusters (e.g., *str-*) or multisyllabic words (e.g., *refrigerator*). We discuss the ways of analyzing phonological behaviors in more detail in the next section. In Table 5-3, we present a brief case summary. This child's speech was assessed using the Goldman-Fristoe Test of Articulation as well as a spontaneous speech and language sample.

Analyzing Speech

In severely impaired individuals, regardless of age or etiology, the SLP describes the range of behaviors used for intentional communication (e.g., gestures, sign language, use of vision in gaze, or overall body orientation). In addition, types of behaviors (such as vowel vocalizations or ability to use fingers to point) that are not intentionally used for communication must be described. The presence of these behaviors is important for planning where to start a treatment program designed to move toward intentional communication in these severely involved clients.

Table 5-3   Steps Involved in the Evaluation of a Child with an Articulation Disorder

Davey was referred for speech and language evaluation when he was 3 years and 10 months old. His mother's concern was that his speech was difficult to understand. His siblings understood his speech as did his mother. However, his father did not understand his speech and neither did his teachers and peers at school. He was becoming frustrated when others did not understand him. A parental interview revealed nothing remarkable in Davey's developmental history except frequent sore throats and ear infections.

Davey's speech evaluation consisted of several parts. The clinician administered the Goldman-Fristoe Test of Articulation, obtained a speech and language sample in the context of play with age-appropriate toys, conducted a hearing screening, and an oral mechanism exam. The evaluation confirmed that Davey's speech was unintelligible approximately 70% of the time to the unfamiliar listener. In addition to phonological errors, the clinician observed that Davey's speech was hyponasal. We discuss the results of the speech evaluation in more detail subsequently.

Davey passed his hearing screening, but in the oral-peripheral examination the clinician observed that Davey's tonsils were extremely inflamed and referred the mother to her pediatrician for follow-up.

The clinician analyzed Davey's speech sample in several ways. Davey obtained a score in the ninth percentile for his age on the Goldman-Fristoe Test of Articulation. This indicated that his articulation skills were less well developed than other children his age. Some examples of Davey's productions on the Goldman-Fristoe included the following:

Telephone	/t Elwə pod/
Gun	/dʌd/
Cup	/tʌp/
Chicken	/tItə/
Zipper	/dIpə/
Lamp	/wæp/
Plane	/peId/
Drum	/dʌp/

The clinician followed up with analyses of Davey's phonetic inventory and substitution and omission patterns. She found that he did not yet use many sounds that were expected for his age. For example, he did not yet use /k/ or /g/ sounds, suggesting that he had difficulty producing sounds that required him to raise the back of his tongue. She also found that he systematically simplified words using several phonological processes including fronting (the substitution of /t/ sounds for /k/ sounds) and consonant cluster reduction ("st" becomes "s" in *stop*). Most of Davey's errors appeared to be developmental in nature, but some of his substitution patterns could be attributed to hyponasality (e.g., the substitution of /b/ for /m/ and /d/ for /n/).

The focus of intervention with Davey was on the development of velar sounds /k/ and /g/. Follow-up with Davey's pediatrician led to a referral to the ear, nose, and throat specialist. Soon after intervention began, Davey had his tonsils and adenoids removed. After he recovered from his surgery, his speech was no longer hyponasal and the substitution errors that could be attributed to hyponasality were no longer observed in his speech. At age 4 years and 6 months, Davey was dismissed from intervention. His speech was intelligible at least 90% of the time. He did not yet produce sounds such as /r/ or /th/. However, because these are later-occurring sounds, they were not of concern. Follow-up evaluations at 6 months and 1 year later revealed that he continued to develop speech normally and was acquiring the remaining sounds and clusters that would be expected.

In individuals who use vocalization for communication, the SLP may employ either phonetic or phonological analysis, depending on the nature of the child's disorder or delay. The clinician is seeking to (1) describe typical patterns of speech production skills and (2) compare those skills to an age-appropriate group of children to plan treatment. The clinician may also employ information about etiology (if it is known) to understand the nature of the client's production deficits. For example, a child with a high-frequency hearing loss may have difficulty with producing sounds such as /s/ that are high in the acoustic frequency spectrum. A child with a cleft palate may have trouble with sounds that require a buildup of oral pressure as a result of impaired ability to close the opening between the nose and mouth during speech production.

As has been noted, speech consists of sounds and sequences of sounds used to communicate. Speech analysis consists of describing consonant and vowel sounds the client can produce and how they are used in sequences (i.e., "b," "a," and "t" can be combined to produce *bat*). In every case, the client's skills are compared to those of his or her peer group (i.e., 5-year-olds are compared to other 5-year-olds, adult speakers to other adults) to determine whether the patterns are different enough from the comparison group to warrant treatment.

An analysis of articulation skills focuses on how the three major peripheral body subsystems (articulatory, phonatory, and respiratory) work together to produce speech. The SLP describes articulation skills (articulatory), vocal fold coordination with articulators (phonatory), and breath support (respiratory) for speech. Specific to articulation, the SLP records in detail the way(s) in which the tongue, jaw, lips, and palate work together to produce speech sounds and sequences and describes patterns of differences from the comparison group. A clinician may note that all sounds made with the tongue tip are deleted and substituted by sounds made with the lips (e.g., /d/, /s/, and /r/ are produced as /b/ /m/, and /w/). Traditional methods of describing articulation skills include the descriptors of *substitution, omission, and distortion.* **Substitutions** are when one sound is produced or substituted for another sound (i.e., the child says "bog" for dog). **Omissions** occur when a sound is left out of a word (i.e., the client says "to_" for top). **Distortions** are sounds produced in a recognizable inaccurate manner (i.e., a "slushy" sounding /s/ sound). Regarding phonation, the clinician describes the use of the vocal folds to produce sound. The client may use voiced sounds (where the vocal folds are vibrating while the client moves the articulators) for all voiceless sounds because he or she does not have good control in coordinating phonation and articulation. Because the vocal folds are always vibrating, the client produces all voiced sounds. Respiratory or breath support for speech production is also an aspect of analysis. Most clients who have difficulty producing adequate breath support for speaking are more severely involved (e.g., children with cerebral palsy who have poor general muscle control). In general, an analysis of articulation skills focuses on patterns of difference in the ways the child uses his or her body to produce sounds and sequences. You can see an example of the results of the analysis of articulation skills in Table 5-3.

Phonological analysis focuses on a description of how the child's speaking reflects underlying mental representations and or rules for producing speech. Emphasis is placed on the client's *knowledge* of the speech sound system rather than any deficit in *behavior* implied by articulation analysis. Many systems of phonological analysis are employed currently. Two of the most prevalent analysis systems make use of distinctive features and phonological processes.

One method of phonological analysis is called phonological process analysis (Hodson, 2004). Recall that phonological processes are phonological rules for the way sounds are combined into words. One example of a phonological process is *final consonant deletion* in which *ball* becomes "ba" because the child is not yet proficient at putting final sounds on words. *Reduplication* is a phonological process in which the child says the same syllable twice to produce a word with more than one syllable (e.g., *bottle* becomes "baba"). Phonological process analysis was used with the child in Table 5-3 as a supplement to analysis of his articulation skills.

Other Testing

In addition to assessment of speech production skills, the SLP may complete an **oral-peripheral examination** to evaluate the structure and function of peripheral articulators (i.e., tongue, lips, and palate), if the child is capable of complying with the tasks. Again, very young or severely impaired children may not be able to comply with the tasks required in the oral-peripheral examination. A *hearing test* is essential to rule out sensory deficit as the cause of the speech disorder or delay. The clinician may administer a variety of tests and observe other aspects of language skills, depending on the SLP's assessment of the child's communication abilities (see the section on co-occurring disorders). In the case study presented in Table 5-3, you can see how the results of the oral-peripheral examination and the hearing screening were used in conjunction with the results of the speech assessment.

Treatment

Treatment for articulation and phonological disorders centers on teaching the child to use sounds and sound sequences of his or her language like that expected for peers in the community. The overall goal of treatment is speech that is easily understandable. The clinician employs assessment data to plan specific goals and treatment techniques for remediation. The clinician uses either articulation or phonologically oriented treatment approaches based on understanding of the nature of the child's disorder determined during assessment and analysis.

Generally, articulation-based approaches focus more on repetitive motor practice with feedback and attention to how the body is used to produce sounds. For example, a child might be provided with cues to help him or her identify the correct place or manner of articulation. Some examples of cues include touching the alveolar ridge with a tongue blade to help children feel where their tongue needs to go to produce alveolar sounds such as a /t/ or /d/. To indicate the length of a sound such as an /s/, the clinician may run a finger up the child's arm. Practice of the speech sounds is usually conducted in short words in activities that provide the child multiple opportunities to produce the target sound at the beginning, middle, and end of words. Then, clinicians work with children on saying the target sound correctly in phrases and sentences. This helps the children incorporate their new articulatory pattern into connected speech.

Phonological approaches emphasize the use of speech sounds and syllable sequences (Hodson, 2004) to communicate ideas (Gierut & Morrisette, 2005). Many phonological approaches deemphasize repetition and feedback on motor performance. One such approach, the metaphon approach, relies on building children's metaphonological awareness of speech sounds. This is a way of increasing the child's knowledge of the phonological system. For example, if the child had difficulty with sounds such as /s/ and /sh/, the clinician might use the analogy that these are hissing sounds to help the child focus on the high-frequency, fricative aspect of these sounds. Children would do intervention activities in which they had to identify the target in the context of games with everyday sounds before turning their attention to speech.

In another phonological approach, called contrast therapy, children are shown pairs of pictures that differ from each other by one sound. The pictures are usually selected to demonstrate a distinctive feature or a phonological process that has been determined to be deficient or absent in the child's phonology. For example, children who do not have the feature +/– voicing might work on producing pairs of words that differ only on the voicing feature such as *pin–bin, pit–bit, fan–van,* and *sip–zip.* Children who present unusual final consonant deletion processes might work on producing pairs that include words with and without final consonants such as *no–nose, see–seed, tea–team,* and *me–meet.* The key to the contrast approach is to select multiple contrastive pairs that demonstrate the distinctive feature or the phonological process that is problematic for the child.

The area of developmental speech disorders is one of the oldest within the scope of practice of the SLP. The examples here are intended to provide you with a glimpse of the many well-developed intervention approaches available to the clinician. See Bernthal and Bankson (2004) for a review of techniques and approaches.

Service Delivery

In general, service delivery for articulation and phonological disorders differs dramatically depending on the setting and the age and severity of the child's speech delay or disorder. Infants who do not develop consistent use of vocalization abilities for communication are often served in *early intervention* programs for birth to 3-year-old infants. These infants must be helped to begin using their voice to communicate ideas before they can begin to work on specific sounds and to learn how to use these sounds in words. In *public school educational settings* (children ranging in age from 3–17), a considerable percentage of the caseload may consist of children who have difficulty with articulation or phonological skills. These children need remediation to help build their ability to produce all the sounds of their language. They also need to learn how to combine the sounds they can produce correctly into words. Children served in public school settings may have mild, moderate, or severe disorders, and they may have a wide variety of etiological factors. Children may be served in *medical settings* such as hospitals or community clinics. Clients in these settings tend to have more severe disorders and sometimes require a major commitment to intervention services to improve their speech intelligibility.

SUMMARY

Articulation and phonological disorders are a core aspect of the SLP's caseload regardless of work setting. From infants who do not begin to talk as expected to the 70-year-old who has had a stroke and is difficult to understand, clients of all ages and severity levels have problems with intelligibility of oral communication. The clinician may be able to link the client's disorder to a specific etiology, or the client may be considered functionally disordered if a cause is not apparent.

Assessment procedures must be tuned to the age or developmental stage of each client. However, for all clients, it is crucial to assess speech intelligibility in spontaneous communication if at all possible. For every client, it is important for the clinician to describe how the individual produces consonants, vowels, and sequences of sounds in various words. There are different types of treatment approaches for articulation disorders and phonological disorders. In all cases of articulation and phonological disorder, the goal of treatment is for the client to produce speech that is intelligible to everyone in his or her daily environment.

BOX 5-7 Case Study

Quincy is 5½ years old and is in kindergarten at a local public school. He was referred to a university speech and hearing clinic because his family felt that his speech was difficult to understand most of the time. Children did not make fun of him at school, but he was reluctant to talk to unfamiliar people because they often could not understand him. He had no history of ear infections or any significant illness. Speech delay was his "only problem in development," according to his family.

Although he could produce most English consonants and vowels, he did not use these sounds accurately when he spoke. He omitted consonants at the ends of words (e.g., "hi_" for *hit*). He also substituted early developing sounds for sounds that occur later in development (e.g., "<u>d</u>it" for *sit*) and left out sounds when two consonants should be produced (e.g., "_top" for *stop*). His speech had a "choppy" quality where all his words were emphasized equally. In single words, Quincy was considered easier to understand, but as his sentences got longer, he made more and more sound errors. He also did not include words like *a* or *the* in his sentences and did not use the sounds needed for plurals (e.g., he produced *dogs* as "do_ _" or "dog_").

Quincy went to therapy twice weekly for 2 years at the university clinic where he was evaluated. Within 1 year, he was considered about 50% intelligible to his friends and teachers and 80–90% intelligible to his family. At the end of the second year, when he was 7 years old, he was dismissed from therapy because he was 100% intelligible with all listeners. He was very well liked and talkative with friends and family when he was dismissed from therapy.

STUDY QUESTIONS

1. What is the difference between an articulation disorder and a phonological disorder?

2. How do mild, moderate, and severe articulation/phonological disorders differ from each other?

3. What is the difference between articulation or phonological *delays* and *disorders*?

4. What are the three possible etiologic categories for articulation disorders? Give one example of each.

5. How might articulatory or phonological disorders be related to language disorders?

6. What assessment methods are routinely used during the evaluation of articulatory and phonological disorders?

7. Describe an approach to speech analysis that would be appropriate for an articulatory disorder. Which analysis approach might be used if the clinician suspects that the child has a phonological disorder?

8. Describe one therapy approach for articulation disorders and one approach for phonological disorders.

KEY TERMS

Articulation
Articulation disorder
Consonant cluster
Distinctive features
Distortion

Intelligibility
Omission
Oral-peripheral examination
Phonological disorder
Single-word articulation test

Speech delay
Speech disorder
Spontaneous speech and
    language sample
Substitution

REFERENCES

Bernthal, J. E., & Bankson, N. W. (2004). *Articulation and phonological disorders* (2nd ed.). Boston: Allyn & Bacon.

Chomsky, N., & Halle, M. (1968). *The sound pattern of English.* New York: Harper & Row.

Davis, B. L. (2005). Clinical diagnosis of developmental speech disorders. In A. G. Kamhi & K. E. Pollock (Eds.), *Phonological disorders in children: Decision making in assessment and intervention.* Baltimore, MD: Brookes.

Davis, B. L., & Bedore, L. (2008). *Developmental speech disorders.* San Diego, CA: Plural.

Gierut, J. A., & Morrisette, M. L. (2005). The clinical significance of optimality theory for phonological disorders. *Topics in Language Disorders, 25,* 266–280.

Gildersleeve-Neumann, C., Stubbe-Kester, E., Davis, B. L., & Pena, E. (2008). Phonological development in three- to four-year-old children from bilingual Spanish/English and monolingual Spanish and English environments. *Language, Speech, & Hearing Services in Schools, 39,* 314–328.

Goldman, R., & Fristoe, M. (1986). *Goldman Fristoe test of articulation.* Circle Pines, MN: American Guidance Service.

Hodson, B. (2004). *Hodson assessment of phonological patterns* (3rd ed.). Austin, TX: Pro-Ed.

SUGGESTED READINGS

Ball, M., & Kent, R. (1997). *The new phonologies: Developments in clinical linguistics.* San Diego, CA: Singular.

Kamhi, A. G., & Pollock, K. E. (Eds.). (2005). *Phonological disorders in children: Decision making in assessment and intervention.* Baltimore, MD: Brookes.

Kent, R. D. (Ed.). (2004). *The MIT encyclopedia of communication disorders.* Cambridge, MA: MIT Press.

McLeod, S. (Ed.). (2006). *The international guide to speech acquisition.* Clifton Park, NY: Thompson Delmar Learning.

Munson, B., Edwards, J., & Beckman, M. E. (2005). Phonological knowledge in typical and atypical speech and language development: Nature, assessment, and treatment. *Topics in Language Disorders, 25,* 190–206.

Velleman, S. L. (2003). *Childhood apraxia of speech resource guide.* Clifton Park, NY: Delmar/Thomson/Singular.

Vihman, M. M. (1996). *Phonological development: The origins of language in the child.* Oxford, England: Basil Blackwell.

chapter six

Laryngeal and Orofacial Disorders

RODGER DALSTON AND THOMAS P. MARQUARDT

LEARNING OBJECTIVES

1. To learn the causes and characteristics of phonation disorders.

2. To understand the embryologic basis of cleft lip and palate.

3. To know the effects of velopharyngeal incompetence on speech production.

4. To understand the purposes, procedures, and goals for evaluation of phonation and resonance disorders.

5. To understand the role of the speech-language pathologist on a team dedicated to the care of individuals with oral-facial clefts and individuals with phonation disorders.

In Chapter 4, you learned about the structures and functions of the speech production mechanism. That is, you learned how we develop an energy source for speech (respiration), create an acoustic sound source at the larynx (phonation), couple the oral and nasal cavities to ensure appropriate resonance (velopharyngeal closure), and modify the shape of the oral cavity to produce the speech sounds of our language (articulation). In this chapter, we consider disorders of phonation (voice disorders) and velopharyngeal closure (resonance disorders) that result from dysfunction at strategic points in the speech production mechanism: the larynx and the velopharynx.

VOICE DISORDERS

Everyone has probably experienced laryngitis at one time or another. This condition results from acute trauma to the vocal folds from screaming at a sports event or rock concert, for example. The vocal fold tissues become swollen (**edema**) causing a change in voice quality. The affected individual sounds hoarse and, if severe enough, may experience a complete loss of voice (**aphonia**).

Hoarseness is one of a number of judgments people make when assessing the quality of a person's voice. Typically, speech-language pathologists use three descriptors: harsh, breathy, and hoarse.

A **harsh** voice is associated with excessive muscle tension. You can simulate this quality by speaking as if you are absolutely furious but want to control your temper and not yell. The vocal folds are pressed together tightly with a quick release during each cycle of vibration; the walls of the throat are tightened to amplify the high-frequency components of the voice.

A **breathy** voice is produced with a partial whisper. The vocal folds are brought together so that they vibrate, but a space between them remains. Air passing through the space creates a fricative noise that is superimposed on the vocal tone. The larger the space between the folds, the greater the fricative noise and the breathier the phonation. If the space is wide enough, the vocal folds are not drawn into phonation and the only sound produced is fricative noise (**whisper**).

A voice that is both harsh and breathy is termed **hoarse**. It results from irregular vocal fold vibrations, typically from differences in the mass and shape of the two folds. Hoarseness can be the sign of a serious laryngeal pathology or simply the result of laryngitis associated with the common cold.

Laryngitis is one of a number of problems that can adversely affect vocal fold function. Some voice disorders result from tissue enlargement, while others are the result of a reduction in tissue (**atrophy**). Some are caused by increased muscle activity (**hyperfunction**), while others may be caused by reduced muscle activity (**hypofunction**). An abnormal degree of muscle activity may be the result of nervous system damage or psychological factors. Each of these categories has a number of conditions associated with it and is not mutually exclusive. For example, increased muscle activity may, and frequently does, result in tissue changes. We begin with a discussion of voice disorders (Table 6-1) and then will discuss how such problems are identified and evaluated.

BOX 6-1   Overview of CD-ROM Segments

The principal aim of this chapter is for you to develop an understanding of voice disorders resulting from vocal fold dysfunction and to learn about speech and resonance problems caused by inadequate velopharyngeal closure. The first segment shows normal vocal fold vibration based on visualization of the larynx by means of videostroboscopy. The following six segments reveal various vocal fold pathologies resulting from abuse, cancer, and neurological disorders. Comparison of normal vocal fold vibration with vibration of the abnormal folds provides information on the effects of various disorders on voice production. Additional video segments show the use of an electrolarynx for individuals who have had the larynx removed because of cancer and a morphing sequence showing the embryological development of the face. Interruption of this developmental process can result in orofacial anomalies of the face and palate.

Segments

6.01 Videostroboscopy, an instrumental technique that allows the larynx to be visualized, is used to show vocal fold vibration in the normal larynx.

6.02 Nodules, located near the middle of the membranous vocal folds, interfere with vocal fold closure and affect voice quality.

6.03 A large fibrous polyp interferes with normal vocal fold production and vibrates at a frequency different from the vocal folds.

6.04 Papillomas are shown on the vocal folds. Vibration of the vocal folds and voice quality are affected by the presence of abnormal tissue.

6.05 Carcinoma, a progressive malignant condition, is shown in the larynx. The presence of the tumor produces a severe voice disorder characterized by hoarseness.

6.06 A unilateral recurrent nerve paralysis affects vocal fold adduction. The resulting abnormal vocal fold production and voice disorder shown in this video segment are marked by breathiness.

6.07 Spasmodic dysphonia characterized by involuntary adduction of the vocal folds is shown for a speaker with the disorder.

6.08 Use of an electrolarynx is shown in this segment. The electrolarynx is used by individuals who have had their larynx surgically removed because of cancer.

6.09 A morphing sequence depicting embryologic development of the human face.

Table 6-1 Some Disorders of Voice

Discrete Tissue Changes	**Neurogenic Voice Problems**
Nodules	Peripheral paralysis or paresis
Polyps	Pyramidal disturbances (e.g., stroke,
Papilloma	pseudobulbar palsy)
Cysts	Extrapyramidal disturbances (e.g., parkinsonism,
Hematomas	spasmodic dysphonia, essential tremor)
Cancer	**Myopathic Voice Problems**
Contact ulcers	Myasthenia gravis
Granulomas	Myotonic muscular dystrophy
Diffuse Tissue Changes	**Nonorganic Voice Problems**
Laryngitis	Stage fright
Laryngeal bowing	Muscle tension dysphonia
Sulcus vocalis	Conversion aphonia/dysphonia
Gross Structural Changes	Ventricular phonation
Mechanical, thermal, or chemical trauma	Mutational falsetto (puberphonia)
Cricothyroid ankylosis	
Laryngeal web	
Larynx removal (laryngectomy)	

VOCAL FOLD ABNORMALITIES THAT AFFECT VOICE

A variety of structural changes in the vocal folds can affect the voice. We discuss several of the more commonly occurring conditions to serve as examples of these types of disorders.

Nodules

Nodules are the most common form of vocal fold abnormality seen by otolaryngologists and are found in approximately 20% of patients who present with a voice problem. Nodules are frequently called "screamer's nodules" because they are often found in children and mothers who scream at their children. However, nodules can develop in persons who do not scream but who abuse their vocal folds in other ways (Table 6-2). Misuses may or may not be traumatic to a particular speaker, whereas abusive vocal behavior almost always is traumatic.

Nodules are much like calluses that develop on the vocal folds in response to trauma, much as calluses develop on the hands of a day laborer or a member of a rowing team. Although such growths protect underlying tissue from further abuse, their presence on the vocal folds adversely affects voice production.

Nodules form in pairs at the point of maximum contact along the length of the vocal fold where the amplitude of vibration is greatest. This point is one third of the distance from the front to the back of the folds.

If you think of nodules as calluses, you can understand why surgical removal is not the preferred treatment. Calluses on the hand disappear if the abusive behavior is

Table 6-2 Some Misuses and Abuses of the Larynx

Misuses (behaviors that may or may not be abusive)	Abuses
Persistent use of glottal attack	Excessive, prolonged loudness
Anterior-posterior laryngeal squeezing, which is seen as approximation of the epiglottis and the arytenoids cartilages	Excessive speaking during periods of swelling, inflammation, or other tissue changes
Puberphonia (maintaining prepubescent voice)	Excessive speaking or singing while in a smoke-filled and/or noisy environment
Persistent glottal fry	Excessive speaking or singing while using irritants, such as tobacco, alcohol, or any number of drugs that affect fluid balance
Speaking with inadequate breath support	
Lack of pitch variability	Prolonged singing without appropriate training
Excessive talking	Excessive coughing and throat clearing
Ventricular phonation	Yelling and screaming
Aphonia/dysphonia of psychological origin	Noise making (e.g., toy or animal sounds)
Loudness variations effected by glottal, rather than respiratory, adjustments	Grunting (during exercise and weight lifting)

Source: Adapted from Case, J. L. (1996). *Clinical management of voice disorders.* Austin, TX: Pro-Ed.

eliminated. Similarly, if the patient alters his or her phonatory behavior to eliminate vocal abuse, the nodules will almost always be eliminated.

A number of potentially useful techniques can be employed for voice disorders related to laryngeal hyperfunction, such as vocal nodules (Table 6-3). Similar patients may respond differently to the techniques; it is the responsibility of the speech-language

Table 6-3 Facilitating Techniques for Extinguishing Inappropriate Laryngeal Behaviors

For All Disorders	Focus:
Counseling	Horizontal focus
Ear training	Vertical focus
Feedback	Glottal fry
For Hypofunction	Massage
Altering habitual loudness	Open-mouth approach
Pushing/pulling	Respiration training
Half-swallow, boom	Inhalation phonation
Head positioning	Warble
For Hyperfunction	Hierarchy analysis
Progressive relaxation	Establishing a new pitch
Yawn–sigh, nasal/glide stimulation	**For Psychogenic Problems**
Elimination of hard glottal attack	Digital manipulation
Chant–talk	Masking
	Warble

Source: Adapted from Boone, D. R. & McFarlane, S. C. (1994). *The voice and voice therapy.* Englewood Cliffs, NJ: Prentice-Hall.

pathologist and patient, working as a team, to experiment with a variety of techniques to determine which is most effective. Enlisting the patient as a partner in this exploratory process is empowering for the patient and can be an important part of the therapeutic process.

It is not possible to discuss each of the techniques listed in Table 6-3, but we describe two to give you a sense of how different these techniques can be. First, the *yawn–sigh* technique takes advantage of the fact that the vocal folds are apart (abducted) during a yawn and that they are not fully adducted (closed) during a sigh. For an individual who produces too much compression of the vocal folds during phonation, a yawn–sigh can be a useful way of helping the patient to hear and to feel voice produced with little or no untoward tension. The patient next works to extend the breathy phonation into a progression of vowels, consonant vowel syllables, words, phrases, and sentences. The contrastive use of breathy versus hypertensive voice is frequently useful in helping the patient to become aware of, and successfully modify, the abusive phonatory pattern.

Vertical focus, in contrast, is an attempt to divert a patient's attention (and hence tension) away from the larynx. One approach is to ask the patient to produce a nasal consonant such as /m/ while lightly touching the sides of the nose with the thumb and index finger. Do it yourself. What did you feel? If you did it correctly, you should have felt the nostrils vibrate in response to the production of a nasal tone. Now remove your fingers and try to perceive that vibration within the nose. Encouraging a patient to do so, using a wide variety of words, phrases, and so on, helps turn their attention away from the larynx, thereby increasing the likelihood that laryngeal muscle tension will diminish.

Polyps

Polyps are another relatively common form of vocal abnormality found in approximately 10% of patients with a voice disorder. Polyps are much like blisters that assume one of two basic shapes. Some are like small balloons connected to the vocal fold by a narrow stalk or foot (pedunculated); others are spread over a relatively large area of the vocal fold (sessile).

Most clinicians believe that polyps develop from vocal abuse, abuse that may be a one-time occurrence. By contrast, vocal nodules develop over time. Another difference is that a relatively hard nodule on one vocal fold tends to cause a nodule on the other fold. However, a soft, pliable mass on one vocal fold does not tend to irritate the other fold so that polyps typically are unilateral. Because a polyp may impede full closure of the vocal folds during phonation, the voice tends to be breathy or hoarse. In some cases, the two vocal folds, because they are substantially different in mass, may vibrate at different rates causing a double voice (**diplophonia**).

Polyps are most typically treated by speech-language pathologists whose goal it is to identify causative behaviors, such as yelling and excessive throat clearing, and help the patient eliminate them. Long-standing polyps that do not respond to voice therapy may be surgically removed.

Contact Ulcers

Contact ulcers and the granulomas that develop at sites of ulceration arise at the vocal processes (on the vocal folds between the arytenoids cartilages). This site is farther back than the midpoint of the membranous folds where nodules and polyps typically form. Contact ulcers develop from a number of disparate causes including: (1) excessive slamming together of the arytenoids cartilages during the production of inappropriately low pitch, (2) frequent nonproductive coughing and throat clearing, (3) gastric reflux resulting in acidic irritation of the membrane covering the arytenoids cartilages, and (4) intubation trauma that can occur during surgery under anesthesia.

Speech-language pathologists work with patients who present with the first two causes because they are habit patterns amenable to treatment. They may also work with patients whose contact ulcers result from gastroesophageal reflux disease or intubation trauma. But in these cases their role is to help patients adjust to the resultant hoarseness in a way that does not make the problem worse and prolong the recovery process.

Papillomas

The human papillomavirus causes warts that can occur on any skin or mucous membrane surface. Most are not life threatening and are easily treated. However, when they occur on the vocal folds, they can grow so large that they compromise the airway, making breathing difficult. Children with laryngeal papillomas are thought to contract the virus at birth from genital warts in the mother.

Fortunately, laryngeal papillomas are uncommon. The incidence in the United States is approximately 7 cases per million people per year. It also is fortunate that the body develops some immunity to warts, and they usually go away without treatment. However, surgical removal is necessary in the case of papillomas whose size threatens the airway. Such growths tend to recur, necessitating repeated surgical procedures. Repeated surgery increases the likelihood of significant scar tissue formation that can adversely affect the vibratory activity of the vocal folds. In addition to postoperative voice therapy, an important role served by the speech-language pathologist is detecting **dysphonia** in undiagnosed children and making an appropriate medical referral. Children with papillomas may go undetected because some professionals assume incorrectly that the child's hoarseness is caused by vocal nodules. This mistake occurs because the vast majority of children with a hoarse voice have vocal nodules, not papillomas.

Carcinoma

Cancer of the larynx affects approximately 11,000 new patients each year and constitutes approximately 10% of the patients seen for voice problems by otolaryngologists. Approximately 75% of cancers are found on the vocal folds, although they may appear above or below the folds. Unlike polyps and nodules that arise from acute or chronic physical trauma, respectively, laryngeal cancer frequently arises from exposure to inhaled smoke that may occur over years.

For a reason that is not well understood, coincident smoking and alcohol consumption dramatically increase the chance of developing laryngeal cancer. That is, there appears to be an additive effect when drinking and smoking coexist. It is not unusual to find that many patients with laryngeal cancer report a history of smoking and moderate to heavy drinking.

Squamous cell carcinomas are malignant tissue changes that arise in the epithelial portion of the outermost area of the vocal folds. These malignant cells can invade the muscle of the vocal folds and, like other forms of cancer, can migrate (**metastasize**) to other locations within the body, increasing the threat to life.

Patients with extensive laryngeal carcinomas may be candidates for complete removal of the larynx because of the life-threatening nature of cancer. With new advances in treatment, only about 15–20% of laryngeal cancer patients now undergo total laryngectomy. For those who must undergo this radical procedure, it is the responsibility of the speech-language pathologist to provide preoperative and postoperative counseling, coupled with postoperative therapy intended to optimize the communication abilities of the patient.

VOICE DISORDERS RESULTING FROM NEUROLOGICAL IMPAIRMENT

Damage to the nervous system can cause muscle weakness (paresis) or a total inability to contract one or more muscles of the larynx (paralysis). Approximately 8–10% of patients seen for voice problems by ear, nose, and throat physicians are found to have laryngeal muscle weakness or paralysis. An example of such a disturbance is adductor paralysis resulting from damage to the recurrent laryngeal nerve (RLN).

Paralysis

The vagus, or 10th cranial nerve, was described in Chapter 4, Speech Science. The RLN of the vagus innervates all the intrinsic laryngeal muscles except for the cricothyroid. The superior laryngeal nerve (SLN) innervates the cricothyroid muscle.

The RLN, because of its location, is prone to damage during neck and chest surgery. If the nerve is damaged on one side, the fold cannot be completely adducted and voice quality will be breathy. Therapy may involve attempts to increase the closing

BOX 6-2   Examples of Normal and Abnormal Vocal Fold Vibration

In CD-ROM segment Ch.6.01, a speaker with normal vocal fold function is shown during speaking and singing. Compare the vocal fold vibration and voice quality of this speaker to the speaker with vocal nodules in Ch.6.02. Where are the vocal nodules located? How is voice quality different for the speaker with nodules? How is vocal fold vibration different for a speaker with a vocal polyp shown in Ch.6.03? Is the polyp on the right or the left vocal fold? Compare vocal fold vibration and voice quality for speakers with papillomas (Ch.6.04) and carcinoma (Ch.6.05). Which of the two speakers has the most hoarseness? Why?

function of the unaffected fold. Recall that one function of the larynx is to close off the airway to allow for stabilization of the thorax. Such a maneuver may be of value in stimulating the unaffected side to "overadduct" and come into contact or approximation with the paralyzed fold. If this or similar techniques are unsuccessful, patients may be referred for surgical care.

Surgery in the case of unilateral vocal fold paralysis involves physically moving the affected vocal fold closer to midline so that the unaffected fold can contact it during phonation. Such surgery is performed under local anesthesia so that the patient is able to phonate as the fold is moved toward midline (medialized). The surgeon continues to move the fold medially until optimal voice is obtained.

While unilateral vocal fold paralysis is fairly uncommon, it is fortunate that bilateral paralysis is even less frequent. Such a disturbance typically results from central nervous system damage. If neural input to both recurrent laryngeal nerves is eliminated, both folds assume a static position partway between being fully abducted (open) and fully adducted (closed). The folds assume a position such that the space between the two folds (glottis) is compromised and may result in difficulty breathing (**dyspnea**). Surgery may be necessary to create an open airway sufficient for breathing. Patients with bilateral RLN impairment but normal SLN function retain reasonably good voice and vocal range. The **paramedian** (half-open) position of the folds makes it fairly easy for the exhaled airstream to draw the folds into vibration. In addition, the pitch range tends to remain fairly normal because the SLN innervates the cricothyroid muscle responsible for pitch adjustments. Individuals with damage to the SLN have problems adjusting pitch because this nerve controls the cricothyroid muscle, which is important in tensing the vocal folds. Which aspects of phonation are affected is dependent on which nerves are damaged.

Spasmodic Dysphonia

Spasmodic dysphonia (SD) is a rare disorder, probably affecting no more than 1–2 people per 10,000 in the United States. It was originally thought to be of psychogenic origin because patients with SD have less difficulty during singing and improvement in the voice occurs when pitch is raised. Moreover, some patients report that the condition arose coincident with an emotional event in their lives. Nevertheless, SD is accepted as a neurological problem involving a disturbance in the basal ganglia that causes disordered muscle tonicity (dystonia).

There are two types of SD. In the most frequent type (*adductor spasmodic dysphonia*), the patient experiences abrupt, uncontrolled (spasmodic) contractions of the adductor muscles resulting in a "strain-strangle" voice quality. In contrast, *abductor spasmodic dysphonia* causes inappropriate contraction of the laryngeal abductor muscles. Inappropriate **abduction** of the vocal folds causes the patient's speech to be interrupted by periods of aphonia.

The preferred method of treatment for SD is repeated injections of botulinum toxin (BOTOX) into the muscles of the larynx. The toxin reduces contraction of the affected muscles but does nothing to address the basal ganglia deficit creating the problem. For this reason, once the BOTOX effects disappear, the condition reappears.

Shortly after BOTOX injections for adductor SD, the patient presents with a breathy voice quality. Thereafter, the voice normalizes and then eventually reverts to the pretreatment strain-strangle quality. The entire cycle from injection to relapse usually occurs over a period of 3 to 6 months, after which another BOTOX injection may be recommended.

The role of the speech-language pathologist is to work with the patient prior to and following medical intervention. The intent of therapy is to help the patient accept the breathiness that occurs following administration of the BOTOX and teach the patient various techniques that may prolong the "normal voice" phase.

VOCAL ABNORMALITIES UNRELATED TO STRUCTURAL CHANGE

Most voice disorders are related to tissue changes in the larynx or abnormal changes in the nervous system. However, a number of disturbances can occur in the absence of underlying pathology. One you may have experienced, perhaps during public speaking, is the "shaky" voice that accompanies stage fright. This condition results from a perfectly normal fight-or-flight reaction to danger whether real or imagined. Other disorders may be more significant.

Conversion Aphonia/Dysphonia

A patient may report a total loss of voice (aphonia) or an extremely abnormal voice (dysphonia) and yet a thorough medical examination fails to uncover an organic cause for the problem. The existence of a psychogenic cause for the disorder may be suspected, particularly if the patient is able to produce normal phonation during such vegetative functions as coughing, gargling, or laughing.

Voice problems of this sort frequently have a sudden onset, and a careful interview of the patient and family often reveals previous occurrences of the problem. In many cases, voice is restored within an hour or less. However, the underlying cause of the problem has not been addressed, and referral to a mental health clinician may be indicated in some, but not necessarily all, cases.

Puberphonia

Puberphonia, also known as mutational falsetto, involves the continued use of a high-pitched voice by a postpubertal male. As with conversion disorders, patients with mutational falsetto typically cough at a pitch level that reflects the more natural vibratory

BOX 6-3 Examples of Vocal Fold Disorders Associated With Neurological Deficits

CD-ROM segment Ch.6.06 shows vocal fold vibration for a speaker with a paralyzed vocal fold. What type of voice quality disorder is apparent? CD-ROM segment Ch.6.07 shows vocal fold vibration for a patient with spasmodic dysphonia. How is voice quality different for the two neurological laryngeal disorders?

frequency of the vocal folds. The condition may be the result of unresolved psychological issues, or it may be a learned behavior. In either case, the abnormal voice is readily amenable to correction by a speech-language pathologist and in fact is one of the most easily corrected psychogenic voice disorders.

Muscle Tension Dysphonia (MTD)

Individuals with muscle tension dysphonia (MTD) display disordered voices that are caused by inordinate tension in the laryngeal muscles. The condition appears to result from the simultaneous contraction of the muscles that close (adductor) and open (abductor) the vocal folds. Muscles that attach to the larynx and to some other structure (**extrinsic laryngeal muscles**) may also hypertense and develop "knots" that may benefit from laryngeal massage.

The voice of MTD patients is usually quite hoarse, and patients frequently report fatigue and laryngeal discomfort. The classic description of such patients is hard-driving, upwardly mobile, Type A executive types whose hypertensive lifestyles are mirrored in their voices. Of course, many MTD patients do not have such classic personality profiles.

Whatever the cause of MTD, voice therapy directed toward facilitating a reduction in muscle tension can have a dramatic effect upon these individuals. However, as with all other voice cases, patients must be motivated to change and be willing to use strategies mutually agreed upon with the speech-language pathologist.

THE VOICE EVALUATION

Voice disorders are best managed by the joint efforts of a team. The core elements of such a team are the otolaryngologist and speech-language pathologist. In the ideal situation, which is most often realized in a hospital setting, these professionals evaluate the patient together. More often, patients are referred to the speech-language pathologist by a physician, a school nurse, or the patients themselves. In all cases, it is incumbent on the speech-language pathologist to ensure that a trusted otolaryngologist is involved in evaluation and treatment planning because some laryngeal pathologies can be life-threatening.

Patient Interview

The interview is intended to provide extensive information concerning the patient and the problem. In addition to gathering basic demographic data, such as age and gender, it is important to thoroughly explore the patient's health history, family situation, dietary habits, use of stimulants, and the level of concern regarding the voice problem. An example may help you understand why the interview and the information it provides are important.

A 62-year-old woman was self-referred for what she described as a "frightening voice." The woman indicated that when speaking with people, she frequently was asked if she was choking. She said it frequently felt as if someone was strangling her while she was speaking.

The interview revealed that the condition began following the death of her sister 6 months before and had been getting progressively worse. She noted that her voice improved when she sang or spoke at a higher than normal pitch level, and it was worse when she spoke on the phone. The patient denied ever having experienced anything like this in the past and her husband confirmed the report. Further discussion revealed that the family physician had examined the larynx with a laryngeal mirror and reportedly found nothing wrong. After considerable probing, the husband reluctantly revealed that his wife had been referred to a psychiatrist by her family physician. However, the referral was rejected and the patient became tearful when this topic was broached.

At first glance it might appear that the patient's voice disorder is the result of a psychological problem. However, you may have identified one or more of a number of clues in the preceding paragraph that suggest otherwise. First, the descriptive terms "choking" and "strangling" indicate the possibility of a neurological disorder such as spasmodic dysphonia. It is not unusual for this condition to be first observed following an emotional trauma, and it is easy to see why it frequently is thought to be a psychiatric disorder. A diagnosis of spasmodic dysphonia may not be substantiated by a cursory examination of the larynx because special equipment is necessary to uncover the laryngeal behaviors characterizing this condition. This equipment rarely is available to the family physician but is routinely used by ear, nose, and throat physicians.

Perceptual Assessment

During the interview, the patient may describe his voice problem using a number of terms. The characteristics that a patient reports are known as *symptoms*. The nine primary symptoms are hoarseness, fatigue, breathiness, reduced pitch range, lack of voice (aphonia), pitch breaks or inappropriately high pitch, strain/strangle, tremor, and lump in the throat (globus). Voice characteristics that can be observed or tested by a clinician are known as *signs*. Some symptoms such as high pitch and hoarseness are signs, whereas other symptoms such as "something in my throat" and "fatigue" are not. The task of the perceptual assessment of the evaluation is for the clinician to use listening skills to identify the presence and magnitude of the signs of a voice problem. Specifically, the clinician makes judgments regarding the pitch, loudness, and quality of the voice during a variety of tasks. A high-quality tape recording of the patient is made using a sample of speech. Typically, this includes the patient's name, the recording date, sustained vowel productions, counting, reading, singing, spontaneous conversation, and pitch and loudness glissandos (rapid sliding up and down a range).

Voice Quality

Numerous terms are used to describe abnormalities of voice, but we can describe voice quality disorders using three: breathy, harsh, and hoarse. If the vocal folds vibrate but are not completely closed, the voice sounds *breathy*, and the acoustic output from the larynx is characterized by a spectrum of tones (voice) superimposed on a noise spectrum (whisper). Now assume that you have a large growth on the medial aspects (inner surface) of your vocal folds. It should be apparent that the presence of such a growth would make it difficult to close the glottis completely. Because such a growth would cause an undesirable quality in the voice (breathiness), there is a natural tendency to increase vocal fold tension in an effort to eliminate that quality by forcing the vocal folds together. In fact, what happens is that vocal fold tension is introduced without the desired result of eliminating the breathiness. This combination of vocal fold tension causing harshness, coupled with breathiness, is what we perceive as *hoarse*.

An individual who does not have an irregularity of the medial margin of the vocal folds, and hence no breathiness, but who phonates with inappropriate vocal fold tension produces a tense voice we describe as *harsh*. An example of a condition characterized by a harsh voice quality is MTD in which both the closing and opening muscles of the larynx are hypertensed. Hypertensive laryngeal function is often accompanied by pharyngeal (throat) muscle tension. Given the inappropriate amount of tension in the vocal folds, such speakers run the risk of traumatizing the folds and causing the development of tissue changes.

In judging the pitch, loudness, and quality of a patient's speech, clinicians use scales for grading the parameters of interest. One of the more commonly used scales is called equal-appearing-interval scaling. Most scales of this type use 5, 6, or 7 steps between polar opposites, such as high and low pitch, or between normal and severely impaired along a continuum such as hoarseness. For example, a 6-point scale regarding hoarseness might use the following assignments:

1 = normal voice quality
2 = mild hoarseness
3 = mild to moderate hoarseness
4 = moderate hoarseness
5 = moderate to severe hoarseness
6 = severe hoarseness

Equal-appearing indicates that the clinician feels confident in stating that the psychophysical distance between mild and moderate is equal to the perceptual distance from moderate to severe. Assuming this confidence is justified, and it may not be, the data collected can be analyzed using relatively powerful statistics.

Instrumental Evaluation

A voice evaluation that does not include instrumental assessment is considered a screening procedure. Data from instrumental techniques are an important way of confirming and extending information obtained by listening to the voice. They also are an extremely valuable means of documenting change, should the patient be enrolled in voice therapy.

Videoendoscopy enables the clinician to visualize the vocal folds and surrounding area using a camera and light source. **Stroboscopy** is a slow motion technique that allows clinicians to examine closely the movement characteristics of the vocal folds; therewith abnormalities can be detected that otherwise may have gone unnoticed.

Another instrument in wide use is the **Visipitch**. This instrument provides objective data regarding a number of acoustic parameters including the patient's fundamental

> **BOX 6-4**   **Examples of Videoendoscopy of the Larynx**
>
> CD-ROM segments Ch.6.01 through 6.07 are videoendoscopic movies of the vocal folds. Review these segments again to see how this technique provides a dynamic view of vocal fold vibration.

frequency and phonatory range, voice intensity, and the relative amount of spectral noise in the speech signal. Data about pitch instability (jitter), for example, obtained using Visipitch may be helpful in providing additional information about judged hoarseness of a speaker.

Disposition

Once the voice evaluation is complete, the task of the speech-language pathologist is to make recommendations regarding referrals and the need for treatment, if any. Among all patients seen, some of the most challenging can be those who have laryngeal cancer, and for whom the medical treatment involves surgical removal of the larynx (**laryngectomy**).

LARYNGECTOMY

The larynx sits at the top of the trachea, or windpipe, and serves as a protective valve as well as a sound generator. Surgical removal of the larynx requires that the trachea be redirected to an opening on the front of the neck known as a tracheal **stoma** (Figure 6-1).

This causes alteration in a number of functions. For example, because the cleansing action of the nose is eliminated by this redirection of the breath stream, **larygectomees** (people who have had a laryngectomy) routinely wear some protective device over the stoma to ensure that foreign matter does not enter the lungs. This device may be a simple gauze pad or it may be a plastic valvular device that serves as an airway protector at the same time as it facilitates phonation.

The loss of the ability to phonate can be devastating. Those of you who have had a bad case of laryngitis have surely experienced short-term frustration in being unable to communicate verbally, but how would you feel if you thought that inability would be total and forever? Now try to understand the impact of knowing that your sense of smell and taste will be compromised, your daily hygiene routine will be increased, showering will require special precautions to protect your airway, and swimming will no longer be possible.

If you are able to comprehend the emotional effects of losing the larynx, you can readily see why speech-language pathologists play such an important role in the counseling of patients both before and after surgery. We also play a major role in ensuring that these individuals do, in fact, regain the ability to communicate verbally. We do so by working with patients to help them adopt one or more communication options.

Artificial Larynx

In anticipation of laryngectomy surgery, the speech-language pathologist will work with patients to familiarize them with two types of artificial larynx they may choose to use after surgery. One of these involves a hand-held battery-activated diaphragm that creates a sound source that, when held up to the air, actually sounds quite obnoxious. However, when held against the neck, it produces a spectrum of tones that can be modulated by the articulators to produce intelligible speech.

In the immediate postoperative period, the throat area is quite tender, particularly if the patient has undergone radiation therapy. As a consequence, a different type of artificial larynx frequently is recommended immediately after surgery. The principal difference is that the sound generated by this device is presented directly to the mouth by means of a small tube making it available for articulatory modulation.

Some laryngectomees are quite pleased with these mechanical devices and choose not to explore other options. On the other hand, many patients dislike the artificial, mechanical quality of voice and the "hassle" of dealing with a device that can be misplaced or lost.

Esophageal Speech

One option for speech production after laryngectomy is to force air down into the esophagus and then release the impounded air pressure in such a way as to cause the vibration in the walls of the esophagus. During **esophageal speech**, air is actively injected down the esophagus past an area variously known as the **neoglottis**, the **pseudoglottis,** or the **pharyngeal-esophageal (PE) segment**. When the impounded air is released, it passes by the PE segment and draws the walls of the esophagus into vibration, much like air passing through the (true) glottis causes vibration of the vocal folds. Because the esophageal walls are much larger in mass than the true vocal folds, esophageal speech is quite low-pitched, and because there is little voluntary control of the muscles in this area, pitch variability is limited. Similarly, utterance length and loudness variation are limited by the small amount of air that can be injected at one time.

Trachoesophageal Speech

In trachoesophageal speech, air is routed from the lungs into the esophagus via a trachoesophageal speech prosthesis (see Figure 6-1). This is possible because patients

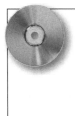

BOX 6-5   Demonstration of an Electrolarynx

CD-ROM segment Ch.6.08 shows an artificial larynx being used for speech production. The electrolarynx produces sound that is transmitted into the vocal tract and shaped into sounds and words by the speaker. How is the sound of the electrolarynx different from that produced by the vocal folds?

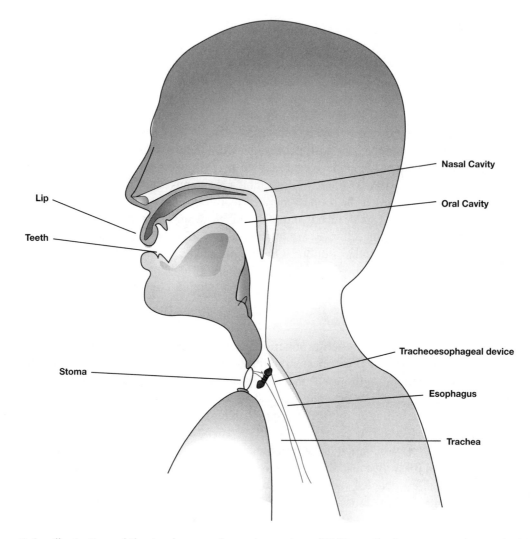

Lip

Teeth

Stoma

Nasal Cavity

Oral Cavity

Tracheoesophageal device

Esophagus

Trachea

Figure 6-1 Illustration of the tracheoesophageal puncture (TEO) surgical reconstruction technique following total laryngectomy. Note the position of the silicone prosthesis in the surgically created tunnel between the trachea and esophagus. Collar on both the esophageal and tracheal sides of the prothesis ensures stable fit of the appliance.

undergo an additional surgery to create a small opening between the trachea and esophagus in which the prosthesis is inserted. To force air from the trachea into the esophagus, the laryngectomee must either cover the hole (stoma) on the front of the throat with a finger or be fitted with a tracheostomal valve. Such a valve automatically shuts as exhaled lung pressure increases in anticipation of speech onset. The volume and pressure of shunted air available for vibration of the neoglottis is limited only by the respiratory capabilities of the individual. Therefore, the patient can produce longer phrases with greater pitch and loudness variability than esophageal speakers can. Not all laryngectomees are candidates for tracheoesophageal speech, but, when appropriate, it provides the most natural speech with the least therapy.

Whichever speaking method is adopted by a patient, the speech-language pathologist plays a critical role in the rehabilitation of these individuals. Our principal reward is knowing that we have helped our patients resume their reliance on the spoken word for human interaction.

Cleft Lip and Palate

We now turn our attention to disorders that result from disturbances to another valve important for speech production, the velopharyngeal mechanism. Velopharyngeal activity enables us to open the port between the nose and mouth for production of nasal consonants and to close it for production of all other speech sounds. Children born with a cleft in the roof of the mouth may have difficulty producing the sounds of English except for the nasal consonants (e.g., /m/, /n/) because of problems closing the velopharyngeal valve.

ORAL-FACIAL CLEFTS: AN OVERVIEW

Oral-facial clefts are the fourth most frequent birth defect. The condition occurs in approximately 1 out of every 750 live births among European Americans. For reasons that we do not fully understand, clefts of the lip and/or palate occur about half as often among African Americans and almost twice as often among Asian Americans.

Approximately 25% of affected individuals have clefts involving either one or both sides of the lip. If the cleft extends all the way up to the base of the nose, there also may be a notch in the alveolar ridge. Twenty-five percent of individuals have clefts of the palate only. Some palatal clefts are so minimal that special equipment is needed to detect them; others may be extremely wide defects that involve almost the entire roof of the mouth. The remaining 50% of affected children have clefts of both the lip and palate.

At about 6 weeks after conception, the structures that will form the roof of the mouth and the face have grown close together and unless disturbed will begin the process of uniting with one another to form the palate and lip. The entire process is completed by 9 weeks.

A relatively early disruption of this normally occurring process can result in a complete cleft of the palate that may extend through the lip on one side (**unilateral**) or both sides (**bilateral**). (See Figure 6-2). A complete unilateral cleft of the lip and palate is shown in Figure 6-2A; a complete bilateral cleft of the lip and palate is shown in Figure 6-2B.

Because union of the lip occurs after palate formation begins, it is possible for a child to be born with an intact palate but a cleft of the lip. The extent of lip involvement may be limited to a notch in the red part of the lip, or it can involve the entire lip, up through the base of the nose and back into the alveolar ridge on one or both sides.

Clefts involving only the lip may affect facial appearance and have consequences for social interaction, but they do not adversely affect speech unless the alveolar ridge

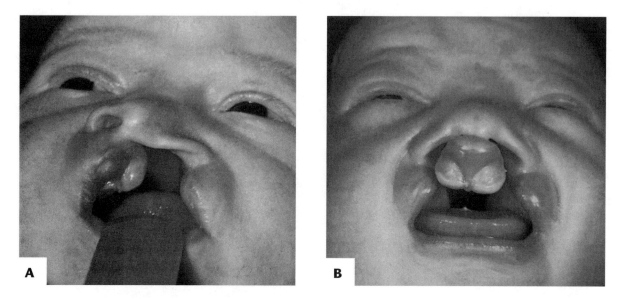

Figure 6-2 Unilateral (A) and bilateral (B) complete cleft of the lip and palate. *Source:* Courtesy of Leonard V. Crowley, MD, Century College

is involved. However, unoperated clefts of the palate make it impossible for the individual to impound air for the production of consonants such as /s/ and /b/. Also, vowels, in particular, are compromised by the introduction of unwanted resonances in the nasal cavity.

HOW CLEFTS OF THE LIP AND PALATE DEVELOP

To understand the genesis of cleft lip and cleft palate, you need to understand what happens during embryologic development of the outer face and palatal vault area. Tissue in the area that will eventually give rise to the midportion of the upper lip grows downward and laterally to meet tissue growing in from the side. These tissues eventually touch one another and join to form the intact upper lip. If they do not, the result is a cleft on one side or both sides of the lip.

The sequential development of the palatal vault begins earlier (week 6) and ends later (week 9) than development of the lip. It begins when a small triangular wedge of tissue (premaxilla) that will eventually become the area housing the upper four front teeth fuses with horizontally oriented shelves of tissue known as the palatine processes of the maxilla (Figure 6-3). Behind the premaxilla, these palatine processes fuse with one another in a front-to-back sequence. If this process is disturbed at any time, a cleft of the palate results. If these processes never begin to fuse, the result is a complete cleft of the palate. Otherwise, the cleft is incomplete. If the palatal cleft co-occurs with a cleft of the lip, the lip involvement may either be on one side or the other (a right or left unilateral cleft of the lip and palate) or it may involve both sides of the lip (a bilateral cleft of the lip and palate).

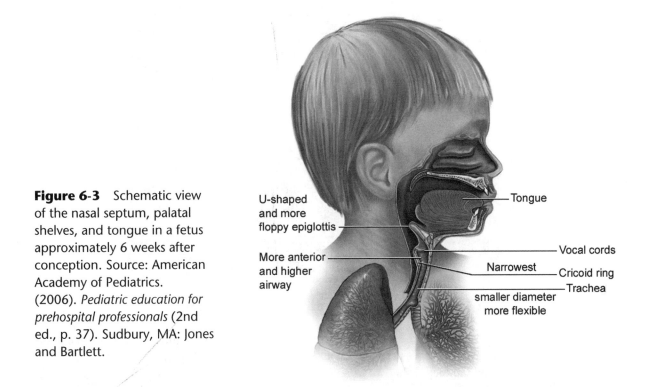

U-shaped
and more
floppy epiglottis

More anterior
and higher
airway

Tongue

Vocal cords

Narrowest

Cricoid ring

Trachea

smaller diameter
more flexible

Figure 6-3 Schematic view of the nasal septum, palatal shelves, and tongue in a fetus approximately 6 weeks after conception. Source: American Academy of Pediatrics. (2006). *Pediatric education for prehospital professionals* (2nd ed., p. 37). Sudbury, MA: Jones and Bartlett.

BOX 6-6   Morphing Sequence of the Embryological Development of the Human Face

CD-ROM segment Ch.6.09 can greatly facilitate your understanding of lip formation during embryologic development. The morphing sequence shows the events in formation of the human face during weeks 4 through 8 following conception. The last image in the sequence is a 1-year-old child. Once you have viewed the entire video segment, scroll back slowly toward the left. When you do this, you will be better able to appreciate the fact that some children with disturbed facial development present with widely spaced eyes and low-set ears. You also can tell that clefts of the upper lip appear to the left and/or right of midline.

Patients differ in the extent of palatal clefting. Palatal union proceeds from front to back; the child with a cleft of the palate only shown in Figure 6-4 experienced a disturbance later in development than the two children in Figure 6-4. In some cases almost all of the hard palate and almost all of the soft palate forms normally and the child has a submucous cleft. This type of cleft has three characteristics including: (1) a notch in the hard palate (not visible but can be palpated with a gloved finger), (2) abnormal orientation of the soft palate muscles causing the middle of the velum to be quite thin and bluish in color, and (3) **bifid** (split) **uvula**.

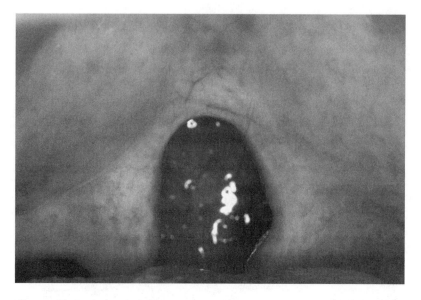

Figure 6-4   Palatal clefting. *Source:* © EH Gill/Custom Medical Stock Photo

In rare cases, the hard palate and the entire mucous membrane have formed completely, leaving only the palatal musculature malformed. This form of cleft is well hidden and, as such, is known as an *occult cleft*. Although the condition is difficult to see, it can result in the same type of speech problems that accompany more involved palatal clefts; that is, the muscular malformation makes it difficult or impossible for the patient to elevate the velum up and back against the **posterior pharyngeal wall (PPW**; back of the throat).

Palatopharyngeal Inadequacy

Another physical condition that adversely affects speech but that is not a result of a cleft is congenital palatopharyngeal inadequacy. This problem may be caused by a congenitally short soft palate or an enlarged pharynx. It may also be caused by a shortening of the muscles at the sides of the pharynx that may tether the velum so that it cannot elevate to the back wall of the throat (PPW). Sometimes these conditions are not obvious early in life because the soft palate can come into contact with the adenoids to close off the nose from the mouth for production of nonnasal speech sounds. However, when the adenoids shrink with maturation or are removed as a result of repeated ear infections, the velum may be unable to reach the PPW, making velopharyngeal closure difficult or impossible. The effect is to cause speech to sound hypernasal with emission of air on consonants requiring impounded air pressure in the mouth.

Surgical Care and the Role of the Speech-Language Pathologist

Clefts of the lip usually are repaired surgically within the first 3 months of life and clefts of the palate at approximately 12 months of age. The type of lip surgery (**chelioplasty**)

and palate surgery (**palatoplasty**) chosen depends on the nature of the cleft and the individual preference of the surgeon. Approximately 80–90% of patients who undergo primary repair of the palate will have adequate velopharyngeal closure. The other 10–20% may need to undergo secondary physical management. Figure 6-4 shows a postoperative picture of a child with a repaired unilateral cleft of the lip.

THE SPEECH OF CHILDREN WITH CLEFT LIP AND PALATE

If a child is unable to close off the nose from the mouth during the production of nonnasal speech sounds, two problems arise. First, the production of the vowels will be accompanied by inappropriate resonances associated with coupling of the oral and nasal cavities (**hypernasal**). In addition, attempts at producing consonants will result in the audible escape of air through the nose (**nasal emission**). Take a moment and try to say the word *puppy* while lowering your soft palate. If you are successful, you will hear frictional noise emanating from your nose during production of each /p/. This frictional noise is the result of the emission of air from the nasal cavity. Types of malformations effecting closure for speech production are shown in Figure 6-4.

Children with palatal clefts whose surgery is not successful frequently produce sounds like /p/ in an atypical manner. They tend to occlude the airway behind the

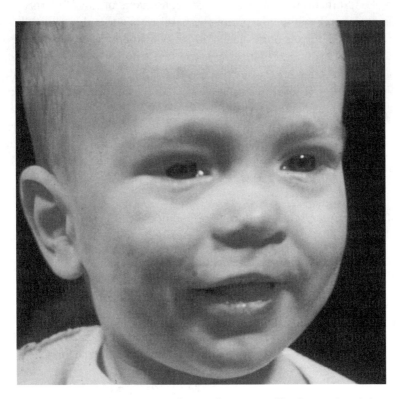

Figure 6-5 Postoperative view of a patient who underwent Millard Rotation Advancement repair of a unilateral cleft lip. *Source:* Courtesy of Leonard V. Crowley, MD, Century College

velopharyngeal port and substitute **glottal stops** or **pharyngeal fricatives** for stop (plosive) consonants. Glottal stops are like little coughs produced at the larynx, whereas **pharyngeal stops** are produced by making and then releasing a contact between the base of the tongue and the back of the throat. Individuals with velopharyngeal impairment may also omit fricative sounds (e.g., /s/, /z/, and "sh") or produce them by retracting the base of the tongue near the back of the throat to create a constriction through which the air is forced, thereby creating fricative noise. Table 6-5 lists a number of speech errors typically observed in the speech of children with cleft lips and palates.

When children develop these **compensatory articulations** for stops and fricatives, they become the purview of the speech-language pathologist. However, it is unreasonable to expect a child to develop oral pressure consonants if the velopharyngeal mechanism remains inadequate. At the same time a child may not be attempting to close the velopharyngeal port if all pressure consonants (stops and fricatives) are glottals or pharyngeals. In some cases, a clinician may opt to see a child for therapy in an attempt to establish oral consonants. If oral consonant articulations emerge but are accompanied by nasal emission, secondary physical management would appear to be indicated. If they emerge as acceptable oral productions, the child has been spared additional surgery or prosthetic management.

Children with repaired cleft palates may also have nasal structure distortions that make it difficult to produce the nasal consonants of English (/m/, /n/, and /ŋ/). That is, the speech will be devoid of the nasal resonances that normally characterize these sounds and vowels immediately adjacent to them because of nasal obstruction. They will sound **hyponasal (denasal)**. If you said "Mother knows many songs" and produced a stop consonant at the same place as the nasal consonant (/b/ for /m/, /d/ for /n/, and /g/ for /ng/), it would be produced as "Buther dowes bedy sogs." In other words, the phrase would sound hyponasal.

Children born with cleft lip and palate, then, may be hypernasal as the result of inadequate velopharyngeal closure and denasal as the result of nasal structure distortions. That is, the affected individual may not be able to produce rich nasal resonances

Table 6-4   Malformations Adversely Affecting Velopharyngeal Closure

Cleft Lip	**Complete Lip and Palate**
Partial	Unilateral
Complete	Right
No alveolar ridge involvement	Left
Alveolar ridge involved	Bilateral
Cleft Palate	**Congenital Velopharyngeal Inadequacy**
Occult submucous	**Congenitally Short Soft Palate without**
Submucous	**Clefting**
Incomplete	**Megapharynx**
Complete	**Posterior Faucial Pillar Webbing**

during nasal consonants but also may be unable to keep from producing some nasal resonance during vowels, which should be produced wholly in the oral cavity. That is why some individuals can be both hypernasal (on vowels) and hyponasal (on nasal consonants).

MANAGEMENT OF PATIENTS WITH ORAL-FACIAL CLEFTS

Children born with cleft lip, cleft palate, or both should be evaluated and treated by a team of specialists with particular expertise in this clinical area. The ideal team is transdisciplinary and the team members work cooperatively and efficiently because each fully understands the treatment priorities of the others. Not all cleft palate teams have these professional resources. To be listed as a cleft palate team in the directory of the American Cleft-Palate Craniofacial Association (1-800-24-CLEFT), a team need only have a speech-language pathologist, a surgeon, and a dentist as active members. However, more comprehensive teams include specialties such as audiology, neurology, and prosthodontics, among others.

Speech Assessment

The responsibility of the speech-language pathologist on a cleft palate team is to decide whether a patient with less than optimal speech would benefit most from intensive speech therapy or secondary physical management. The three critical elements in cleft palate assessment are articulation testing, examination of the speech production mechanism, and estimates of nasality.

Articulation Testing

Speech assessments are usually conducted by administering single-word articulation tests and by collecting speech samples during conversations with children. In children with a history of cleft palate, particular attention is paid to the production of speech sounds that require the development of intraoral pressure such as stops, fricatives, and

Table 6-5 Types of Compensatory Articulations Frequently Observed in the Speech of Individuals With Velopharyngeal Impairment

Misarticulation	Description
Glottal stop	Plosive release of air pressure built up below the glottis (similar to a light cough)
Pharyngeal stop	Plosive release of air pressure built up below contact between the base of the tongue and the posterior pharyngeal wall
Pharyngeal fricative	Frication caused by forcing air through a constriction between the base of the tongue and the posterior pharyngeal wall

affricates because compensatory articulations such as glottal stops and pharyngeal fricatives are expected if there is inadequate velopharyngeal closure. However, the child may also have a phonological delay in addition to difficulty producing speech sounds because of inadequate velopharyngeal closure. The two types of speech sound disorders are not mutually exclusive, and the speech-language pathologist needs to make a judgment about why and in which ways speech sound development is delayed or deviant.

Examination of the Speech Production Mechanism

Examining the speech structures and their functioning during nonspeech and speech tasks is part of the assessment of all children and adults with articulation disorders. The examination is undertaken to determine the anatomic and functional integrity of the speech production system. The speech-language pathologist views the face, teeth, hard palate, tongue, and velopharynx using a penlight and makes judgments about individual structures and the relationship of structures at rest and during nonspeech and speech activities to answer the questions "Do the structures appear normal?" and "What is the potential effect of any structural and/or functional deficits on speech production?"

Listener Judgments of Nasality

Most speech-language pathologists make perceptual judgments about the acceptability of children's nasal resonance as they listen to their conversational speech. These judgments have good face validity; that is, they appear intuitively to be a true indicator of the communicative significance of impaired velopharyngeal function. However, they tend to be somewhat unreliable, and the degree of reliability seems to vary depending on the parameter being assessed. Moreover, listener judgment variability seems to be a particularly troublesome problem in clinical settings where treatment decisions typically are made. There are several reasons for listener judgment errors including the lack of a linear relationship between perceived nasality and the area of the velopharyngeal port deficit, increased estimates of hypernasality with increased numbers of articulation errors, the listener's personal biases, and past experiences of the listener in making perceptual judgments. In general, the reliability of subjective judgments can be improved by training and by pooling judgments from multiple listeners.

Compensatory articulations usually are easy to discern, although they may be difficult to eliminate. Conversely, hypernasality can vary over a wide range, and mild degrees of hypernasality may be difficult to identify and quantify. Therefore, most clinicians augment perceptual assessments of speech with information from instruments that are designed to measure nasality.

Instrumental Assessment of Nasality

Instrumentation has been developed in an attempt to provide valid and reliable measures of velopharyngeal inadequacy to overcome some of the shortfalls attendant to the use of perceptual ratings. Information obtained from these measures is intended to supplement, rather than supplant, impressions obtained by speech-language pathologists in the diagnostic process.

One such instrument is the **Nasometer**. This device records oral and nasal components of a person's speech sensed by microphones on either side of a sound separator that rests on the patient's upper lip. The patient is asked to produce a series of sentences without nasal consonants. In the absence of nasal consonants, little acoustic energy would be expected to be picked up by the nasal microphone with most of the acoustic energy coming from the mouth. A computer processes signals from the nasal and oral microphones; the resultant signal is a ratio of nasal to nasal-plus-oral acoustic energy. The ratio is multiplied by 100 and expressed as a percentage, known as a nasalance score. In general, the score for individuals with normal velopharyngeal function is less than 20, the score for individuals with mild hypernasality is in the high 20s and low 30s, and those with more significant degrees of hypernasality may receive scores in the 40s and 50s.

Secondary Surgical Management

After careful consideration of the perceptual and instrumental data, the treatment team may decide that the patient is a candidate for additional surgery to improve velopharyngeal closure. Two secondary procedures typically utilized are the **pharyngeal flap surgery** and the **superior sphincter pharyngoplasty**.

Velopharyngeal closure involves upward and backward movement of the velum and medial (inward) movement of the lateral pharyngeal walls. If a patient has a short soft palate but good lateral wall movement, he or she would benefit from a pharyngeal flap, in which a flap of tissue from the back wall of the throat is raised and inserted into the velum. This provides for a constantly present veil over the velopharyngeal port. When the lateral walls of the velopharynx are relaxed, the patient can breathe through the nose and can also produce nasal consonants. When complete velopharyngeal closure is desired, the well-functioning lateral walls can move in against the sides of the velum and flap.

If a patient has good velar length and movement, but reduced lateral pharyngeal wall activity, a superior sphincter pharyngoplasty would appear to be the method of choice. In this case, the posterior faucial pillars are cut free and swung up into the area of velopharyngeal closure. They are sutured together to form a purse string in that area. Their added bulk is intended to ensure that the reduced lateral wall movement is adequate to effect closure.

Prosthetic Management

Most patients requiring additional physical management after primary palate repair are treated surgically. However, some patients may not be good surgical risks and may be treated prosthetically.

Patients who have a short soft palate or a deep **nasopharynx** may be candidates for a speech bulb. The front part of this appliance is similar to the acrylic retainer worn by patients who have undergone orthodontic treatment. Extending back from that retainer is a connecting piece that has a mass of acrylic attached to it that is shaped to fill the velopharyngeal space that the patient is unable to eliminate during attempts at closure.

Patients who have adequate soft palate length but inadequate muscle control to close the velopharynx may be candidates for a palatal lift appliance (Figure 6-6). The primary difference in this appliance is that a broad, spatula-like shelf of acrylic extends back from the retainer portion of the appliance. This part of the appliance lifts the weak (flaccid) velum and places it in a static position of the PPW.

The advantages of the prosthetic appliances is that (1) the patient does not have to undergo surgery; (2) the appliances can be adjusted as many times as necessary to provide the optimum speech result; and (3) the prosthesis can be discarded if the final result in unsatisfactory. There also are a number of disadvantages, including (1) they require daily care for proper oral hygiene; (2) they may be difficult to retain in the mouth if velar movement is extensive; (3) they require periodic follow-up to ensure maintenance of a good fit; (4) they usually cannot be worn while eating; and (5) children may lose them. In general, surgical intervention is usually the preferred method of treatment of velopharyngeal impairment.

SUMMARY

This chapter addressed the characteristics, evaluation, and treatment of voice and resonance disorders. Voice disorders arise from changes in the structure and function of the larynx and result from a variety of causes. Abuse results in the formation of new tissue that changes the vibratory pattern and interferes with vocal fold closure. Neurological disorders may paralyze muscles of the larynx so that the vocal folds cannot be closed for phonation or fully opened for breathing. Cancer of the larynx frequently requires that the vocal folds be removed and an alternative sound source for speech be

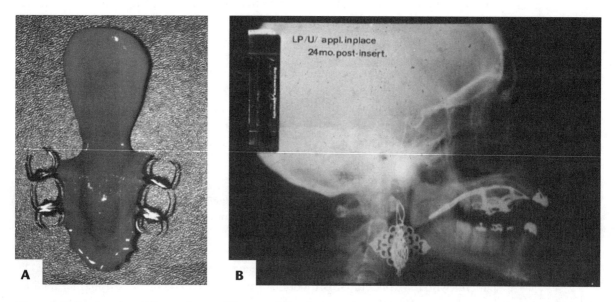

Figure 6-6 A palatal lift appliance (A) and a lateral x-ray view (B) of a patient wearing that appliance. *Source:* Photo courtesy of Dr. Rodger Dalston

developed. Psychological disorders may cause voice disorders, but there is no physical basis for the problems with phonation.

Primary perceptual characteristics of voice disorders are breathiness, harshness, and hoarseness. Perceptual analysis of these signs, direct visualization of the vocal folds by **endoscopy**, the results of a medical evaluation, and a comprehensive case history provide the information necessary to diagnosis the disorder and to develop a treatment program for voice disorders. Treatment depends on the type and severity of the disorder and requires the collaboration of the speech-language pathologist and other healthcare professionals. In cases of abuse, therapy focuses on reducing the abusive phonation pattern. Paralysis may require medical intervention to provide improved vocal fold closure. Psychologically based disorders may necessitate referral to other healthcare professionals for counseling. The ultimate goal of intervention is improved phonation for speech production.

Most voice disorders are acquired. In contrast, resonance disorders in cleft lip and palate are congenital. All consonants, with the exception of nasal consonants such as /m/ and /n/, have oral resonance, which is accomplished by actions of the velum and the pharynx. Children with cleft lip and palate often have large openings into the nose because of missing palatal bone and/or velopharyngeal insufficiency that cause varying degrees of hypernasality and nasal emission of air. These children tend to have difficulty with the production of pressure consonants (fricatives and stops). Clefts of the lip and/ or palate are treated through surgical procedures and, in some cases, the insertion of prosthetic devices. Some children require additional surgery to reduce nasality. Speech-language pathologists conduct assessments of children's speech to evaluate the functional outcomes of surgery and to determine whether there is a need for speech therapy.

BOX 6-7 Case Study of Speaker Following Laryngectomy

Mr. Jackson was a merchant marine who had worked for many years on ships that traveled to Asia. Following several months of increasing hoarseness, he was diagnosed with carcinoma of the larynx and underwent a complete laryngectomy followed by radiation treatment. Initially, he used writing and gesturing to communicate and then began therapy to develop esophageal speech. Speech development was very slow. Mr. Jackson had difficulty generating a consistent esophageal sound source and sounds were short in duration. Part of his difficulty learning esophageal speech was attributed to tissue changes in the neck associated with radiation. He tried several electrolarynges including a Western Electric neck device and a Cooper-Rand intra-oral electronic larynx. The Western Electric device was difficult for Mr. Jackson to use because the neck irritation from radiation made use of the neck device uncomfortable. He found the Cooper-Rand device, however, more acceptable because the electronic sound source is provided through a tube placed in the oral cavity. With several weeks of additional therapy, Mr. Jackson was able to communicate effectively with family, friends, and strangers. However, he was not able to return to work as a merchant marine because of the physical limitations caused by the laryngectomy.

STUDY QUESTIONS

1. What are three alternatives for producing oral speech following surgical removal of the larynx?

2. What is the difference between hypernasality and hyponasality?

3. An individual with a paralyzed vocal fold is breathy. Why?

4. What speech sounds are easiest to produce for a person with velopharyngeal inadequacy?

5. What is meant by "secondary management" of individuals with repaired cleft palate?

6. What are three characteristics of submucous cleft palate?

7. What is a primary medical treatment for spasmodic dysphonia?

8. Why do some children with repaired cleft palate produce pharyngeal fricatives?

9. How are vocal polyps different from vocal nodules?

10. How is therapy for hyperfunctional voice disorders different from therapy for hypofunctional voice disorders?

KEY TERMS

Abduction	Glottal stops	Paramedian
Aphonia	Harsh	Pharyngeal-esophageal (PE) segment
Atrophy	Hoarse	Pharyngeal flap surgery
Bifid	Hyperfunction	Pharyngeal fricatives
Bilateral	Hypernasal	Pharyngeal stops
Breathy	Hypofunction	Posterior pharyngeal wall (PPW)
Chelioplasty	Hyponasal (denasal)	Pseudoglottis
Compensatory articulations	Laryngectomee	Stoma
Diplophonia	Laryngectomy	Stroboscopy
Dysphonia	Metastasize	Superior sphincter pharyngoplasty
Dyspnea	Nasal emission	Unilateral
Edema	Nasometer	Uvula
Endoscopy	Nasopharynx	Visipitch
Esophageal speech	Neoglottis	Whisper
Extrinsic laryngeal muscles	Palatoplasty	

SUGGESTED READINGS

Brown, W. S., Vinson, B. P., & Crary, M. A. (1996). *Organic voice disorders: Assessment and treatment*. San Diego, CA: Singular.

Bzoch, K. R. (1997). *Communicative disorders related to cleft lip and palate*. Austin, TX: Pro-Ed.

Colton, R., & Casper, J. K. (1996). *Understanding voice problems: A physiological perspective for diagnosis and treatment*. Baltimore, MD: Williams & Wilkins.

Dworkin, J. P., & Meleca, R. J. (1997). *Vocal pathologies: Diagnosis, treatment and case studies*. San Diego, CA: Singular.

Moller, K. T., & Starr, C. D. (1993). *Cleft palate: Interdisciplinary issues and treatment*. Austin, TX: Pro-Ed.

Shprintzen, R. J., & Bardach, J. (1995). *Cleft palate speech management: A multidisciplinary approach*. St. Louis: Mosby.

chapter seven

Fluency Disorders

COURTNEY T. BYRD AND RONALD B. GILLAM

LEARNING OBJECTIVES

1. To identify and describe the primary behaviors of stuttering: single-syllable-word repetitions, syllable repetitions, sound repetitions, inaudible and audible sound prolongations.

2. To differentiate between primary and secondary stuttering behaviors.

3. To differentiate between stuttering-like and non-stuttering-like speech disfluencies.

4. To learn what may contribute to the onset, development, and maintenance of stuttering.

5. To learn about the characteristics of chronic stuttering.

6. To learn about the assessment procedures used in most stuttering evaluations.

7. To differentiate between the two primary types of treatment for stuttering: stuttering modification versus fluency shaping.

8. To understand how the treatment of children who are beginning to stutter differs from the treatment of adolescents and adults who are chronic stutterers.

Imagine yourself sitting in a restaurant. You overhear the man at the table next to you trying to order dinner. The man says, "I'll have, um, the, uh, spa, spa, spa (long pause) spaghetti (audible breath) and m-----meatballs." During the long pause after the third "spa," you can't help but notice that his lips are protruding and quivering. Then, when he says *meatballs*, he holds the /m/ for about a second and his eyelids flutter a little before he gets the rest of the word out. The waitress looks surprised, smiles in an awkward, uncomfortable sort of way, and hurries off. You may feel sorry for him or perhaps even embarrassed for him. You might think he looks and sounds really nervous. You may even assume that he isn't very smart. However, if this person is like many other people who stutter, you will have formed the wrong impressions. He may be a software developer, an architect, a real estate agent, or a college professor. He probably has a wife, children, and a number of close friends. It is likely that he had some speech therapy that has helped him lessen his stuttering even though he still stutters in some speaking contexts.

Imagine another scenario where you are at a family gathering with your preschool child. You ask him to tell your family what happened when he went fishing with his dad. He turns to everyone and opens his mouth as if to say the word but no sound comes out. His face becomes increasingly tense until the initial sound of the word finally bursts out so loudly that it startles your child and his listeners. You find yourself overwhelmed with fear because this is at least the fifth time he has had this type of speech breakdown in the past week. Your mother quickly tells your son to "take a deep breath and say it over again." Your child does what he is asked yet this time he seems to get stuck even worse than before. After several tries, he just looks at you and your family members in desperation and cries, "Why can't I talk?" How do you respond to this question? Why can't your child talk? Is it because of something you did?

This chapter reviews some of the more important findings about stuttering in children and adults and summarizes best practices in assessing and treating individuals who stutter. We begin with a discussion of fluency, normal disfluency, and stuttering. Then, we examine what is currently known about the development of stuttering in children and the factors that contribute to persistent stuttering in adolescents and adulthood. Finally, we look into the ways that speech-language pathologists (SLPs) assess and treat stuttering.

THE NATURE OF FLUENT SPEECH

Most children and adults speak with relatively little effort. Their speech is produced at a rate that makes it easy for listeners to perceive what they are saying, and their words flow together evenly. The term **fluency** is used to describe speech that is effortless in nature. It is easy, rhythmical, and evenly flowing.

Speakers do not speak in a perfectly fluent manner all the time. Sometimes they repeat phrases (*My paper, my paper* is right here). Sometimes they interject fillers (My paper is, *um*, right here), pause in unusual places (My [pause] paper is right here), or revise their sentences (*My paper, that paper I wrote last week*, is right here). The term **disfluency** is used to describe speech that is marked by phrase repetitions, interjections, pauses, and revisions like the ones just listed. Listen carefully to a friend during a

BOX 7-1 Overview of the CD-ROM Segments

The CD-ROM that accompanies this book contains six short video segments of an adult who stutters. The first two segments demonstrate types of stuttering. Later you will use these segments to practice identifying stuttering. The other segments depict stuttering therapy. Two segments show an approach to therapy called stuttering modification, and two segments demonstrate an approach to therapy called fluency shaping. You should watch all the segments before you read the remainder of this chapter. That way, you will have an idea about what stuttering looks like and how it can be changed.

Segments

Ch.7.01. The individual is talking to a speech-language pathologist about one of his early speech therapy experiences. He is not employing any strategies to reduce or modify his stuttering.

Ch.7.02. The individual reads a short passage from an article without using any strategies to reduce or modify his stuttering.

Ch.7.03. The speech-language pathologist teaches the stutterer to "cancel" moments of stuttering. This is part of a technique called speech modification.

Ch.7.04. The stutterer practices a speech modification strategy called pull-outs. This technique is also one of several intervention strategies that are referred to as speech modification approaches.

Ch.7.05. The speech-language pathologist teaches the individual how to use a fluency shaping strategy that involves letting out a short breath before saying the first sound, slowing down the rate of speech, and saying sounds gently.

Ch.7.06. The stutterer practices fluency shaping controls while reading a short passage about stuttering.

phone conversation or to your professors as they lecture. You might be surprised at the number of disfluencies you hear. It is normal for speakers to produce speech disfluencies some of the time.

Some individuals have an unusual number of speech disfluencies or produce types of speech disfluencies that differ from the ones previously listed. The disfluencies that commonly occur in the speech of people who stutter but rarely occur in the speech of people who do not stutter include repetition of single-syllable words (*My, my* paper is right here), syllable repetitions (My *pa-pa*per is right here), or sound repetitions (*M, m, m*y paper is right here). They may also prolong some sounds a little longer than usual (*M---y* paper is right here) and this prolongation may be audible or inaudible. An inaudible sound prolongation where the mouth is in position for the sound for an extended period of time but no sound is coming out is also commonly referred to as a block. These speech disfluencies produced by people who stutter interfere with their ability to communicate effectively and may cause the speakers to have negative emotional reactions to their own speech. These individuals have a condition called **stuttering**, which is the most common form of fluency impairment.

Stuttering is not the only type of fluency disorder. Some individuals speak disfluently as a result of psychological trauma, neurological disease, or brain injury. This type of stuttering is referred to as **acquired (or neurogenic) stuttering**, and it typically has a sudden onset in adulthood. Table 7-1 compares and contrasts acquired versus developmental stuttering. Other individuals have a condition called **cluttering**, which is characterized by very rapid bursts of dysrhythmic, unintelligible speech.

WHAT IS STUTTERING?

Table 7-2 lists the basic facts of stuttering. Guitar (2005) has proposed a three-part definition of stuttering. First, stuttering is characterized by an unusually high frequency or duration of repetitions, prolongations, and/or blockages (tense moments when voicing

Table 7-1 Developmental versus Acquired Stuttering

Developmental Stuttering	Acquired Stuttering
Accounts for vast majority of stuttering cases.	Accounts for small percentage of stuttering cases.
Onset is typically before 7 years of age.	Onset is typically in later life.
Onset is usually gradual.	Onset is usually sudden.
No known psychological and/or physical trauma.	Related to some psychological or physical trauma.

Table 7-2 Basic Facts of Stuttering

- About 1% of school-age population stutters.
- Five percent of the population report that they have stuttered for a period of 6 months or more at some point in their lives.
- On average, 3 boys for 1 girl stutter.
- For 50% or more of people who stutter, some other family member also stutters.
- Ninety percent have begun to stutter by 7 years of age.
- For about 70%, onset of stuttering is gradual.
- Speech at stuttering onset typically includes physically non-tense repetitions of sounds and syllables, but can include physically tense sound prolongations and/or blocks.
- At least 50% of children who stutter exhibit improvement in speech without treatment (i.e., spontaneous recovery).

and/or the flow of air is interrupted) that interrupt the flow of speech. Second, these interruptions are often combined with excessive mental and physical effort to resume talking. People who stutter sometimes report that they lose their train of thought when they concentrate too much on ways to avoid stuttering, and they often tighten their speech musculature and push harder to escape from moments of stuttering. Ironically, avoidance and escape behaviors that are meant to decrease speech disfluencies often have the opposite effect; they actually increase speech disfluencies. Third, some young children, many older children, and most adults who stutter have negative perceptions of their communication abilities because of their inability to say what they want to say when they want to say it. Worse, some people who stutter develop unusually low self-esteem because they internalize the negative reactions of others.

Primary Stuttering Behaviors

There are primary and secondary stuttering behaviors. The **primary stuttering behaviors**, sometimes referred to as "core behaviors," are the stuttering-like speech disfluencies that were mentioned earlier (i.e., repetitions, prolongations, and blocks). It is not unusual for normal speakers to repeat phrases or whole words, to interject fillers like *uh* and *um*, or to pause to collect their thoughts before continuing. People who stutter tend to have somewhat different kinds of speech disfluencies. They may produce three or four rapid repetitions of sounds at the beginning of words or even within words (*baseb,b,b,ball*). They may also produce **prolongations** in which they hold out or prolong a sound for an unusually long period of time. Say the word *van*, but keep saying just the /v/ out loud for 2 or 3 seconds before you move into the "-an." That's a prolongation.

There is another type of speech disfluency, commonly called an inaudible sound prolongation or a block, that rarely is heard in the speech of people who do not stutter. Blocks are silent prolongations. People who stutter sometimes feel like they become stuck as they are producing sounds. When this happens, they hold the articulators in place to say the sound, but the articulators are so tense that they do not allow any sound to come out for an unusually long time (1 or 2 seconds). Imagine you are going to say the word *car*. Put the back of your tongue up against the posterior part of your hard palate and hold it there tightly. At the same time, push with your diaphragm so that your breath is trying to get out. It can't because your tongue is "blocking" the air from being released. Keep pushing your breath against your tongue for a few seconds, and then release the tongue so that you say the word *car* with a hard /k/. The breath should tumble out all at once, and the word should be pronounced a little louder than usual. That is what it feels like to have a controlled (voluntary) block. Imagine how frustrating it might be if that often happened when you did not want it to.

Secondary Stuttering Behaviors

Secondary stuttering behaviors are counterproductive adaptations that people who stutter make as they try to get through primary stuttering behaviors or to avoid them altogether. There are many different kinds of secondary stuttering behaviors. We have seen people who stutter blink their eyes, open their jaws, purse their lips, change words, insert *uh* right before a word that they anticipate stuttering on, flap their arms, and even stamp the floor with their feet. Unfortunately, as these compensations become more and more automatic, they also become less and less successful ways to escape or avoid stuttering. Soon, the secondary behaviors are as distracting, or in some cases even more distracting to the listener, than the primary stuttering behaviors.

Incidence and Prevalence of Stuttering

How common is stuttering? There are two ways to answer this question. You could consider the percentage of individuals who stutter at any given point in time. This percentage is referred to as the prevalence of stuttering. You might also want to consider the percentage of the population that has stuttered at any point during their lives. This percentage is called the incidence of stuttering. Bloodstein and Bernstein Ratner (2008) provide an extensive review of the literature and report that approximately 1% of the population stutter at the present moment (the prevalence of stuttering), and that approximately 5% of the population report that they have stuttered for a period of 6 months or more at some point in their lives (the incidence of stuttering). If you could round up all these people, you would probably find that most of them are males. Across all ages of stutterers, there are approximately three male persons who stutter to every female person who stutters.

INDIVIDUALS WHO STUTTER

Individual Variability

Not all individuals stutter in the same manner or with the same frequency. People with mild stuttering have fleeting speech disfluencies, and these may occur only in the most stressful of speaking contexts. Typically, the duration for such disfluencies averages less than 3 seconds, but in some cases an instance of speech disfluency can last much longer. In addition, these disfluencies may occur in 20% or more of the words that are spoken. Most individuals who stutter fall between those extremes, and the severity of their stuttering may change somewhat over time. For example, some people who stutter report they experience periods of time when they are relatively fluent and other periods when they are disfluent. These peaks and valleys of fluency and stuttering tend to be one of the most frustrating aspects of this disorder.

Despite the considerable degree of individual variation between and within people who stutter, some generalizations apply to many individuals who stutter. For those

---

BOX 7-2 Identify Primary and Secondary Stuttering Behaviors

Watch CD-ROM segments Ch.7.01 and Ch.7.02 again. Look for repetitions, prolongations, and blocks. Are there instances of stuttering in which the individual combined repetitions and blocks? What secondary behaviors can you identify?

individuals who are cognitively aware of their stuttering, their speech disfluency tends to be worse when they put the most pressure on themselves to be fluent. However, for young children who stutter, it is difficult to determine whether the pressure to be fluent exists and, if indeed it does exist, whether the pressure is internally or externally driven. Nevertheless, for both children and adults stuttering tends to more commonly occur during productions that include critical content that must be communicated in one or two words (saying one's name, ordering in a restaurant), when speaking in long and complex utterances, when speaking to authority figures (e.g., professors, parents, bosses), or when something needs to be said in a hurry.

An interesting phenomenon of stuttering is that certain types of speaking tend to induce fluency. Most people who stutter are notably fluent when they sing, when they use pretend voices, when they are engaged in choral reading (as often happens during church services), or when they talk to babies or animals. There are at least a few possible explanations for this marked difference in fluency in these speaking situations. First, there is an apparent lack of bidirectionality. Bidirectional communication refers to spoken communication that goes back and forth between the speaker and listener. How many animals talk back? How many babies are able to carry on a conversation? Another explanation is propositionality. None of these situations require the speaker to convey critical new or meaningful information to a listener. Also, in singing and choral reading, speech is not only slow, but the syllables tend to be linked together more smoothly. As we discuss in more detail later, some therapy approaches are based on the fact that slower rate and smooth transitions between syllables and words induce fluency in most stutterers. Thus, another explanation could be the reduced complexity in motor planning and execution across these tasks. Given the diversity of explanations for where and when stuttering is least likely to occur, it should not surprise you that there is also diversity in the theories related to the onset and development of stuttering. We address this issue in further detail later when we discuss the cause of stuttering.

Differences Between Individuals Who Do and Do Not Stutter

In a number of areas, apart from fluency, people who stutter differ from people who do not stutter. Individuals who stutter tend to have more negative concepts of themselves as speakers, and they have higher levels of concern about their speech. This difference in communication self-concepts seems reasonable because there have been many instances in which people who stutter knew what they wanted to say, but they could not say it in the fluent manner that they would have liked. In addition, some listeners form negative impressions about people who stutter. It is no wonder people who stutter might feel less confident about their communication skills, and this ultimately might affect their self-concept in general.

There are also subtle differences in the language abilities of people who do and do not stutter. Language involves formulating what is going to be said and organizing the words and sentences that are needed to express one's thoughts. These functions are dynamically related to speech, which involves planning, initiating, and executing the motor movements that produce words and sentences. Difficulties formulating messages and organizing the words and sentences that best express those messages could affect speech production. For example, one might expect greater frequency of stuttering on words within long, grammatically complex sentences than on words within short, grammatically simple sentences. This is especially true for children who are in the process of learning language (Logan & Conture, 1995). In addition, adults who stutter are more likely to stutter on complex words that express the main idea or that are critical to the communication context. Clearly, stuttering tends to increase in relation to the complexity and importance of the information that is being expressed.

Results from some studies further suggest that differences in the motor systems of people who stutter interfere with their ability to react rapidly. Rapid motor responses are tested by presenting a cue (a visual picture or an auditory sound) and asking individuals to respond as quickly as they can by saying a word, producing a vowel sound, closing their lips, or just tapping a finger. In all of these response conditions, people who stutter tend to have slower response times than people who do not stutter. Studies of speech samples reveal similar findings. Even when they are not stuttering, individuals who stutter sometimes have slower voice onset times (the time between the release of a consonant at the beginning of the vowel as in the syllable / pa/), longer vowel durations, and slower transitions from one sound to the next. The implications of these findings are that people who stutter have less efficient motor systems, and these differences may contribute to the development and/or the continuation of stuttering.

Finally, people who stutter appear to use their brains a little differently during speech production. Recall from Chapter 4, Speech Science, that the left hemisphere is usually dominant for speech and language functions. Individuals who stutter present more right hemisphere activity during speech than do people who do not stutter. For example, Fox and his colleagues (1996) compared positron emission tomography scans of people who do and do not stutter. People who stutter presented greater activation of speech motor and language-processing areas in the right hemisphere, more activation in the cerebellum (which is responsible for coordination and smooth muscle actions), and less activation in the left hemisphere language-processing areas than did people who do not stutter. They also found that the individuals who stutter demonstrated more left hemisphere activation during their fluent speech than they did during stuttered speech. Recent research lends additional support to this hemispheric difference during language-based tasks that do not require speech production. Results like these suggest that people who stutter may be using the right hemisphere for functions that are better handled by the left hemisphere. The participants in these studies were adults who stutter. With more research, we hope to learn more about the potential similarities or, perhaps, differences in the brain functions of children who stutter.

Taken together, these results suggest that stuttering is related to emotional, conceptual, linguistic, and motor performance. Given the rapid advances that are occurring in brain imaging technology, it is likely that important discoveries about the systems and processes underlying stuttering will be made in the near future.

THE CAUSE OF STUTTERING

Research has yet to reveal the exact cause of stuttering. Over the years, many theories have been advanced to explain stuttering. Some theories that seemed to be reasonable explanations of stuttering at one time have been shown to be false. Table 7-3 lists the common myths about stuttering. We discuss two of these myths about the cause of stuttering, and then summarize current thinking about the reasons why people stutter.

Myth: Stuttering Is a Nervous Reaction

Many people assume wrongly that stuttering results from excessive nervousness. We have heard parents and well-meaning friends say things like, "Just relax, there's nothing to be nervous about" when someone is disfluent. Unfortunately, these are not helpful comments. Many studies have shown that, in general, individuals who stutter are not more anxious than are individuals who do not stutter. Nervous disorders and other psychiatric disabilities are not more common in people who stutter than they are in the general population. Finally, relaxation-based therapies have not been particularly helpful for stutterers. For example, people who stutter may stutter even though they are completely relaxed. The results of these studies suggest that people who stutter are not generally more anxious or nervous than people who do not stutter. However, nobody doubts that increased levels of anxiety may lead to increased speech disfluencies in individuals who stutter. The key point, however, is that stuttering is not the result of a nervous condition.

Myth: Stuttering Is Caused by Overly Sensitive Parents

In the 1940s, an influential researcher named Wendell Johnson developed the Diagnosogenic Theory, which purported that stuttering was caused by parents who were unnecessarily concerned about normal speech disfluencies their children produced. These parents were thought to have diagnosed their children as stutterers, this diagnosis was conveyed to the child, and the child then became concerned about these

Table 7-3 Common Myths of Stuttering

- People who stutter are more introverted than people who do not stutter.
- People who stutter are more anxious and nervous than people who do not stutter.
- Parents of children who stutter are more anxious and sensitive than parents of children who do not stutter.
- People who stutter have lower intelligence than people who do not stutter.
- People who stutter have less self-confidence than people who do not stutter.
- People who stutter are more deceitful than people who do not stutter.
- People who stutter are more sensitive than people who do not stutter.

behaviors (the speech disfluencies) and tried to avoid them. This theory, in particular, was the intellectual springboard for many studies of the parents and families of children who stutter. Some of the more consistent results relating to similarities and differences between the families of stuttering and nonstuttering children are summarized in Table 7-4. Most researchers and clinicians agree that parent reactions do not cause stuttering, although parents' behaviors may exacerbate stuttering and/or facilitate fluency in young children who stutter.

Current Thinking About the Etiology of Stuttering

Current models of stuttering depict the disorder as arising from complex dynamic relationships between internal (neurological and cognitive) factors and external conditions. The internal factors include inherited traits, temperament, cognitive abilities, language abilities, information processing mechanisms (attention, perception, memory, and reasoning), and speech motor control. The external conditions include culture, parental expectations, childrearing practices, educational experiences, and relationships with siblings and peers. It is important to understand that the sets of factors that may prompt the onset and development of stuttering in one person are not necessarily the same factors that prompt stuttering in someone else.

THE DEVELOPMENT OF STUTTERING

This section provides more information about the kinds of factors that may influence the development of stuttering. Please keep in mind as you read this section that the data to support theoretical assumptions about the etiology of stuttering are limited and that, currently, the etiology of stuttering remains unknown.

Early Stuttering

Recall that normal speech is not completely fluent. Given the difficult motor patterns that must be refined during speech development, it should not be surprising that the

Table 7-4 Similarities and Differences Between Families of Stuttering and Nonstuttering Children

Similarities	Differences
Socioeconomic status and number of siblings	Children who stutter are more likely to grow up in less harmonious, less sociable, and less close families.
Parent personalities and emotional adjustment	Parents of children who stutter are more anxious about their children's speech development.
Parent's general attitudes about childrearing	Parents of children who stutter are more likely to be overprotective.
Parent's speech style and rate of speech	Parents of children who stutter sometimes criticize their children's disfluent speech.

speech of preschool-age children is often marked by phrase repetitions, interjections, revisions, and pauses. These disfluencies can occur in as many as 10% of the words that children speak. For the majority of children, the amount of disfluency declines over time. Unfortunately, some children's speech disfluencies increase in frequency and their speech contains more sound repetitions, prolongations, and blocks. These types of disfluencies are commonly referred to as stuttering-like disfluencies, and most children who stutter present three or more of these per 100 words (Conture, 2001). This proportion of stuttering-like disfluencies rarely occurs in the speech of children who do not stutter. In addition, some children who stutter may evidence feelings of frustration about their speech and may also begin to develop secondary stuttering behaviors. Behaviors that indicate the beginning of stuttering are listed in Table 7-5.

For some children stuttering seems to evolve over time before they or their listeners notice it. Other children's stuttering seems to be noticed within the first day of onset. Some parents have reported that their child's stuttering developed within a day or two. Occasionally, parents report that their child was relatively fluent one day and exhibited many stuttering-like behaviors the next.

Genetic Influences

Could stuttering be a trait that is inherited? In a review of genetic studies of stuttering, Felsenfeld (1997) concluded that approximately 15% of the first-degree relatives (fathers, mothers, sisters, brothers, sons, daughters) of people who stutter were current or recovered stutterers themselves. That means that the likelihood of stuttering is three times greater for a person who has a first-degree family member who stutters. Because relatives of people who stutter are generally at greater risk for stuttering than relatives of people who do not stutter, it is likely that some aspect of the disorder, perhaps

Table 7-5 Indicators of Early Stuttering in Children

- An average of three or more sound repetitions, prolongations, or blocks per 100 words.
- An average of three or more stuttering-like disfluencies (i.e., single-syllable-word repetitions, syllable repetitions, sound repetitions, prolongations, or blocks) per 100 words.
- Seventy-two percent or more stuttering-like disfluencies per total disfluencies.
- Twenty-five percent or more of the total disfluencies are prolongations or blocks.
- Instances in which repetitions, prolongations, or blocks occur in adjacent sounds or syllables within a word.
- Increases in the rate and irregularity of repetitions.
- Signs of excess tension or struggle during moments of disfluency.
- Secondary behaviors such as eye blinks, facial tics, or interjections immediately before or during disfluencies.
- Feelings of frustration about disfluencies.

something like a predisposition for stuttering, may be inherited. Researchers have yet to discover a gene that carries stuttering, and studies of stuttering in families have not revealed a clear line of genetic transmission. Other developmental and environmental factors must interact with a predisposition for stuttering for the disorder to develop.

Environmental Demands and the Capacity for Fluency

There are many theories to describe the etiology of stuttering; however, we do not have evidence to support any one theory. Nevertheless, some theories are more frequently used to describe stuttering than others are, with the Demands and Capacity Model (DCM) perhaps being the most frequent. Starkweather (1987) has suggested that disfluencies are likely to occur in children's speech when there is an imbalance between the demands for fluency and the child's capacity to produce fluent speech. Four interrelated mechanisms contribute to the capacity for fluency: neural development that supports sensory-motor coordination, language development, conceptual development, and emotional development.

Recall from Chapter 4 that the brain is composed of millions of interconnected neurons. As brain cells proliferate and differentiate, they create neural networks, some of which support motor coordination. In a process known as **neural plasticity**, neural circuits organize and reorganize themselves in response to interactions with the environment. But the environment is not all that matters for brain organization. Inheritance probably plays an important role in the rate of development and the patterns of neural development that occur. Slowed neurological development and/or less efficient patterns of neural activation could result in a diminished capacity for producing fluent speech. When this reduced capacity is combined with the child's perception of excessive environmental demands, disfluency is the likely result. For example, if two parents are in a hurry to go somewhere at the same moment their child is trying to tell them something, the child might feel undue pressure to talk faster than his motor speech capabilities will allow. This disparity between the child's desire to talk faster to meet his parents' needs (who are in a hurry at that moment) and his ability to talk fast may be likely to result in disfluent speech.

Children tend to be disfluent when they are not sure what to say or when they must expend a great deal of mental energy to solve a conceptual problem. For example, a child may want to tell her parents about a recent experience. To do so, she needs to weave together a series of sentences that represent the multiple events that were involved and the sequence in which they occurred. The demands inherent in formulating and organizing the story might exceed the child's linguistic and conceptual capacities to do so. This creates a situation in which speech disfluency is quite likely.

Emotional constancy also contributes to speech fluency and disfluency. Some children are inherently more sensitive than others, and some children are more likely than others to be disfluent in response to emotional stress. Imagine a child with a sensitive temperament who spilled ice cream in the living room, even though he knew there was a household rule not to take food out of the kitchen. A parent might ask this child to explain why he took food into the living room when he knew he was not supposed to. The child who stutters, sensing that his parent is displeased, might not be able to produce fluent speech under this emotional circumstance.

The demand–capacities explanation of the development of stuttering accounts for the fact that some children who are raised in relatively high-demand environments do not stutter, whereas other children who are raised in what appear to be less demanding environments might. The nature of the environment is not the critical factor in and of itself. What matters most for the development of stuttering is the balance between children's perception of the demands that are present in their environment and their motoric, linguistic, cognitive, and emotional resources for meeting the demands they place on themselves. Even in an environment that most people would consider to be relatively undemanding, increased disfluencies would be expected to occur in children who have extreme motoric, cognitive, linguistic, and/or emotional restrictions on their ability to produce fluent speech. All this being said, it is important to remind you that this is still speculation because the cause (or perhaps causes) of stuttering has yet to be discovered.

The Influence of Learning

Recall that children's brains are relatively plastic, meaning that experiences excite individual neurons and influence connections between networks of neurons. For some children, demand and capacity imbalances that contribute to increased disfluency may occur in many circumstances with many different listeners. When multiple experiences occur over time, as might happen during repeated instances of speech disfluency, new neural groups that are related to speech disfluency may form, grow, and strengthen.

In some instances, children's speech disfluencies may be more physically tense than they are in other instances. Children remember many aspects of their experiences, especially the ones that are distinct in some way. Children would be likely to recall instances when a speech disfluency was particularly tense or when they had an increased emotional reaction to a disfluency. Brains are good at spotting similarities across situations. Over a relatively short period of time, children may be likely to recognize subtle similarities in speaking contexts that induced more emotion or more tense disfluencies. Recognizing these similarities could prompt children to anticipate difficulties in speaking contexts that share common characteristics. This kind of anticipation is likely to heighten muscle tension, which then increases the likelihood of tense disfluencies and struggle. In this way, disfluency and struggle in a few situations may potentially lead to a pattern of disfluency and struggle in many situations.

Consider the earlier example of a child who wanted to tell her parents about an experience she had. Her story was disfluent, partially because the linguistic and cognitive requirements of storytelling were too demanding given the child's level of development. If this happened a few times, the child might begin to associate storytelling with disfluency. This association contributes to anticipation, which leads to heightened levels of neurological activity and increased muscle tension, which increases the likelihood of tense disfluencies. It is not long before tense speech disfluencies and negative emotional reactions become associated with storytelling in many contexts. Our brains work so efficiently that patterns of behavior, even undesirable patterns such as stuttering, can strengthen and stabilize rather quickly.

FACTORS THAT CONTRIBUTE TO CHRONIC STUTTERING

Fortunately, stuttering resolves in 60–80% of the individuals who stutter during childhood. The resolution of stuttering often occurs before adolescence. The resolution of stuttering is probably related to growth spurts in developmental domains such as speech motor control, language, cognition, and temperament. Rapid developments in these domains could increase the capacity for fluency, thereby leading to a sudden reduction in stuttering. Such growth spurts can shift demands and capacities for fluency into greater balance. This new balance results in greater fluency, which begins to break down neurological and behavioral patterns of speech disfluency.

Unfortunately, many children continue to stutter into adolescence and adulthood. The term **chronic stuttering** is often used to refer to these individuals. The following section summarizes some of the factors that contribute to chronic stuttering.

Contributing Factor: Negative Feelings and Attitudes

People who stutter often report that they are frustrated and embarrassed by their inability to say what they want to say in the way they want to say it. Adolescents and adults often feel their stuttering is out of their own control; it is something that happens to them rather than something that they do. Some people who stutter may also feel self-conscious about their speech. They may have been teased by classmates as children or laughed at as they struggled to get a word out. People sometimes avoid the person who stutters because they have negative preconceptions of people who stutter as being less intelligent or excessively nervous. They may be unsure about how to respond when the person is disfluent. They may wonder whether they should look away or finish the word for the stutterer. Unfortunately, avoiding talking to people who stutter, looking away when they stutter, and finishing their stuttered words contribute to feelings of shame and embarrassment about stuttering that people who stutter experience. Table 7-6 offers general guidelines for the listener when talking with a person who stutters.

Table 7-6   How to Interact With a Person Who Stutters

- Maintain reasonable eye contact.
- Do not finish his or her words, sentences.
- Do not interrupt.
- Pay attention to what the person is saying, not how he or she is saying it.
- Pause at least 1 second prior to responding.
- Do not allow common stereotypes to override your opinion of the person who stutters.

Above all, it is important for listeners to pay attention to what is being said, not how it is being said. Listeners should be careful not to finish the sounds, words, and sentences of the person who stutters even if they are certain they know what the person is struggling to say. In the end, the best help listeners can provide to the person who stutters is to let him or her know that they have the patience to wait and the desire to hear the words of the person who stutters as that person says them, not as the listener predicts they will be said.

Contributing Factor: Avoidance

Individuals who stutter sometimes avoid stuttering by changing the words they plan to say as they talk. A person who stutters that we knew believed that he tended to stutter more on words that contained the voiceless -*th* sound, so he decided to change his productions to avoid saying words that included that sound. For example, when making arrangements for a date, he told his friend, "I'll pick you up at six, uh, make that half past six." This word change was a way to avoid saying the /th/ sound in the phrase *six-thirty*.

Another way people who stutter keep from stuttering is to avoid speaking situations in which they believe they will stutter. Some people who stutter simply refuse to answer the telephone, introduce themselves, ask questions, or speak in front of groups of people. Unfortunately, avoidance of any type adds to feelings that stuttering is controlling the individual rather than the other way around. In therapy, it is difficult to make changes in the speech pattern of someone who consistently avoids talking. As we discuss later, an important aspect of therapy involves getting the person who stutters to deal constructively with his fear of stuttering by facing his stuttering head-on.

Contributing Factor: Difficulties With Speech Motor Control

Some people who stutter evidence unusual patterns of breathing, vocalizing, and speaking even when they are not stuttering. They may tense the muscles in their chest, neck, larynx, jaw, and/or face before they start to talk, and they may maintain excess tension in these areas while they are speaking. Some individuals who stutter have inadequate breath support for speech because they inhale too little air or exhale too much air before speaking. There are reports of people who stutter whose rate of speech is very uneven. They speed up excessively when they think they are going to be fluent and slow down excessively when they anticipate stuttering. Overly tense musculature, breathing that is too shallow or too deep, and uneven rates of speech create a system that is conducive to stuttering.

Contributing Factor: Difficulties With Language Formulation

Although motoric aspects (e.g., speech motor control of articulation, phonation, and respiration) of stuttering have received considerable attention over the past 20 years, recent research indicates that linguistic variables such as phonology, semantics, and syntax may also contribute to childhood stuttering. For example, children whose stuttering persists exhibit poorer scores on measures of phonology than children who recover from stuttering. People who stutter are also reportedly slower than people who do not stutter at tasks related to word retrieval. In addition, people who stutter exhibit increased stuttering with increased grammatical length and complexity. Furthermore, Arndt and Healey (2001) found that half of 467 children who stutter that they tested presented with some type of concomitant disorder, with 32% presenting with phonological disorders, 35% presenting with language disorders, and 33% presenting with both phonological and language disorders.

The next section concerns the clinical management of stuttering. We begin by examining methods that are commonly used to assess stuttering. Then, we discuss the two principal approaches to treating stuttering, known as speech modification and fluency shaping, and the ways these approaches are applied to beginning stutterers and chronic stutterers.

ASSESSMENT OF STUTTERING

Evaluations of individuals who are excessively disfluent are designed to determine whether the person is a stutterer, to describe the patterns of disfluency that are exhibited, and to determine what therapy procedures to use. It is critical for clinicians to remember that their primary concern is to serve the needs of the client. Clinicians should always ask individuals and/or their family members what they want to learn from the evaluation. Then, clinicians should do their best to collect the information necessary to respond to the individual's and his or her family's concerns.

Cultural Considerations

It is more and more common for clinicians to assess and treat clients and families who are members of ethnic and cultural groups that differ from their own. When this occurs, clinicians need to be sensitive to cultural issues that can affect childrearing practices, conceptions about disabilities, and interaction patterns. Clinicians will want to find out as much as possible about the cultural values and norms that affect communication. Clinicians should never assume that the communication traditions and patterns from one culture are more *correct* than those from another culture. Careful observation and family interviews are necessary for all evaluations. These assessment strategies are especially critical when the clinician is conducting an assessment of a child or an adult from a different cultural group.

Language Considerations

Although more research is needed, the general consensus is that if you present with developmental stuttering, you will stutter in both your native language and your second language (see Van Borsel, Maes, & Foulon, 2001, for a review). The amount and types of stuttering may vary across these languages and, thus, assessment as well as treatment should allow for adequate evaluation of stuttering across languages as well as adequate practice of fluency-facilitating techniques in each language.

Assessment Procedures and the Information They Yield

We have characterized stuttering as a dynamic interaction between internal processes and environmental conditions. Table 7-7 lists the procedures that are typically used to evaluate the internal and external factors that may contribute to stuttering.

Interviews and Case History

Evaluations should begin with a thorough case history. When assessing children, clinicians collect most of the history information from parents. When assessing adults, clinicians collect history information from the client. The clinician should always ask questions about other family members who stutter, changes in the rate and nature of disfluency over time, and perceptions about the person's fluency at the time of the evaluation. It is also a good idea for clinicians to interview family members and teachers of preschool- and school-age children about their perceptions of the individual's speech and their reactions to speech disfluencies. The case history should reveal information about environmental conditions, reactions to speech disfluency, the consistency of speech disfluency behaviors across situations, and changes in disfluencies over time.

Table 7-7 Assessment Procedures That Provide Information About Factors That Contribute to the Development and/or Continuation of Stuttering

Factor	Assessment Procedure
Internal Processes	
Genetic influences	Case history, family interview
Language ability	Language testing, language sample analysis
Temperament	Interviews, questionnaires, and observations
Cognitive ability	Screening and/or observation
Attitudes	Questionnaires
Avoidance	Speech sample
Speech motor control	Speech sample
External Conditions	
Culture	Interviews and observations
Parental attitudes and child-rearing practices	Parent interviews
Family interactions	Family interviews, observations
Educational experiences	Teacher interviews

Speech Samples

Stuttering evaluations should include the collection and analysis of speech samples from a variety of speaking contexts including dialogue, monologue, and oral reading. Some clinicians use a commercially available test for collecting and analyzing speech samples called the Stuttering Severity Instrument-3 (Riley, 1994), which is often abbreviated as the SSI-3. To administer the SSI-3 examiners obtain speech samples in reading and conversation contexts. Reading passages are provided, and the conversation sample is obtained while the patient and the examiner converse about familiar topics such as school, jobs, recent holidays, favorite TV shows, or current movies. The SSI-3 can be used to make judgments of stuttering severity. We use it to augment information we obtain from patient interviews, speech samples, and other speech and language tests.

Measures of Stuttering

At minimum, clinicians measure the frequency of certain types of stuttering. To do this, we select a 10- to 15-minute segment of conversation that seems to be representative of the individual's fluency and disfluency. We transcribe (write out) what the individual says, using conventional spelling, until we have at least a 100-word sample. From this 100-or-greater-word sample, we need to calculate the following: (1) percentage of total disfluencies/total words; (2) percentage of stuttering-like disfluencies/total words; (3) percentage of stuttering-like disfluencies/total disfluencies. Table 7-5 indicates the percentages associated with these formulas that are indicative of stuttering. To measure the percentage of total disfluencies per total words, we count the number of words that would have been spoken if there were no disfluencies. Then, we count the number of words that contained **non-stuttering-like disfluencies** (phrase repetitions, revisions, and interjections) and **stuttering-like disfluencies** (single-syllable-word, sound, and syllable repetitions; prolongations; and blocks). The percentage of total disfluencies is simply the total number of words containing non-stuttering-like and stuttering-like disfluencies divided by the total number of words. This calculation yields a proportion. To convert the proportion to a percentage, simply multiply the proportion by 100. For example, in a sample with 400 total words, we counted 46 words that contained non-stuttering-like and stuttering-like disfluencies. Dividing 46 by 400 and then multiplying by 100, the percentage of total disfluencies per total words, was 11.5. To calculate the percentage of stuttering-like disfluencies per total words you complete the same steps with the exception that only the stuttering-like disfluencies are counted. For example, in that same 400-word sample, 34 of the words contained stuttering-like disfluencies. Dividing 34 by 400 and then multiplying by 100, the percentage of stuttering-like disfluencies was 8.5. Note that both of these values are higher (worse) than the frequency of disfluencies noted in stuttering (Table 7-5). This doesn't mean that the individual who was assessed is definitely a stutterer. The correct interpretation of these data is that the individual presents with indicators of stuttering-like behavior. In addition to the total disfluencies and total stuttering-like disfluencies per total words, we also need to determine how many of the disfluencies produced were stuttering-like in nature.

Thus, we need to calculate the percentage of stuttering-like disfluencies per total disfluencies. In that same 400-word sample, 34 of the 46 disfluencies were stuttering-like. Dividing 34 by 46 and then multiplying by 100, the percentage of stuttering-like disfluencies per total disfluencies is 74.

We also describe the kinds of disfluencies that are present. Table 7-8 can be used for this purpose. We make a tic mark in the number box corresponding to each type of disfluency we observe. Then, we total the number of disfluencies. To calculate the percentage of each disfluency type, simply divide the number of disfluencies of each type by the total number of disfluencies and multiply that proportion by 100. This enables the evaluator to determine the relative percentage of types of disfluencies. Recall that prolongations and blocks often comprise 25% or more of the total disfluencies of children and adults who stutter.

Additional measurements that should be completed include the average number of times the stuttered moment is repeated (i.e., iterations), the average duration of the stuttered moments, and the types as well as percentage of stuttering moments that are accompanied by secondary behaviors. Iterations obviously apply only to sound, syllable, and monosyllabic whole-word repetitions. To calculate the average number of iterations, the clinician examines each moment of stuttering, counts how many times that moment was repeated (e.g., *sh-sh-sh-shopping* = 3 iterations), and then averages those numbers. To determine the average duration of the stuttered moment, the clinician can use a stopwatch and simply time how long each individual moment lasts,

Table 7-8 Types of Speech Disfluencies

Description	Number	Percentage
Typical (Non-stuttering-like) Disfluencies		
Phrase repetitions		
Revision		
Interjections		
Subtotal		
Atypical (Stuttering-like) Disfluencies		
Single-syllable-word repetitions		
Syllable repetitions		
Sound repetitions		
Prolongations		
Blocks		
Subtotal		
TOTAL		

and then calculate the average. Finally, to complete a thorough analysis of the secondary behaviors, the clinician should first describe any nonspeech (e.g., eye blinks; jaw, lip, and neck tension) or speech behaviors (e.g., pitch rises) that co-occur with the moment of stuttering. The SLP should then calculate how many moments of stuttering are accompanied by a secondary behavior, divide that by the total number of disfluent moments, and multiply by 100. This calculation provides the percentage of stuttering moments that are accompanied by secondary behaviors.

Consistency and Adaptation

Some clinicians ask individuals who stutter to read a short passage over and over again. People who stutter tend to stutter on the same words from the first reading of a passage to the second reading of the same passage. This is known as **consistency**. For example, across these two repeated readings of the same material, people who stutter will likely stutter on the same words over and over. It is not unusual to find that at least 60% of the words that were stuttered in the second reading were also stuttered in the first reading.

In addition, as people who stutter read the same passage over and over (beyond two times), they also tend to stutter less on successive readings. This effect is called **adaptation**. There is often the greatest reduction after the first two times a passage is repeated, after which the percentage of adaptation gradually decreases. By the fifth reading most of the reduction in disfluencies has occurred.

Screening

As with every evaluation, the clinician needs to ensure that hearing sensitivity is within normal limits and that the structure and function of the oral mechanism are adequate to support speech. This means that, at minimum, the client should receive a hearing screening and an oral mechanism screening. We also make informal judgments about the individual's voice quality.

Speech and Language Testing

Speech and language difficulties may contribute to the onset and/or exacerbate stuttering in children and adults; thus the speech and language skills of people who stutter

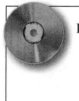

BOX 7-3 Frequency and Types of Disfluencies

Watch CD-ROM segments Ch.7.01 and Ch.7.02 again. This time, use Table 7-8 to calculate the frequency of disfluencies. Does this stutter present more or less than three within-word disfluencies per 100 words? Also, calculate the percentage of each type of disfluency. Are 25% or more of the moments of stuttering prolongations or blocks?

need to be formally assessed. The tests typically used assess receptive and expressive vocabulary, receptive and expressive language skills, and articulation abilities.

Feelings and Attitudes

We mentioned earlier that negative feelings and attitudes about communication contribute to the continuation of stuttering and can interfere with success in therapy. Clinicians can administer a number of scales to assess attitudes and feelings related to stuttering. Many of these scales are available in the books that appear on the list of suggested readings at the end of the chapter. Clinicians usually administer these scales to get a sense for the extent to which negative attitudes and feelings contribute to stuttering behaviors. This can be useful information for planning treatment because different treatment approaches address feelings and emotions to different degrees. Also, some informal measures are particularly successful with children, including having the children draw pictures of how they feel when it is hard to talk, list things they like and don't like about talking, engage in puppet shows role-playing reactions to communication breakdowns, and so forth.

Diagnosis and Recommendations

Clinicians should hold a feedback conference with the individual and/or the family after the assessment data have been analyzed. Clinicians should begin the feedback conference with a review of the assessment questions. The clinician should describe the characteristics of the individual's disfluencies and should indicate whether a diagnosis of stuttering is warranted. Information that reveals excessive amounts of concern by the individual, his parents, and/or his teachers; high rates of disfluency that vary little across situations; and a pattern of increasing struggle is indicative of a serious situation that requires immediate therapeutic attention. In these cases, the clinician should work with the individual and the family to devise a treatment plan that is well suited to the client's abilities and needs.

TREATMENT

We noted earlier that stuttering resolves in 60–80% of the individuals who have the disorder. This probably occurs most often in children who have been stuttering for a relatively short period of time. Adults who receive treatment are not "cured" often, but it does happen. Unfortunately, we do not know how often it happens. The good news is that many children, adolescents, and adults who receive treatment become fluent to the point where they can communicate effectively.

There are two types of treatment for stuttering. Table 7-9 compares and contrasts stuttering modification versus fluency shaping therapy. **Stuttering modification** procedures help the stutterer change or modify his stuttering so that it is relaxed and easy. **Fluency shaping** procedures establish a fluent manner of speaking that replaces stuttering. One of the main differences between these two approaches is focus on attitudes and emotions related to stuttering. Stuttering modification therapy has such a focus, but fluency shaping therapy does not. Thus, many clinicians combine aspects of

Table 7-9 Stuttering Modification versus Fluency Shaping

Stuttering Modification	Fluency Shaping
Client is taught to stutter less and more easily.	Client is taught to have stutter-free speech.
Speech is more natural.	Loss of speech naturalness.
Considerable focus on attitudes and negative reactions to speaking situations.	Little to no attention given to attitudes, negative reactions, etc.

stuttering modification and fluency shaping in their therapy. This section summarizes two well-known stuttering modification and fluency shaping approaches and describes one method for integrating stuttering modification and fluency shaping procedures.

Stuttering Modification Therapy

Stuttering modification therapy is used to teach the person who stutters to change the way he stutters. Charles Van Riper is probably the best-known proponent of stuttering modification therapy. His approach (Van Riper, 1973) to treatment is frequently referred to by the acronym MIDVAS, which stands for motivation, identification, desensitization, variation, approximation, and stabilization. Table 7-10 lists the phases in MIDVAS, their primary focus, and some of the procedures that are used. The primary goal of Van Riper's therapy is to help stutterers acquire a speech style that they find to be acceptable.

Van Riper believed that attitudes and feelings about stuttering play a critical role in the development of the disorder, in its continuation, and in its remediation. In fact, four of the six stages of the MIDVAS approach (motivation, identification, desensitization, and stabilization) relate primarily to the ability of the person who stutters to deal with his own stuttering and the consequences of his stuttering in a rational manner.

The hallmarks of Van Riper's approach are the modification procedures that are taught in the approximation phase. Van Riper proposed a three-step sequence for teaching stutterers how to stutter in a relaxed, controlled manner. First, people who stutter are taught to stop as soon as a stuttered word is completed, pause, and then say the word again in an easy (though not necessarily fluent) manner. This technique is called **cancellation**. When they have mastered cancellations, they are taught to ease their way out of repetitions, prolongations, and blocks. This strategy is called a **pull-out**. Finally, people who stutter are taught to modify their stuttering before it occurs. That is, when they anticipate stuttering on an upcoming sound or word, they form a **preparatory set** in which they ease their way into the word that they thought they would stutter on.

Fluency Shaping Therapy

Fluency shaping therapy is used to teach a new speech style that is free of stuttering. There are many different fluency shaping procedures, but most involve slower rates of speech, relaxed breathing, easy initiation of sounds, and smoother transitions between words. For example, Neilson and Andrews (1992) describe an intensive 3-week fluency shaping therapy program. During the first week, stutterers are taught a new way of

Table 7-10 A Summary of Van Riper's Approach to Stuttering Modification Therapy

Phase	Focus	Primary Procedures
Motivation	Prepare the client emotionally and mentally for the steps that follow.	1. Client teaches clinician to stutter. 2. Discuss client's feelings. 3. Explain the course of therapy.
Identification	Help the client understand and explain exactly what he does and how he feels when he stutters.	1. Client describes his stuttering in detail. 2. Speech assignments in which the stutterer observes listener reactions.
Desensitization	Reduce the client's fears, frustrations, and embarrassment about his stuttering.	1. Freezing—extending a moment of stuttering 2. Pseudostuttering (fake stuttering) in public
Variation	Teach the client to change his stuttering patterns.	Speech assignments in which the stutterer explores different ways of stuttering in public
Approximation	Teach the client new responses that reduce stuttering.	1. Cancellations 2. Pull-outs 3. Preparatory sets
Stabilization	Help the client become his own clinician.	1. Practice techniques on feared words in feared situations 2. Practice placing fake stuttering into fluent speech

BOX 7-4   Comparing Cancellations and Pull-outs

CD-ROM segments Ch.7.03 and Ch.7.04 show a stutterer practicing cancellations and pull-outs. Notice the differences between the two procedures. In cancellations (segment Ch.7.03), stuttering is modified after a stuttered word is completed. In pull-outs (segment Ch.7.04), stuttering is modified within the moment of stuttering. What does this stutterer do to modify his stuttering?

speaking in group and individual sessions. People who stutter slow their rate of speech down to 50 syllables per minute by extending the duration of consonants and vowels. (Try this yourself; you will find that it is very difficult to continue this abnormally slow rate of speech for very long.) They also learn to use a relaxed breathing pattern before they phonate, to initiate voicing in a very gentle manner, to use soft articulatory contacts during speech, to use constant voicing between syllables, and to move smoothly from one word to the next. When these skills are mastered at one speaking rate, the stutterer is allowed to speed up in 10 syllables per minute intervals. Once the individual reaches a rate of 100 syllables per minute, Neilson and Andrews teach appropriate speaking styles that incorporate such aspects as phrasing, rhythm, loudness, body language, and eye contact. They also teach stutterers how to use slower and smoother speech when they anticipate stuttering. In this way, individuals who stutter learn their new speech style in small increments.

During the second and third weeks of intervention, stutterers engage in "transfer" activities in which they use their new speech style in a variety of speaking situations outside the clinic. These outside activities help stutterers generalize their new way of speaking to the kinds of speech situations they routinely encounter in their everyday lives. Difficult speaking situations such as giving a speech, introducing oneself to a stranger, giving on-the-street interviews, and calling a radio talk show are practiced during the third week of therapy. To institute a new speech style, Neilson and Andrews give their clients repeated and varied opportunities to use fluent speech style in real speaking contexts.

Integrating Stuttering Modification and Fluency Shaping Methods

One of the major differences between stuttering modification and fluency shaping methods is that in fluency shaping the focus is only on speech production whereas in stuttering modification focus is also on attitudes and beliefs about speech production. Like Van Riper, most clinicians also believe that individuals who stutter need assistance with reducing their negative emotions about stuttering, their worries about listener reactions, and their tendencies to avoid stuttering. For this reason, many SLPs believe that it is best to combine stuttering modification and fluency shaping techniques in therapy. People who stutter are shown how to alter their speech style so that they are more likely to be fluent, but they are also taught how to modify their speech when they encounter moments of stuttering.

Therapy for Children Who Stutter

Therapy for children between 3 and 8 years of age involves many of the basic concepts and procedures from stuttering modification and fluency shaping approaches. Most

---

BOX 7-5   Examples of Fluency Shaping

CD-ROM segment Ch.7.05 shows a stutterer learning a fluency shaping strategy. In segment Ch.7.06, he practices this speech style during oral reading. Compare the speech in segments Ch.7.01 and Ch.7.02 to the speech in segments Ch.7.05 and Ch.7.06. Do you notice a difference between rate of speech, the onset of phonation, and the transitions between words? Does the speech in segments Ch.7.05 and Ch.7.06 sound "natural" to you?

clinicians utilize fluency shaping approaches somewhat more than stuttering modification because young children may not be developmentally ready for the amount of self-awareness that is required for stuttering modification. Clinicians frequently use the term "turtle talk" to describe the slower and easier fluency shaping speech style. Often, clinicians teach turtle talk in a step-by-step fashion, starting with single words, and then advancing to short repeated phrases (e.g., "I have a _____."), short imitated sentences, longer imitated sentences, and finally multiple connected sentences in conversations and storytelling. Clinicians also teach the client different ways of talking (e.g., smooth versus bumpy speech) so that they can indirectly learn how to modify their speech production.

It is critical that clinicians who work with young children involve families in the therapy process as much as possible. Clinicians have to make sure parents understand exactly what will be done in therapy and enlist parental support in the therapy process. Clinicians help parents increase factors that induce fluency (such as slower speech) and decrease factors that disrupt fluency at home (such as rapid rates of speech). Clinicians also invite parents to attend treatment sessions with their children so that they can learn the fluency shaping and stuttering modification techniques that their children are using. In addition, clinicians counsel parents about their feelings related to the child's stuttering and educate them about stuttering in general and how it is specifically related to their child. In fact, of the treatments currently available for young children who stutter, the singular approach that has been investigated the most thoroughly and that appears to be the most effective (though additional research is needed) is the Lidcombe Program (Harris, Onslow, Packman, Harrison, & Menzies, 2002; Miller & Guitar, 2008). This program essentially trains the parents to treat the child's fluency; parents learn how to help their child modify the stuttering through acknowledging/praising fluent moments and having the child correct or repeat fluently any stuttered moment.

An additional, though admittedly less researched approach, is one based on the previously described DCM. For this approach, the parents are also trained to work with their child, but the focus is more on the parent changing his or her speaking style than on the parent requesting that the child do so. Specifically, the parent learns how to use a slower rate, to pause prior to responding to the child, to reduce the number of questions, and so forth; all of these strategies are presumed to reduce any communicative demands placed on the child.

Interestingly, a study was recently completed that compared the Lidcombe Program to the DCM approach, and the results indicated that both approaches resulted in similar, significant reductions in disfluency (Franken, Kielstra-Van der Schalk, & Boelens, 2005). Yaruss, Coleman, and Hammer (2006) also completed a study that investigated a DCM-based approach referred to as family-focused treatment and reported significant reductions in speech disfluency. Although more investigations are necessary, at the very least, these results support the assumption that parental involvement in the intervention process and parental commitment to helping their child become more fluent are significant factors in the child's success in reducing or eliminating stuttering-like disfluencies.

SUMMARY

In summary, stuttering may be the result of an imbalance between internal processes (e.g., inherited traits, speech motor control, language development, cognitive development, and temperament) and external conditions (e.g., culture; parent, sibling, and peer interactions; and educational experiences). The relationships between these internal and external factors are dynamic, meaning that they vary from individual to individual, and they even vary within a single individual over time.

After stuttering develops, certain factors may serve to exacerbate the problem. These factors include negative feelings and attitudes, methods for avoiding stuttering, inefficient language formulation skills, and maladaptive speech motor control processes that affect respiration, phonation, and articulatory rate. We pointed out that some children may inherit traits that can possibly contribute to the development of stuttering. These traits could relate to delayed neurological maturation or the development of inefficient neurological networks. Subtle neurological deficiencies and delays could affect various aspects of development, including language, cognition, temperament, and speech motor control. As we discussed, environmental demands that exceed children's capacities for dealing with the requirements of the moment may also result in disfluency. However, it is important to remember that we do not know the cause (or possibly causes) of stuttering and that there is a strong need for further research into the nature of this complex disorder.

During assessment, clinicians evaluate the internal and external factors that contribute to stuttering, determine the need for therapy, and plan intervention. If therapy is provided, clinicians usually combine aspects of stuttering modification and fluency shaping intervention. When the person who is being treated is a child, it is critical to involve the parents in the treatment process.

BOX 7-6 Personal Story

Geoff Coalson, the person shown in the video clips, spent most of his school-age and adolescent life searching for the "cure" to his stuttering. He tried every technique from easy onset to purchasing the SpeechEasy device. The therapy program that proved to be most effective for him lasted for 9 months and consisted of both fluency shaping and stuttering modification techniques. Geoff had to practice each technique in those speaking situations that were least to most difficult for him. Through this program Geoff also had to learn to disclose his stuttering to others and to use voluntary stuttering to further desensitize himself to his stuttering. During this therapy experience, Geoff shared and explored his feelings of anger, guilt, and shame about his stuttering until he was finally able to reach true acceptance, not just of his stuttering, but of himself. Upon reflection of his journey, Geoff realized that, for him, the only way to transcend stuttering was to take an active role in learning about stuttering and to be an active participant in his stuttering treatment. Geoff has said that there was a time in his life when stuttering threatened to rob him of his dreams; however, stuttering now serves as the main inspiration of his dreams. Geoff is currently studying to receive his doctoral degree in speech-language pathology with hopes that one day he can help other people like him to transcend their stuttering.

STUDY QUESTIONS

1. Give an example of the following primary behaviors of stuttering: single-syllable-word repetition, syllable repetition, sound repetition, prolongation, and block.

2. What are the incidence and prevalence of stuttering? What do differences between incidence and prevalence suggest about the likelihood of recovery from stuttering?

3. List two basic facts about stuttering.

4. What is the difference between primary stuttering behaviors and secondary stuttering behaviors?

5. What are two myths about the etiology of stuttering?

6. Identify environmental/external conditions and individual capacities for fluency that may affect the development of stuttering.

7. What factors may contribute to chronic stuttering?

8. What types of assessment procedures are used in most stuttering evaluations?

9. During an evaluation, why is it important to measure the attitudes and feelings about communication of the person who stutters?

10. Describe cancellations, pull-outs, and preparatory sets.

11. What are the differences between stuttering modification and fluency shaping approaches to the treatment of stuttering?

12. What are some general guidelines to adhere to when interacting with a person who stutters?

KEY TERMS

Acquired (or neurogenic) stuttering
Adaptation
Cancellation
Chronic stuttering
Cluttering
Consistency
Disfluency

Fluency
Fluency shaping
Neural plasticity
Non-stuttering-like disfluencies
Preparatory set
Primary stuttering behaviors

Prolongations
Pull-out
Secondary stuttering behaviors
Stuttering
Stuttering-like disfluencies
Stuttering modification

REFERENCES

Arndt, J., & Healey, C. E. (2001). Concomitant disorders in school-age children who stutter. *Language, Speech, and Hearing Services in Schools, 32,* 68–78.

Bloodstein, O. (1995). *A handbook on stuttering* (5th ed.). San Diego, CA: Singular.

Bloodstein, O., & Bernstein Ratner, N. (2008). *Stuttering: The search for a cause and cure.* Boston: Allyn & Bacon.

Conture, E. G. (1990). *Stuttering* (2nd ed.). Englewood Cliffs, NJ: Prentice Hall.

Conture, E. G. (2001). *Stuttering: Its nature, diagnosis, and treatment.* Needham Heights, MA: Allyn & Bacon.

Felsenfeld, S. (1997). Epidemiology and genetics of stuttering. In R. F. Curlee & G. M. Siegel (Eds.), *Nature and treatment of stuttering: New directions* (2nd ed., pp. 3–23). Boston: Allyn & Bacon.

Fox, P. T., Ingham, R. J., Ingham, J. C., Hirsch, T. B., Downs, J. H., Martin, C., et al. (1996). A PET study of the neural systems of stuttering. *Nature, 382,* 158–162.

Franken, M., Kielstra-Van der Schalk, C. J., & Boelens, H. (2005). Experimental treatment of early stuttering: A preliminary study. *Journal of Fluency Disorders, 30,* 189–199.

Guitar, B. (205). *Stuttering: An integrated approach to its nature and treatment* (3rd ed.). Baltimore, MD: Williams & Wilkins.

Harris, V., Onslow, M., Packman, A., Harrison, E., & Menzies, R. (2002). An experimental investigation of the Lidcombe Program on early stuttering. *Journal of Fluency Disorders, 27,* 203–214.

Logan, K., & Conture, E. (1995). Length, grammatical complexity, and rate differences in stuttered and fluent conversational utterances of children who stutter. *Journal of Fluency Disorders, 20,* 35–61.

Miller, B., & Guitar, B. (2008). Long-term outcome of the Lidcombe Program for early stuttering intervention. *American Journal of Speech-Language Pathology, 18,* 2–33.

Neilson, M., & Andrews, G. (1992). Intensive fluency training of chronic stutterers. In R. Curlee (Ed.), *Stuttering and related disorders of fluency* (pp. 139–165). New York: Thieme.

Riley, G. (1994). *The Stuttering Severity Instrument for children and adults* (3rd ed.). Austin, TX: Pro-Ed.

Starkweather, W. (1987). *Fluency and stuttering.* Englewood Cliffs, NJ: Prentice Hall.

Van Borsel, J., Maes, E., & Foulon, S. (2001). Stuttering and bilingualism: A review. *Journal of Fluency Disorders, 26,* 179–205.

Van Riper, C. (1973). *The treatment of stuttering.* Englewood Cliffs, NJ: Prentice Hall.

Wingate, M. (1976). *Stuttering theory and treatment.* New York: Irvington.

Yaruss, S. J., Coleman, C., & Hammer, D. (2006). Treating preschool children who stutter: Description and preliminary evaluation of a family-focused treatment approach. *Language, Speech and Hearing Services in Schools, 37,* 118–136.

SUGGESTED READINGS

Andrews, G., Craig, A., Feyer, A., Hoddinot, S., Howie, P., & Neilson, M. (1983). Stuttering: A review of research findings and theories circa 1982. *Journal of Speech and Hearing Disorders, 48,* 226–246.

Andrews, G., Morris-Yeates, A., Howie, P., & Martin, N. (1991). Genetic factors in stuttering confirmed. *Archives of General Psychiatry, 48,* 1034–1035.

Curlee, R. F., & Siegel, G. M. (Eds.). (1997). *Nature and treatment of stuttering: New directions* (2nd ed.). Boston: Allyn & Bacon.

Onslow, M. (2004). Treatment of stuttering in preschool children. *Behavior Change, 21,* 201–214.

Shapiro, D. (1999*). Stuttering intervention: A collaborative journey to fluency freedom.* Austin, TX: Pro-Ed.

chapter eight

Dysarthria

THOMAS P. MARQUARDT

LEARNING OBJECTIVES

1. To learn the major causes of cerebral palsy.

2. To understand differences between dysarthria in cerebral palsy and in adults.

3. To learn about diseases that cause dysarthria in adults.

4. To understand how dysarthria is identified and treated.

5. To learn about augmentative communication systems.

6. To learn the speech characteristics of different types of dysarthria.

Damage to central and/or peripheral nervous system pathways causes muscle dysfunction, that is, muscle weakness, incoordination, or paralysis. Speech disorders caused by neuromuscular dysfunction are termed **dysarthria**. There are a number of different types of dysarthria; some affect a small part of the speech production apparatus, others the entire system. As a group, the dysarthrias involve all the major subcomponents of speech production: respiration, phonation, resonance, and articulation.

Dysarthria in children most commonly is associated with cerebral palsy; in adults, it results from cerebrovascular or progressive neurological disease. Frequently, the neuromuscular problems that underlie dysarthria cause difficulties in swallowing as well as in speech. This chapter considers speech disorders in cerebral palsy and acquired dysarthria. Dysphagia, or disordered swallowing, is considered in Chapter 9.

CEREBRAL PALSY

Injury to the nervous system that occurs before, at the time of, or shortly after birth can cause cerebral palsy, a syndrome of deficits in visual, auditory, intellectual, and motor functions in the critical early development period for speech and language At the center of the disorder is motor dysfunction. That is, the child's muscles are weak, paralyzed, and/or uncoordinated. Consider this description of cerebral palsy from the standpoint of developing speech and language. A child is born with vision, hearing, cognitive, and neuromuscular disorders. How might this affect speech and language learning?

The primary causes of cerebral palsy are anoxia, in which the brain has a restricted oxygen supply, and trauma, in which the brain is injured. Frequently, the causes are divided into three groups: *prenatal* (before birth), *perinatal* (at the time of birth), and *postnatal* (after birth). Disease or metabolic problems of the mother are prenatal causes of cerebral palsy. If the umbilical cord is wound around the neck causing strangulation, if there is a premature separation of the placenta, or if the birth process is delayed, the infant may be deprived of oxygen at the time of birth. The brain also may be damaged by trauma during the birth process or at a very early age as a result of falls or car accidents. Regardless of the cause, cerebral palsy is the result of nervous system damage, and it has an adverse effect on the development of speech and language skills.

Classification of Cerebral Palsy

There are several ways of classifying cerebral palsy: by the extremities affected (typography), by neuromuscular characteristics, and by severity of the disorder. The following subsections consider each of these classifications and then consider them together.

BOX 8-1   Overview of the CD-ROM Segments

The CD-ROM segments that accompany this chapter include two speakers with dysarthria. The first speaker (segment Ch.8.01) has an acquired dysarthria; the second speaker (segment Ch.8.02) has cerebral palsy. In segment Ch.8.03, the speaker with cerebral palsy demonstrates the use of an augmentative communication device.

Orthopedic Classification

Orthopedic classification is based on the limbs affected. If one limb is involved, it is called *monoplegia*. If both legs are affected, it is termed *paraplegia*. Other terms are used when three limbs (*triplegia*) and four limbs (*quadriplegia*) are involved.

Neuromuscular Characteristics

Cerebral palsy can be classified by underlying neuromuscular characteristics. Damage to the pyramidal tract and the associated extrapyramidal system yields a spastic type of cerebral palsy. **Spasticity** is characterized by an abnormal resistance to muscle lengthening and is produced by a hypersensitivity of muscle stretch reflexes. What this means is that when an attempt is made to stretch out the arm or to flex the leg, the muscles resist the movement. The **hypertonicity** is most prominent in antigravity muscles (muscles that allow us to stand, for example), which leads to a characteristic flexion pattern of the arms and extension pattern of the legs with inward rotation at the knees. The pattern includes arms that are bent upward and legs that are positioned like a scissors with the knees together but the feet spread apart. A feature of abnormal hypertonicity is chronic muscle shortening, which may be accompanied by muscle atrophy (wasting).

Involuntary movements characterized by a writhing and twisting motion typify **athetoid** cerebral palsy. In this case, the primary damage is to the basal ganglia and associated components of the extrapyramidal tract (see Chapter 4 for a review of this tract). The involuntary movements progress from the body outward to the hands and feet, and the child may give the appearance of being in almost constant motion. The involuntary movements are superimposed on and interfere with voluntary purposeful movements. What this means is that when the child tries to reach for an item like a pencil or spoon, the arm may move back and forth and up and down repeatedly until the target is reached and then continue as the item is manipulated.

Ataxic cerebral palsy results from damage to the cerebellum. In ataxic cerebral palsy, the primary neuromuscular features are related not to increased or alternating muscle tone, but to a disturbance in movement coordination. Movements are characterized by errors in their speed, direction, and accuracy. When asked to carry out a rhythmic and precise motor activity like playing on a drum, the child has difficulty not only hitting the drum, but in maintaining the rhythm.

Two other types of cerebral palsy have been identified. Rigid cerebral palsy, with balanced hypertonicity and **rigidity** resulting from increased tone in muscles at both sides of a joint, and **tremor** cerebral palsy, characterized by rhythmic involuntary movements. These types have a low frequency of occurrence and rarely occur alone.

Individuals with cerebral palsy infrequently have features of a single type of the disorder. Most often, spasticity occurs with **athetosis** or with **ataxia**. These types of cerebral palsy co-occur because multiple sites in the motor pathways have been damaged. Although one type of cerebral palsy may predominate, features of the other types of neuromuscular pathology are evident as well. Therefore, descriptions such as "primarily spastic" or "dominant athetosis" are often used as labels.

Severity

Severity ranges from mild to severe and is usually determined by an overall judgment of the level of impairment. This judgment is based on the degree of independence in communication, ambulation, and self-help skills. For example, clinicians ask themselves, "Is the child independent in self-help skills such as walking and feeding?" "What types of special equipment are required?" "Is speech understandable?" Table 8-1 lists the characteristics that are typically associated with mild, moderate, and severe forms of cerebral palsy.

A description of cerebral palsy for any individual is based on the three classification system components. Severe athetoid quadriplegia, mild spastic paraplegia, and moderate ataxic quadriplegia are typical diagnostic descriptions.

Motor Development in Children With Cerebral Palsy

Motor deficits are the focal point of a diagnosis of cerebral palsy, and delayed motor development is most frequently observed in children with the disorder. In general, children with cerebral palsy have developmental delays in sitting, standing, walking, and speech development related to the motor impairment. The basis for delayed motor development is twofold: impaired neuromuscular functioning and abnormal reflexes. Neuromuscular abnormalities in terms of type of cerebral palsy were discussed briefly earlier. These abnormalities have significant effects on motor development. Coupled with abnormal neuromuscular functioning is the lack of inhibition of primitive reflexes and the failure to develop the kinds of higher order reflexes that are seen in adults.

An infant's head movements elicit stereotypical patterns of limb movements. For example, movement of the head to the side elicits a pattern of arm and leg extension on the side to which the head is turned. This reflex, termed the asymmetrical tonic neck reflex, is expected to disappear by the time the infant is a year old. However, the reflex is not inhibited in cerebral palsy, and it interferes with the development of independent limb movements. Consider how difficult it would be to eat if, when your head turned to the right or left, the arm holding the spoon moved away from you. (See Table 8-2 for a brief review of some postural reflexes.)

Table 8-1 Levels of Severity in Cerebral Palsy

Severity Level	Description
Mild	Self-help skills are adequate to care for personal needs, no significant speech problems, ambulates without appliances, no treatment necessary.
Moderate	Speech is impaired and special equipment may be needed for ambulation. Self-help skills are insufficient to meet daily care needs. Habilitation therapy is needed.
Severe	Poor prognosis for developing self-help skills, ambulation, and functional speech even with treatment and the use of adaptive equipment.

Source: Adapted from Rusk, H. (1977). *Rehabilitation medicine* (4th ed.). St. Louis, MO: Mosby.

Table 8-2 Examples of Early Postural and Movement Reflexes

Reflex	Characteristics
Asymmetric tonic neck reflex	Turning the head to the side causes extension of the arm and leg on the side to which the head is turned and flexion of the limbs of the opposite side.
Symmetric tonic neck reflex	Raising of the head results in extension of the arms and flexion of the legs. Legs are extended and arms are flexed when head is lowered.
Positive and negative supporting reactions	Contact of feet with ground causes simultaneous contraction of flexors and extensors of the legs and fixing of joints (positive); relaxation of the extensors of the legs occurs when the infant is lifted from the ground (negative).
Moro reflex	Adduction-extension reaction of the limbs with movement of the supporting surface, loud noise, or blowing on the face.
Neck righting reflex	Rotation of the head results in the rotation of the body as a whole to the side to which the head is turned.

Children with cerebral palsy often fail to develop higher level reflexes related to walking. For example, if you are shoved while standing, you adjust your posture by widening your stance and raising the arm to maintain balance. Children with cerebral palsy may not develop this righting reflex, making it more difficult for them to learn how to walk. Given the importance that reflexes have for development, it is not surprising that children with cerebral palsy nearly always have delays in sitting, standing, walking, and speech development.

Speech and Language Development in Children With Cerebral Palsy

Speech disorders in cerebral palsy result from weakness and incoordination. All aspects of speech production are affected.

Respiration

Respiratory activity is characterized by reduced vital capacity and impaired ability to generate and maintain subglottal pressure (see Chapter 4 for a review of the relationship between respiration and speech). At least part of the reduced respiratory support for speech results from inefficient valving of the outgoing airstream at the glottis, velopharynx, and within the oral cavity by the lips and tongue.

Phonation

Laryngeal functions of children with cerebral palsy often are compromised by changing tonicity. This results in intermittent breathiness and a strangled harshness in voice quality as vocal fold tension decreases and increases. The tension may be so great that phonation does not occur at all even though the child appears to be trying to talk. Timing of respiratory and laryngeal activity also is disrupted. Expiration frequently begins before the vocal folds are closed, causing a loss of air. Errors in the production of the voiced-voiceless distinction in contrasts like /p/ and /b/ and /s/ and /z/ are frequent because of impaired timing in phonation onset.

Resonance

Resonance during speech production is disrupted in cerebral palsy. Netsell (1969) investigated aerodynamic aspects of speech production in cerebral palsy and found a gradual premature opening of the velopharynx during the production of syllables and a break of the velopharyngeal seal during nonnasal productions. These difficulties lead to hypernasality and nasal emission during speech production.

Articulation

Individuals with cerebral palsy frequently have significant articulation problems. The mandible may be hyperextended with the mouth open, making it difficult to round, protrude, or close the lips. The hyperextension of the jaw and abnormal tongue postures prevent precise shaping and constriction of the vocal tract for vowel and consonant production.

Prosody

Utterances in children with cerebral palsy may be limited to one or two words on each breath. Because of poor respiratory control, disrupted timing of respiratory and laryngeal functioning, and poor control of laryngeal tension, intonation and the ability to mark stressed words in an utterance are impaired.

The overall effect of neuromuscular impairment of the speech production components is to reduce the intelligibility of speech. Intelligibility may be so limited that words and phrases are not understandable unless the listener knows the topic.

Speech Development

Speech sound development is delayed in children with cerebral palsy with the highest frequency of errors on fricatives and glides requiring tongue movement. Stops and nasals develop earlier than fricatives, and children with cerebral palsy make fewer errors on voiced consonants than they do on voiceless consonants. In general, the latest

---

BOX 8-2   An Adult With Mild Mixed Dysarthria

In CD-ROM segment Ch.8.03, an adult with mild mixed dysarthria talks about himself. Note that although his speech is intelligible, prosodic aspects of speech production are impaired.

developing sounds in normal children, such as fricatives and affricates, are the most delayed in children with cerebral palsy.

The entire speech production system is affected in many cases of cerebral palsy because of reduced respiratory support and inefficient valving of the outgoing airstream at the glottis, velopharynx, and oral cavity. The developmental course of speech sounds follows what might be expected in normally developing children but at a reduced rate, with articulation errors continuing into adulthood. The melody of speech (prosody) also is affected and, in conjunction with speech sound errors, causes a reduction in speech intelligibility.

Cognitive, speech, and language deficits are interrelated in cerebral palsy. Intelligence and functional motor limitations affect speech and language performance (Pirila et al., 2007). Language deficits are a frequent concomitant of cerebral palsy. Reduced ability to explore the environment because of motor limitations, mental retardation, hearing loss, and perceptual deficits all work to limit the development of vocabulary, grammar, and discourse skills in children with cerebral palsy.

ACQUIRED DYSARTHRIA

Acquired dysarthria differs from cerebral palsy in several respects. In the case of acquired dysarthria, the adult developed speech and language before the onset of the disorder. Therefore, primitive reflexes do not contribute significantly to the speech deficits that are observed. In addition, adult patients usually present sensory problems related to the aging process.

Classification of Acquired Dysarthrias

Historically, acquired dysarthrias were categorized by the causative disease process ("the dysarthria of multiple sclerosis") or the part of the body affected. However, with the seminal work of Darley, Aronson, and Brown (1975), a universal system of classification has been developed based primarily on the underlying dysfunction of muscle that characterizes the disorder. In many cases of acquired dysarthria, the disease progresses and speech becomes increasingly more difficult to understand. (See Table 8-3 for an overview of acquired dysarthrias.)

Flaccid Dysarthria

Interruption of normal input to the muscles from the peripheral nervous system causes muscle weakness and atrophy (wasting), hence the term *flaccid*. Muscles that are cut off from their innervation as a result of peripheral nerve damage are flaccid. They are *hypotoned* (**hypotonicity** is a condition of reduced background electrical activity) and weak. Often, twitching of the muscle fibers occurs with their wasting away (atrophy).

The problem in flaccid dysarthria may be at the motoneuron cell bodies, at the peripheral nerve as it courses to the muscle, at the myoneural junction, or at the muscle fibers themselves. In other words, impulses from the central nervous system are interrupted as they course down to the muscle fibers.

Table 8-3 Types and Characteristics of Acquired Dysarthria

Type	Disease/Disorder	Site of Lesion	Speech Characteristics
Flaccid	• Bulbar palsy • Myasthenia gravis	Lower motor neuron	Audible inspiration, hypernasality, nasal emission, breathiness
Spastic	Pseudobulbar palsy	Upper motor neuron	Imprecise articulation, slow rate, harsh voice quality
Ataxic	Cerebellar damage Friedrich's ataxia	Cerebellum	Phoneme and syllable prolongation, slow rate, abnormal prosody
Hypokinetic	Parkinson's disease	Extrapyramidal system	Monoloudness, monopitch, reduced intensity, short rushes of speech
Hyperkinetic	• Huntington's chorea • Dystonia	Extrapyramidal system	Imprecise articulation, prolonged pauses, variable rate, impaired prosody
Mixed	• Multiple sclerosis • Amyotrophic lateral sclerosis	Multiple motor systems	Speech characteristics dependent on motor systems affected

Motoneurons can be injured by trauma, or they can deteriorate from degenerative disease. The myoneural junction is affected by a disorder called myasthenia gravis, in which neurotransmitter substances are depleted where the nerve endings synapse with muscle fibers. This requires longer than expected periods of time for the junction to restabilize. The individual may have almost normal muscle function following rest, but then will rapidly fatigue with prolonged motor activity. Hereditary conditions such as muscular dystrophy cause the muscle fibers to deteriorate. In this progressive disorder, the muscles become weaker as the disease progresses. Depending on what parts of the motor unit (peripheral nerves and the muscle fibers they innervate) are affected, individuals with flaccid dysarthria demonstrate reduced muscle tone, with atrophy and weakness and reduced muscle reflexes.

The parts of the speech musculature affected by flaccid dysarthria depend on the underlying problem. If a single nerve, such as the hypoglossal nerve (cranial nerve XII, which innervates the tongue), is damaged on one side, the tongue only on that side will be weak or paralyzed. If the brainstem is damaged on one side and involves several cranial nerves, one side of the face, tongue, and palate musculature will be impaired. In conditions such as muscular dystrophy or myasthenia gravis, the entire speech production apparatus is affected.

The speech characteristics of flaccid dysarthria result primarily from weakness. Speech rate is slow with breathy phonation, hypernasality, weak production of stops and fricatives, articulatory imprecision, and reduced phrase length. Reduced breath support resulting from respiratory weakness and air wastage at the glottis, velopharynx, and oral cavity causes phrases to be short, with monoloudess and monopitch.

Spastic Dysarthria

When the pyramidal and extrapyramidal tracts are damaged bilaterally at or near the cortical surface, impaired innervation to the muscles causes them to be weak, hypertoned (too much background electrical activity), and hyperreflexic (**hyperreflexia** is a condition of exaggerated responses to reflex elicitation). When stretched, the muscles contract before releasing with continued extension (spasticity). This leads to the types of muscle spasms that are characteristic of spastic dysarthria. Some atrophy may occur, but it is related to a lack of muscle use because of weakness.

All four limbs of the body are affected in spastic dysarthria as well as the trunk, head, and neck. In contrast to flaccid dysarthria, where muscles of a single speech structure may be completely paralyzed, the whole speech production musculature is affected in spastic dysarthria. Speech is characterized by articulatory imprecision, slow rate, short phrases, and a harsh voice quality. Prosody is affected with reduced loudness and pitch variation.

A variety of conditions can lead to spastic dysarthria. Pseudobulbar palsy, for example, is caused by small strokes in the white fiber pathways beneath the surface of the brain. The individual typically is elderly, with both speech and swallowing problems.

Ataxic Dysarthria

The primary characteristics of ataxic dysarthria relate to coordination. In ataxic dysarthria, movements are inaccurate and dysrhythmic. However, in contrast to flaccid and spastic dysarthrias, reflexes are normal and there is only minimal weakness. Ataxic dysarthria results from damage to the cerebellum, which functions to coordinate the direction, extent, and timing of movements.

Like the other dysarthrias, ataxic dysarthria has a negative impact on speech production. Prosody tends to be monotonous and there are disruptions in stress patterns. Normally stressed syllables are sometimes unstressed and unstressed syllables are stressed. The rate of speech is usually slowed, and vowels, in particular, are increased in duration. The good news for individuals with ataxic dysarthria is that speech intelligibility frequently is only mildly affected. This is quite unlike the speech of individuals with flaccid and spastic dysarthrias, who may have marked difficulty in making themselves understood.

Hypokinetic Dysarthria

In hypokinetic dysarthria, the individual's muscles are hypertoned and rigid, resulting in reduced movement. Many people with hypokinetic dysarthria experience a resting tremor that disappears with voluntary movement. The hand may tremble rhythmically, but the tremor disappears when the person reaches for a spoon. People with hypokinetic dysarthria may have difficulty starting and stopping movements. For example, when trying to move from a chair to another room, the individual begins getting up from the chair, stops, and then starts again to get to a standing posture. Small shuffling steps move him to the next room, but he has to put his hand on the table to stop so that he can sit down. There is an apparent difficulty initiating, continuing, and terminating movements.

Parkinson's disease is the primary example of a disorder that results in hypokinetic dysarthria. Parkinson's disease is caused by a degeneration of dopamine-producing cells of the basal ganglia, which are three large nuclei that are deep within the cerebral hemispheres. The effect of this deficit is a balanced hypertonicity of the musculature and resting tremors of the head and limbs.

The speech movements of individuals with hypokinetic dysarthria are small, but their speech rate sometimes sounds fast. In fact, hypokinetic dysarthria is the only dysarthria in which accelerated movements and short rushes of speech characterize the disorder. Speech melody is flat with monoloudness, monopitch, and reduced intensity.

Hyperkinetic Dysarthria

When the basal ganglia of the extrapyramidal system are damaged, involuntary movements are a telltale sign. In Parkinson's disease, the involuntary movements disappear with movement. In other disorders such as Huntington's chorea and dystonia, however, the involuntary movements are superimposed on voluntary movements of the body. Depending on the underlying cause, the involuntary movements in hyperkinetic dysarthria may be slow or fast, rhythmic or dysrhythmic, involve the entire body or be restricted to a single structure such as the jaw.

Involuntary movements interfere with speech production. Articulation is imprecise in individuals with hyperkinetic dysarthria, and they often have breakdowns in the flow of speech, which sound like hesitations in unusual places. The person with hyperkinetic dysarthria often speaks with short phrases, and there are long pauses while he or she waits for the involuntary movement to subside. After the involuntary movements, the person continues with speech. The voice quality of these individuals may be breathy or strangled sounding depending on the state of the fluctuating tonicity of the laryngeal musculature and the degree of breath support.

Mixed Dysarthrias

Several disease processes affect more than one part of the motor system at the same time. Multiple sclerosis, a disease in which the myelin covering of axons is damaged, may affect the spinal cord, brainstem, cerebellum, cerebrum, or any combination of these structures. Another example of a disease that affects more than one part of the motor system is amyotrophic lateral sclerosis (Lou Gehrig's disease), which damages the upper motor neurons of the pyramidal tract as well as the peripheral motoneurons of the brainstem and spinal cord. How speech production is affected depends on which systems are damaged and may vary from a barely detectable change in speech production in multiple sclerosis to completely unintelligible speech in advanced amyotrophic lateral sclerosis.

BOX 8-3   **Speech Sample for Adult with Cerebral Palsy.**

In CD-ROM segment Ch.8.01, an adult with cerebral palsy answers a series of questions. Can you understand his answers?

ASSESSMENT OF INDIVIDUALS WITH DYSARTHRIA

When assessing an individual with dysarthria, the speech-language pathologist (SLP) needs to evaluate each subsystem of the speech production process—respiration, phonation, velopharyngeal function, and articulation—to determine the type and extent of dysarthria.

The Oral-Peripheral Examination

The SLP determines the anatomic and functional integrity of speech production structures by completing an oral-peripheral examination. What this entails is a careful examination of structures such as the tongue, jaw, and lips at rest and during nonspeech (rounding and spreading the lips, opening and closing the mouth) and speech (saying syllables rapidly) activities. A key element in the evaluation of the individual with dysarthria is the determination of speech intelligibility because it serves as the index of dysarthria severity, progression of the disease, and the effects of treatment.

In addition to the oral-peripheral examination, there are several evaluation protocols for dysarthria. The Frenchay dysarthria assessment (Enderby, 1983) is one such test. It includes tasks to assess reflex and voluntary activities of speech structures during nonspeech and speech activities. For example, in the evaluation of the tongue, the SLP asks the patient to move the tongue in side-to-side and in-and-out movements and to push the tongue against the inside of the cheek on both sides. The SLP may use the assessment findings to assign the individual to a specific dysarthria group such as hypokinetic or ataxic.

Intelligible speech requires a stable subglottal air pressure as a power source for vocal fold vibration and for additional sound sources in the upper airway. Respiratory weakness, except in the severest forms of neuromuscular disease, seldom is the basis for reduced intelligibility. Movements of air that are sufficient to support life are nearly always sufficient for producing short sequences of understandable speech.

The SLP should assess respiration during non-speech- and speech-related tasks. The SLP must carefully observe quiet respiration and respiration for speech for lack of coordination and signs of compensation for muscular weakness. One simple device to evaluate nonspeech respiration is to place a straw in a water-filled glass that has centimeter markings on the side (Hixon, Hawley, & Wilson, 1982). If the patient can blow bubbles in the water with the straw inserted 5 centimeters below the surface for 5 seconds, respiratory function is sufficient for speech.

SLPs evaluate laryngeal function by making subjective judgments of voice quality. They ask patients to produce prolonged vowels during syllable production and during connected speech. The SLP estimates the degree of hoarseness, harshness, breathiness, and fluctuations in voice quality during these activities and others in which the patient is instructed to increase loudness and pitch. See Chapter 6 for a discussion of additional activities that are used to assess voice production.

The SLP also looks for evidence of weakness and/or coordination of the velopharynx. These judgments should be based on physical examination of the mechanism at rest and during production of a prolonged vowel. Nasal emission of air is assessed during the articulation of syllables containing stops and fricatives in connected speech. If the SLP hears nasal emission and hypernasality during speech production, there is probably abnormal function of the velopharynx resulting from weakness and/or incoordination.

The SLP should assess articulatory structures of the upper airway, including muscles of the tongue, jaw, and lips, to determine whether they are weak, atrophic, and/or uncoordinated. The SLP should look for reductions in strength, speed, range of motion, and coordination. The SLP can examine the patient's face at rest and during rounding and retraction of the lips to assess facial weakness. The examiner may ask the individual to hold a tongue depressor between the lips. This is routinely performed on the left and right sides to see if one side is weaker than the other. Asking the individual to alternate lip rounding and retraction at maximum rates may reveal problems with speech and coordination. Similarly, the examiner evaluates jaw strength on each side by attempting to close the jaw after asking the patient to hold the jaw open and by testing the compression of a tongue depressor between the teeth on each side. Requesting up-and-down movements of the jaw provides information on speech and coordination. The SLP tests the tongue by evaluating function during protrusion and retraction, lateral movement, and rapid alternating movements. Based on these systematic observations, the clinician obtains an estimate of the functional integrity of each subcomponent of the speech production system.

The Speech Examination

Several aspects of speech production provide important information about the type and extent of dysarthria. The clinician requests that maximum rates of syllable production be generated using bilabial (/b/, /p/), lingualveolar (/k/, /g/), and linguavelar (/t/, /d/, /s/) consonants plus a vowel. If dysarthria is present, the number of syllables that the individual can produce is decreased compared to normal performance.

Speech samples serve as assessment vehicles to estimate articulatory precision, speech rate, prosodic patterning, and other perceptual features. Typically, the examiner asks the patient to read a standard passage and give a sample of conversational speech. The SLP listens to these samples for evidence of altered speech characteristics that are indicative of dysarthria. Behaviors that indicate dysarthria include slow rate, hypernasality, and harsh voice quality.

SLPs administer several measures of speech intelligibility to individuals who they suspect may have dysarthria. Perhaps the measure most often used is the Assessment of the Intelligibility of Dysarthric Speech (Yorkston & Beukelman, 1981). The patient reads or repeats words and phrases. These speech samples are recorded and are evaluated by a second listener to provide estimates of word and sentence intelligibility. In general, SLPs expect sentences to be more intelligible than words. It is important to point out that the severity of impairment to any major component of the system may have major effects on speech intelligibility. For example, mild weakness of the entire speech production system may result in only mild reductions in intelligibility. Severe impairment in tongue or velopharyngeal functioning, even if the rest of the system is intact, may render speech almost entirely unintelligible.

TREATMENT OF INDIVIDUALS WITH DYSARTHRIA

A team of professionals including physicians, SLPs, occupational therapists, audiologists, special educators, and physical therapists works to help children with dysarthria develop functional independence. Drugs are prescribed to reduce spasticity and involuntary movement; bracing and special seating equipment are useful for preventing contractures and for facilitating sitting and walking; prescriptive glasses and hearing aids may improve sensory functioning; specialized teaching is employed to deal with deficits in attention, memory, and learning; and counseling may help to reduce emotional lability.

Treatment for dysarthria may take several forms. Surgery and drugs are beneficial for some disorders in which dysarthria is a symptom. For example, individuals with Parkinson's disease benefit from the administration of dopamine, which is used to replace naturally produced dopamine, a substance that is required for brain metabolism. Patients with Parkinson's disease do not produce dopamine in sufficient quantities as a result of degeneration of cells in the basal ganglia. The treatment team may prescribe other drugs that serve to reduce involuntary movements or spasticity. In some cases, improved motor performance has been brought about by surgical intervention that destroys a part of the thalamus or a portion of the globus pallidus. Efforts have also been made to transfer fetal brain cells to patients with Parkinson's disease to replace those cells that have been destroyed. An early consideration in dysarthria treatment, then, is the use of drugs and surgery to benefit motor performance.

Surgical and prosthetic management may be used to improve speech performance directly. In unilateral vocal fold paralysis, it may be beneficial to surgically move the fold to the midline so that it can be approximated by the noninvolved fold during phonation. An alternative is to fill the paralyzed vocal fold with Teflon, effectively moving it to a closed position, for better closure during approximation of the unparalyzed fold. For severe velopharyngeal inadequacy, a palatal lift or pharyngeal flap may reduce nasal emission and hypernasality and can result in improved speech intelligibility.

Postural supports are important for children with cerebral palsy and for adults with acquired dysarthrias because it is necessary to place the individual in a better position for speaking. These supports take the form of slings to hold up the arms and adapted wheelchairs for maintaining upright supported posture. For example, an adapted wheelchair in which the head is stabilized may restrict reflex patterns that interfere with voluntary arm movements.

Speech therapy is often geared toward improving speech intelligibility. In children with cerebral palsy, treatment may initially focus on the development of a stable respiratory pattern. For example, the child may be placed in a supine position (on the back) with the legs, arms, and neck flexed. Attention is focused on the sensations associated with a pattern of rapid inhalation followed by prolonged expiration. As the child develops control over the respiratory pattern for speech, he is asked to phonate a prolonged vowel with expiration. When phonation is consistent, superimposing constrictions in the mouth, such as closing the lips, results in the production of the voiced /b/ with a vowel. In general, treatment focuses on the development of coordinated volitional control of the speech production system.

For adults, speech intelligibility can be improved by reductions in speech rate, increases in intensity, and exaggerated articulatory movements during speech production. A particularly effective program for individuals with Parkinson's disease (Ramig, Countryman, Thompson, & Horii, 1995), for example, focuses on talking louder in therapy sessions and in self-practice outside the clinic. Talking louder results in an increase in movement of the speech structures with greater articulatory precision (Fox et al., 2006).

For individuals with good intelligibility, the focus of treatment may change to improving the naturalness of speech. Although their speech may be fully understandable, it calls attention to them because of abnormal intonation or stress. Treatment to improve naturalness centers on feedback during speech production to focus on words that should be stressed and intonation patterns appropriate to the utterance.

Teaching effective strategies such as identifying the topic of a conversation; supplementing speech with gestures and alphabet boards; paying careful attention to the speaker; communicating in quiet, well-lighted settings; and establishing communication rules also are important to overall rehabilitation success (Yorkston, Strand, & Kennedy, 1996). The focus is not only on speech but also on the communicative process and the adjustments the speaker and communication partner make to maximize communication success.

What if intelligible speech is not an option? What if the neuromuscular condition is so severe that the child with cerebral palsy or the adult with acquired dysarthria cannot be understood, even by family members who know him or her well? What can they do to communicate?

AUGMENTATIVE COMMUNICATION

All humans augment their communication with facial expressions and gestures. If you were asked to communicate a message but could use only one word, you would probably use gestures or pantomime to help convey the information. Augmentative communication refers to supplementing or augmenting speech using various techniques and aids. Sometimes the communication system people employ temporarily replaces speech. Examples of these systems include using writing or gestures in a noisy environment. But in contrast to the unimpaired speaker who relies on augmentative communication only in particular situations, individuals with dysarthria or severe language impairments may need to use an augmentative communication system all the time.

Augmentative communication can take various forms. Some systems do not require any type of communication aid or device. Consider the case in which you need to convey three messages without speaking: *stop*, *yes*, and *I don't know*. How would you do it using gestures? The gesture you would probably use for *stop* is holding your hand in a vertical direction palm forward with your arm extended, upward and downward movements of the head for *yes*, and a shrugging of the shoulders for *I don't know*. In this case, you needed no tool or device other than your own body to communicate. But what if you were paralyzed except for movements of your left foot? How would you communicate in this situation? In all likelihood, you would need some type of device to accomplish message transmission. For example, a switch triggered by movements of your foot that moves a cursor on a screen with printed words would allow you to select the word you wanted to communicate. This is an example of an aided augmentative communication because more than your own body is required to accomplish communication. The two systems, aided and unaided, also are different because one is nonelectronic (gestures) and the other is electronic (scanning system).

Based on this short description, it is apparent that augmentative systems are extremely variable and depend on the capabilities of the communicator. They may be as basic as words or pictures on a board that the user employs to communicate everyday needs such as requests for a drink or food, to technologically advanced systems based on speech synthesizers capable of storing hundreds of phrases and words.

Augmentative communication differs in several important respects from oral speech. Augmentative communication is slower. An unimpaired individual might produce approximately 150 words per minute while speaking. With an augmentative system, even when items are directly selected from a picture or word array or from a series of stored phrases on a speech synthesizer, communication is slower. This is particularly true when the individual must use a cursor to scan across a field of possible options. Augmentative communication also introduces other complexities. If the person uses a communication board that requires a communication partner to view it, the communication partner must be positioned behind the user; neither can see the other's face. If the individual uses gestures, then the partner must interpret what the gestures convey; both communicators must know the code. In some environments, it may be difficult to use a speech synthesizer because the output may not be sufficient to overcome background noise.

BOX 8-4   An Adult With Cerebral Palsy

The adult with cerebral palsy shown in CD-ROM segment Ch.8.03 uses an augmentative communication device to respond to questions. View segment Ch.8.02 again and compare the intelligibility of his responses using speech and the augmentative system.

For individuals with dysarthria resulting from cerebral palsy or acquired motor system damage, augmentative communication may be the primary means of conveying messages (see Figures 8-1 and 8-2). No system is ideal, and frequently multiple options are available.

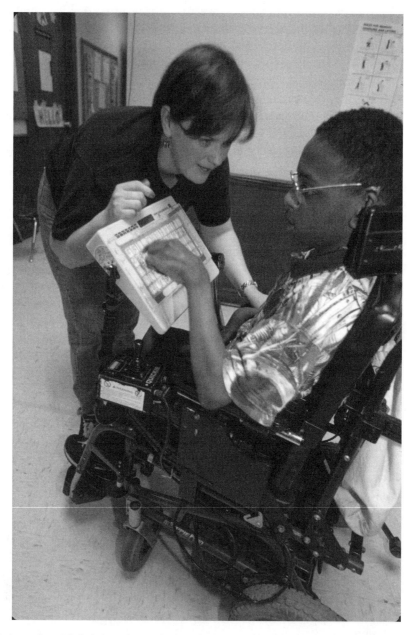

Figure 8-1   Adult male with left facial weakness who uses an augmentative communication system.
Source: © Jeff Greenberg/Alamy

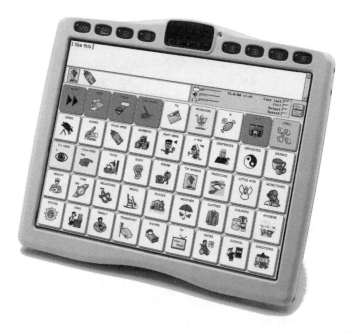

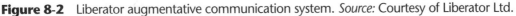

Figure 8-2   Liberator augmentative communication system. *Source:* Courtesy of Liberator Ltd.

To help an individual decide which system to use, SLPs need to assess intellectual, sensory, motor, and academic skills. By knowing which motor behaviors are available, the SLP and patient can decide whether a gestural system is possible or what size the keys on a keyboard need to be for the individual to access a word-based augmentative system. If the individual can read, words rather than pictures can be used on the communication device. SLPs must consider the degree of cognitive functioning to be able to determine whether a symbol system can be used as part of the display and whether the individual is capable of learning how to use the system.

An assessment of the person's communication needs is perhaps as important as his or her abilities. What and how meaning is conveyed by the augmentative communication user depends on the person's age and situation. An 8-year-old child with cerebral palsy may need to communicate in a classroom setting with his teacher and classmates, not only on academic topics such as mathematics and reading assignments, but on social events and activities outside the classroom. The needs of the adult with severe multiple sclerosis may be markedly different. The ability to communicate to meet everyday functional needs and to discuss family issues may be paramount.

The overriding goal is to develop an augmentative system within the capabilities of the user that meets communication needs with maximum efficiency. Few individuals with cerebral palsy are speechless or entirely unintelligible. The augmentative system may be the primary communication mode for some individuals; for others, it serves to supplement speech only in difficult communication situations.

A period of training with the system is essential. For the child or adult who has had limited opportunity to communicate, this training may take the form of demonstrating turn-taking, initiation of communication, and question asking (Lung & Light, 2007). In adults with acquired dysarthria and severely reduced intelligibility, the training may focus on using the procedure of pointing to the first letter of each word verbalized to increase the probability that the communication partner can interpret the content of the intended message. In thinking about augmentative communication systems, it is always important to remember that speech is faster, more flexible, and more efficient. The initial focus of rehabilitation should be to maximize oral speech function and to augment or to substitute an alternative communication system only if necessary.

SUMMARY

Neuromuscular speech disorders result from damage to the motor systems of the central and/or peripheral nervous system. Speech is affected because muscles are weak, paralyzed, or uncoordinated. Although there are similarities between dysarthria in cerebral palsy compared to acquired nervous system damage, children with cerebral palsy demonstrate visual, auditory, and cognitive impairments that have a bearing on the development of their speech and language abilities. This is because the injury or damage responsible for the cerebral palsy occurred near the time of birth. The assessment of dysarthria focuses on speech production but may include language and cognitive assessment because deficits in these domains of communicative functioning also may be associated with the cause of the disorder. The purpose of drug, prosthetic, and behavioral intervention is to maximize the communication ability of individuals with dysarthria. Augmentative communication systems may have an important role in meeting this goal, particularly for the severely impaired individual.

BOX 8-5 Personal Story

Mike was involved in a serious traffic accident and suffered severe brain trauma that left him in a coma for 3 months. Gradually, he recovered and with intensive occupational and physical therapy regained the ability to walk, dress, and feed himself. Six months following the accident he was able to care for himself independently but continued to have cognitive deficits in working memory and executive functioning and his speech was moderately dysarthric with slowed rate, abnormal prosody, reduced intelligibility, and hypernasality. Following intensive speech-language therapy that focused on his speech, he could be understood by his family, friends, and by strangers, but clearly the melody of his speech was altered. Mike returned to the university and completed a degree in psychology and obtained a job supervising dispensing of chemical supplies and has returned to his hobby of painting. Return to CD-ROM segment Ch.8.03 and listen to Mike read a passage. How does his melody differ from normal?

STUDY QUESTIONS

1. Which neuromuscular disorders have involuntary movement? Why?

2. How does the assessment of dysarthria differ for an adult compared to a child?

3. What are the major causes of cerebral palsy?

4. What are two diseases that result in mixed dysarthria?

5. How is speech intelligibility assessed?

6. How does augmentative communication differ from oral speech production?

KEY TERMS

Ataxia (ataxic)
Athetoid
Athetosis (athetoid)
Dysarthria

Hyperreflexia
Hypertonicity
Hypotonicity

Rigidity (rigid)
Spasticity (spastic)
Tremor

REFERENCES

Darley, F., Aronson, A., & Brown, J. (1975). *Motor speech disorders*. St. Louis, MO: W. B. Saunders.

Enderby, P. (1983). *Frenchay dysarthria assessment*. Austin, TX: Pro-Ed.

Fox, C., Ramig, L., Ciucci, M., Sapir, S., McFarland, D., & Farley, B. (2006). The science and practice of LSVT/LOUD: Neural plasticity-principled approach to treating individuals with Parkinson disease and other neurological disorders. *Seminars in Speech and Language, 27*, 283–299.

Hixon, T. J., Hawley, J. L., & Wilson, K. J. (1982). An around-the-house device for the clinical determination of respiratory driving pressure: A note on making the simple even simpler. *Journal of Speech and Hearing Disorders, 47*, 413–415.

Lung, S., & Light, J. (2007). Long-term outcomes for individuals who use augmentative and alternative communication: Part II—communicative interaction. *Augmentative and Alternative Communication, 22*, 1–15.

Netsell, R. (1969). Evaluation of velopharyngeal function in dysarthria. *Journal of Speech and Hearing Disorders, 34*, 113–122.

Pirila, S., van der Meere, J., Pentikainen, T., Ruusu-Niemi, P., Korpela, R., Kilpinen, J., et al. (2007). Language and motor speech skills in children with cerebral palsy. *Journal of Communication Disorders, 40*, 116–128.

Ramig, L., Countryman, S., Thompson, L., & Horii, L. (1995). A comparison of two intensive speech treatments for Parkinson disease. *Journal of Speech and Hearing Research, 39*, 1232–1251.

Rusk, H. (1977). *Rehabilitation medicine* (4th ed.). St. Louis, MO: Mosby.

Yorkston, K., & Beukelman, D. (1981). *Assessment of intelligibility of dysarthric speech*. Austin, TX: Pro-Ed.

Yorkston, K., Strand, E., & Kennedy, M. R. T. (1996). Comprehensibility of dysarthric speech: Implications for assessment and treatment planning. *American Journal of Speech-Language Pathology, 5*, 55–66.

SUGGESTED READINGS

Beukelman, D., Garrett, K., & Yorkston, K. (2007). *Augmentative communication strategies for adults with acute or chronic medical conditions.* Baltimore, MD: Brookes.

Duffy, J. (2005). *Motor speech disorders: Substrates, differential diagnosis and management* (2nd ed.). St. Louis, MO: Elsevier Mosby.

Love, R. (1992). *Childhood motor speech disability.* New York: Macmillan.

McDonald, E. (Ed.). (1987). *Treating cerebral palsy.* Austin, TX: Pro-Ed.

Odding, E., Roebroeck, M., & Stam, H. (2006). The epidemiology of cerebral palsy: Incidence, impairments and risk factors. *Disability & Rehabilitation, 28*, 183–191.

Weismer, G. (2007). *Motor speech disorders: Essays for Ray Kent.* San Diego, CA: Plural.

Wohlert, A. (2004). Service delivery variables and outcomes of treatment for hypokinetic dysarthria in Parkinson disease. *Journal of Medical Speech-Language Pathology, 12*, 235–239.

chapter nine

Dysphagia

DENA GRANOF

LEARNING OBJECTIVES

1. To learn the normal processes involved in feeding and swallowing.

2. To understand the causes of swallowing disorders.

3. To learn clinical and instrumental procedures for evaluating dysphagia.

4. To learn the speech-language pathologist's role in assessing and treating swallowing disorders in children and adults.

Dysphagia (dis-fay-ja) is a difficulty in swallowing or an inability to swallow. A swallowing problem affects a person's ability to eat, which serves two primary purposes: (1) nutrition and hydration and (2) pleasure. To remain healthy, to recover from illness or trauma, or to grow, both of these functions must be achieved in a safe and efficient manner. When patients have dysphagia, they are unable to consume enough food or liquid safely and efficiently. Food plays an important role in all cultures and families and is a significant part of our social interactions. Dysphagia also impairs a person's ability to participate in social gatherings or events.

EXAMPLES OF DYSPHAGIA

The following two case studies illustrate what happens when a person has dysphagia (see Figure 9-1 for a view of the anatomic structures involved in the swallowing process). Ms. T is a 73-year-old woman who recently had a stroke affecting the left side of the brain. The brain damage caused by the stroke impairs the function of the muscles of the face, mouth, larynx, and pharynx. Because of this muscle dysfunction, Ms. T has trouble chewing and moving the food around in her mouth. When she attempts to swallow or move the food from the mouth to the stomach, the weakness of her muscles makes it difficult for her to push the food into the pharynx and then into the esophagus so that it can continue on to the stomach. Some food remains in the part of the mouth that is now paralyzed and no longer has sensation. After every two or three bites, Ms. T coughs because food is going toward the tracheal airway and lungs instead of the stomach.

When the food enters the airway, it is called **aspiration**. Aspiration may occur because the weak and/or paralyzed pharyngeal and laryngeal muscles cannot control the food. Ms. T is able to eat and drink only small amounts at a time. She may not be a "safe" eater because the impaired muscle function may allow food to enter the lungs and cause possible aspiration or choking. Ms. T's nutrition, hydration, safety, and eating pleasure are negatively affected by the symptoms of her stroke.

The second case study is an example of dysphagia in a child. Rebecca is 4 years old and has spastic cerebral palsy. She uses a wheelchair with supports for her head and trunk. She is able to say one word at a time, but because of severe dysarthria, her speech is not very understandable. Rebecca drinks small sips of thickened liquids out of a special cup and eats food that is of a puree or pudding consistency (because of abnormal muscle tone and slow movement). It takes more than an hour for Rebecca to

BOX 9-1   **Overview of CD-ROM Segments**

Normal (CD-ROM segment Ch.9.01) and disordered (CD-ROM segment Ch.9.02) swallowing are shown during modified barium swallow (MBS) studies. Barium swallow studies allow the examiner to view the bolus as it moves from the mouth through the pharynx to the esophagus.

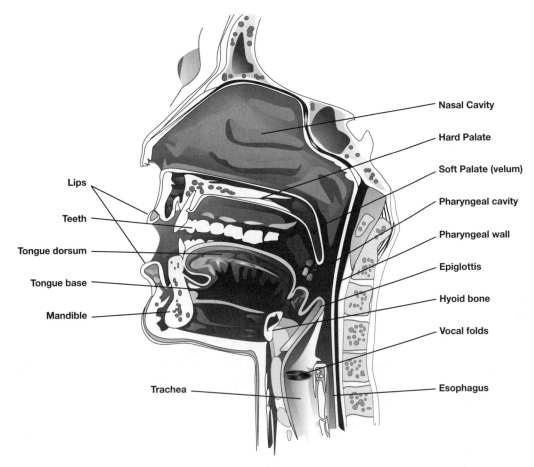

Figure 9-1 Anatomical structures involved with swallowing. *Source:* Chiras, D. D. (2008). *Human Biology* (6th ed., p. 106). Sudbury, MA: Jones and Bartlett.

finish a meal. She frequently coughs and chokes toward the end of her meals. Rebecca has been diagnosed with dysphagia because she is not able to eat enough food to maintain good nutrition for growth or to drink an adequate amount of liquid. Her coughing indicates that some food may be going down her airway.

ROLE OF THE SPEECH-LANGUAGE PATHOLOGIST

For both Ms. T and Rebecca, the speech-language pathologist (SLP) will be an integral part of the dysphagia team that assesses and treats their swallowing problems. SLPs have been involved with swallowing since the 1930s when they treated the feeding problems of children who had cerebral palsy (Miller & Groher, 1993). Over the past 25 years, there has been an expansion of the practice of speech-language pathology into medical settings such as hospitals and nursing homes. Additionally, more multidisabled children are being served in the public schools. According to the 2002 American Speech-Language-Hearing Association Omnibus Survey (American Speech-Language-Hearing

Association [ASHA], 2002), approximately 30% of practicing SLPs are involved in the management of dysphagia. The survey also looked at different employment settings and found that 11.2% of school-based SLPs and 84.3% of hospital-based SLPs regularly served individuals with dysphagia.

For several reasons SLPs are a key part of a dysphagia team. Communication and swallowing problems frequently occur together. A study by Martin and Corlew (1990) surveyed 115 patients at a Veterans Administration medical center. Of these patients, 81% had swallowing problems and 87% of those with swallowing problems also had communication disorders. Similar results were reported in a Rehabilitation Institute of Chicago study (Cherney, 1994) of 973 consecutive referrals to the Department of Communicative Disorders. This study found that 307, or 31.55%, of these patients had dysphagia.

Communication and swallowing problems often co-occur because these two activities share some common structures and functions. Historically, SLPs have been trained to understand the structure and function of the oral mechanism, pharynx, and larynx and to apply this knowledge to the assessment and treatment of speech disorders. These same structures and functions are an important part of the swallowing process; thus, it is more efficient to have one professional managing these overlapping areas. In 1987, the Ad Hoc Committee on Dysphagia Report (ASHA, 1987) set out guidelines regarding the role of the SLP in the area of dysphagia. The report clearly states that dysphagia should be included in the scope of practice and that the SLP should be involved in the evaluation and treatment of dysphagia with or without the presence of a communication disorder.

STAGES OF SWALLOWING

Before examining the reasons for dysphagia and what techniques or skills the SLP uses to evaluate swallowing problems, it is important to understand the normal swallow. The process of swallowing is viewed in terms of different stages. These include an anticipatory stage, oral stage, pharyngeal stage, and esophageal stage.

The Anticipatory Stage

The anticipatory stage of swallowing occurs before the food actually reaches the mouth. Sensory information about what is going to be eaten is provided through vision and smell. These senses allow the person the opportunity to prepare to eat. They help the person "get ready" for the food by understanding what is on the plate and whether it is a desirable thing to eat.

BOX 9-2   A Normal Swallow

CD-ROM segment Ch.9.01 is an MBS study of a normal swallow. Note the rapid movement of fluid from the mouth through the pharynx to the esophagus.

The Oral Stage

The oral stage marks the beginning of events that lead up to the swallow. There are two parts to this stage, and both are under voluntary control. In the preparatory part of the oral stage, a **bolus** (food after it has been chewed and mixed with saliva) is being readied for a safe swallow. Figure 9-2A shows the position of the bolus during the oral stage. Once the food enters the mouth, a labial or lip seal is needed to prevent the food from falling out, and there needs to be an open nasal airway for breathing. The pharynx and larynx are at rest. At the same time, the buccal or cheek musculature prevents the food from falling into lateral sulci, which are the spaces between the cheek and the mandible. The bolus is masticated (chewed) and manipulated by the tongue and jaw in a rotary lateral movement. Sensory input about the taste, texture, temperature, and size of the bolus determines the amount of oral motor movement and strength that are needed. During this process, the back of the tongue is usually elevated to keep the bolus in the oral cavity.

The second part of the oral stage, sometimes called the transport phase, begins when the tongue pushes the bolus against the palate, moving it in a posterior or backward direction toward the pharynx. The size and consistency of the bolus affect the amount of lingual strength that is necessary to complete this movement. The oral stage of the swallow is completed when the bolus passes the anterior faucial arches and enters the pharyngeal area. At this point, the pharyngeal stage of the swallow is triggered.

The Pharyngeal Stage

The pharyngeal stage (see Figure 9-2B) begins with the triggering of the pharyngeal swallow. The two purposes of the pharyngeal stage are to protect the airway and to direct the bolus toward the stomach. The pharyngeal swallow motor pattern is initiated by sensory information sent from the mouth and oropharynx to the brainstem. The swallow is facilitated by both sensory and motor fibers in the cortex of the brain and the brainstem. The part of the brainstem called the **medulla** contains the nuclei for the cranial nerves that control the motor movements of the larynx, pharynx, and tongue. These structures are integral to the swallowing process.

A number of simultaneous physiological events occur as a result of the swallow. The velum elevates and contracts to close off the velopharynx so that food cannot enter the nasal cavity. The larynx and hyoid bone move upward and forward. The larynx closes to prevent food from entering the airway beginning at the level of the vocal folds and moving superiorly or upward to the false vocal folds and then the aryepiglottic folds. As the larynx elevates and moves forward, the epiglottis comes over the larynx to provide additional airway protection.

When the swallow is triggered, pharyngeal **peristalsis** is initiated. The contraction of the muscles of the superior, medial, and inferior pharyngeal constrictors transports the bolus through the pharynx toward the esophagus. These muscles are on the back part of the pharyngeal wall. The upper esophageal sphincter, which is on top of the esophagus, relaxes or opens with the upward and forward movement of the larynx. This allows the food to enter the esophagus.

The Esophageal Stage

The esophageal stage (see Figure 9-2C) begins with the lowering and backward movement of the larynx and resumption of breathing. The upper esophageal sphincter contracts to prevent food from reentering the pharynx. The bolus moves through the esophagus to the stomach in a series of peristaltic waves.

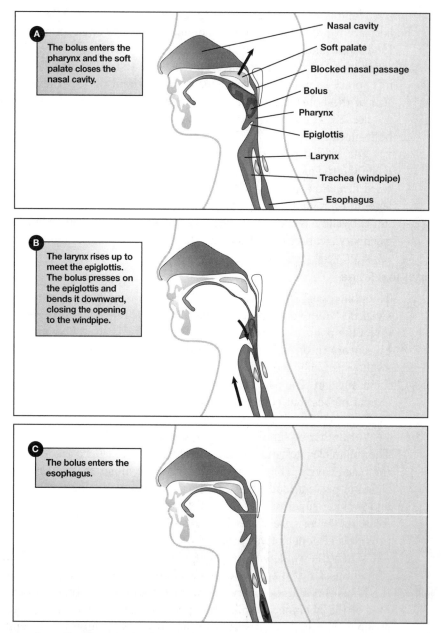

A The bolus enters the pharynx and the soft palate closes the nasal cavity.

- Nasal cavity
- Soft palate
- Blocked nasal passage
- Bolus
- Pharynx
- Epiglottis
- Larynx
- Trachea (windpipe)
- Esophagus

B The larynx rises up to meet the epiglottis. The bolus presses on the epiglottis and bends it downward, closing the opening to the windpipe.

C The bolus enters the esophagus.

Figure 9-2 Stages of swallowing: **A.** Oral stage (parts 1 and 2). **B.** Pharyngeal phase (parts 3 and 4) and **C.** Esophageal phase (part 5). *Source:* Chiras, D. D. (2008). *Human Biology* (6th ed., p. 106). Sudbury, MA: Jones and Bartlett.

DYSPHAGIA IN ADULTS

Swallowing requires both cognitive and motor skills. Cognitively, a person must be able to recognize the need to eat and decide what to eat. The description of the different stages of swallowing indicates that the normal swallow requires an intact motor system. Swallowing is a process of finely coordinated, sequential muscular movements. When an illness or injury affects either the cognitive or the motor skills, there is a high risk for dysphagia. Following is information on some of the most common etiologies of dysphagia in adults and the resultant swallowing problems.

Left Hemisphere Cerebrovascular Accident

Persons who suffer cerebrovascular accidents (CVAs), or strokes, to the left hemisphere of their brain often have an oral stage difficulty resulting from weakened or paralyzed facial musculature including labial, lingual, and mandibular function. There may be a delay in initiating the pharyngeal swallow, which could cause the bolus to be aspirated.

Right Hemisphere Cerebrovascular Accident

Individuals who suffer right hemisphere strokes often have oral stage difficulties resulting from reduction in labial, lingual, and mandibular strength. They also have a delayed pharyngeal swallow, which could cause aspiration. There is a reduction in pharyngeal peristalsis, which contributes to food getting "stuck" in the throat. Cognitive deficits including impulsivity, errors in judgment, and attention difficulties may compound these muscular difficulties.

Brainstem Stroke

Individuals who have brainstem CVAs often have oral stage difficulties resulting from reduced labial, lingual, and mandibular sensation and strength. These persons also have a delayed or absent pharyngeal swallow, causing incomplete laryngeal elevation and closure and reduced upper esophageal sphincter opening. This may result in possible aspiration and an inability for the bolus to enter the esophagus.

Traumatic Brain Injury

Dysphagia symptoms resulting from traumatic brain injury (TBI) vary according to the location and severity of the injury, but problems usually exist at each stage of the swallow. Cognitive deficits in orientation, memory, judgment, attention, and reasoning may affect the person's ability to choose foods, control the rate of eating, and maintain attention to the task of eating. Common oral stage problems include reduced tongue control, abnormal reflexes, and difficulty with chewing. The pharyngeal swallow may be delayed or absent, and pharyngeal peristalsis and aspiration may be reduced.

Dementia

Dementia causes cognitive deficits such as reduced attention, reasoning, judgment, and poor orientation skills. These deficits can significantly affect the initiation of the eating process. There may be an overall reduction in oral awareness, resulting in slow

> **BOX 9-3 A Comparison of Normal and Abnormal Swallows**
>
> View the normal swallow in CD-ROM segment Ch.9.01 again. Now view segment Ch.9.02, which shows an MBS from a stroke patient. Note that the muscles that control swallowing are weak, the time required for the liquid to pass from the mouth to the esophagus is slow, and there is a significant amount of liquid left in the pharyngeal area.

oral preparatory movements. Food may be held in the mouth for an extended period of time and not recognized as something to be swallowed. As a result, pharyngeal swallow is often a delayed. Because dementia is frequently a part of a neurological disease, the muscular deficits of that disease serve to compound the problems of dementia and cause swallowing dysfunction in all of the stages.

Neuromuscular Disease

Multiple sclerosis, amyotrophic lateral sclerosis, Parkinson's disease, myasthenia gravis, and muscular dystrophy are progressive neuromuscular diseases that cause changes in the strength, rate, and efficiency of muscular movements. As these diseases progress or get worse, muscular movements frequently become weak and uncoordinated. This causes difficulty at all stages of the swallow.

Cancer

Cancer can cause several types of swallowing problems. If surgery is necessary to remove a cancerous part of the oral, pharyngeal, or laryngeal structures, the anatomic structures used for swallowing change. The anatomic change has a significant effect on swallow physiology and the way that the bolus is prepared and moved through the pharynx. Radiation often causes tissues such as those in the mouth and throat to become irritated and dry, making swallowing very uncomfortable. Many of the chemotherapy drugs used to treat cancer reduce the patient's immune system and make the patient susceptible to infections. These infections can cause sores in the mouth and throat.

MANAGEMENT OF ADULT DYSPHAGIA

Assessment and treatment of adult dysphagia requires a team approach. The SLP is one part of a dysphagia team that can include occupational and physical therapists, nurses, nutritionists, and a variety of medical doctors such as radiologists, neurologists, gastroenterologists, and pulmonologists. The patient and family are also an integral part of this team. The dysphagia assessment is composed of a number of procedures, including review of the patient's history, a bedside examination, and an instrumental examination. Based on the results of the assessment, the team meets and decides on a treatment plan.

The following case study illustrates assessment procedures, decision making, and formulation of a treatment plan. Tim, a 17-year-old, was involved in a motorcycle accident. He was thrown off his motorcycle while driving around a curve too quickly and sustained a TBI. He was taken by ambulance to the nearest trauma center where he remained unresponsive (in a "coma") for 72 hours. During this period of time, he was nourished through **intravenous (IV)** solutions. Upon awakening, Tim was confused and disoriented; he did not know where he was, how he got there, or the day or time. One side of his body, including his face and neck, had reduced muscle movement and strength. The neurologist assigned to his case requested a dysphagia evaluation. The purpose of the evaluation was to determine whether Tim could begin eating orally again. To make that decision, a number of questions needed to be answered: (1) Are the muscles in Tim's tongue, lips, and jaw able to adequately prepare a bolus? (2) Do the pharyngeal and laryngeal muscles have enough strength and movement to elevate the larynx to close off the airway and direct the bolus to the esophagus? (3) Is Tim aware of the food on his plate and can he feed himself? (4) Can Tim eat safely (without aspiration) and maintain adequate nutrition?

Review of History Prior to the Accident

Upon receiving the referral for a dysphagia evaluation, the SLP needs to collect relevant feeding, behavioral, and medical information. The SLP needs to know whether the patient had swallowing problems prior to the illness or accident. Information about any preexisting illness or trauma is also important. Additionally, the SLP needs to find out what medications, if any, the patient had been taking. This information can be ascertained from both a review of the medical chart and an interview with the patient's family.

Tim was a healthy young man with no history of illness or trauma. Prior to the accident, he had no swallowing or eating problems. In middle school, he had been diagnosed with a mild learning disability and had been on medication to improve his attention.

Current Medical Status

The next step in a dysphagia evaluation is to review the patient's current medical condition. The dysphagia team, including the SLP, needs to know whether the patient is medically stable, the respiratory status, which medications have been prescribed, and the current level of cognitive functioning. The team also needs to know how the patient is currently receiving nutrition. The patient may be eating orally, receiving nutrients through an IV tube (like Tim), being fed through a tube placed in the nose that goes to the stomach (**nasogastric or NG tube**) or by a tube surgically placed directly into the stomach (**gastric or G-tube**). The way in which the dysphagia assessment is structured depends on the answers to these questions. It is more complicated to perform a dysphagia assessment when there are respiratory or cardiac problems. Some medications that are given to patients after a TBI cause drowsiness, and knowledge of this effect will allow the evaluation to be scheduled at an optimal time. If a patient is disoriented and confused, he or she may not understand the instructions of the SLP or even comprehend that food is something to be eaten. If the patient is not currently receiving oral nutrition, there are safety considerations related to the use of food in the assessment. This information is gathered from the medical chart, by consulting with the nurses and doctors on the dysphagia team, and by observing the patient.

Tim was medically stable; however, he was being given a medication to control seizures, which are common after TBI. This medication made him very sleepy. He could not maintain adequate alertness for more than 10 minutes at a time. He was also confused and did not understand why he was in the hospital or why he was unable to get out of bed and walk. He could not remember any of his therapists, nurses, or doctors, even though they were each in his room several times a day. He had not eaten orally in the 3 days since his accident.

Noninstrumental Clinical Exam (Bedside Clinical Assessment)

At this point in the assessment process, the SLP sits down with the patient and assesses his or her ability to take food off the plate, prepare the bolus, and safely swallow in the noninstrumental clinical examination (NICE), also called the bedside clinical assessment (BCA). The SLP evaluates the cognitive and motor skills necessary to perform these actions. The examination procedures are influenced by the information gathered by the review of the patient's medical history and the patient's current medical status.

In Tim's case, the team knows he may have a short attention span and have difficulty following directions. Given his medical history, they expect he will have some motor difficulty with chewing and swallowing. They also know he has not eaten food for 3 days.

First, the SLP observes the patient's level of alertness, ability to follow directions, and any other behaviors that might interfere with the ability to attend to the feeding process. This is followed by an examination of the structure of the oral anatomy. The SLP examines the lips, tongue, cheeks, jaw, palate, and teeth, noting any abnormalities such as scarring or asymmetry.

During the oral-motor examination, the SLP observes the patient's ability to perform the motor movements necessary for a safe and adequate swallow to occur. Based on the SLP's review of the patient's current medical status, food may or may not be used to assess these skills. The SLP observes (1) lip closure and lip strength, (2) jaw and cheek movement and strength, (3) lingual ability to move the food around in the mouth for both bolus preparation and the transporting of the bolus to the posterior of the oral cavity, and (4) initiation of the pharyngeal swallow. Once the bolus moves into the pharyngeal area, it can no longer be directly observed without additional procedures.

As was discussed previously, a safe swallow occurs when the larynx moves upward and forward while opening the upper esophageal sphincter that is at the top of the esophagus. This allows the food to go toward the stomach. The pharyngeal constrictor muscles propel the bolus through the pharynx to the esophagus. Because this cannot be directly observed, the SLP can observe several "signs" to help understand what is happening to the bolus after it moves through the oral cavity. These include (1) watching the neck along with placement of two fingers under the chin to determine whether there is upward and forward laryngeal movement; (2) listening for coughing, which could mean that the bolus or part of the bolus is going down the "wrong way" toward the lungs; (3) and listening for a "gurgly" sound after swallowing, which might indicate that part of the bolus is on the vocal folds.

Pharyngeal stage problems cannot be diagnosed by the BCA. However, the SLP can ascertain an indication of possible pharyngeal stage deficits through the information provided by this evaluation. Weak and uncoordinated oral motor movements may indicate the presence of poor pharyngeal stage movements. The initiation of the swallow may be delayed, which could cause possible aspiration. Laryngeal movement may be judged to be inadequate, which could cause incomplete protection of the airway. The patient may cough after the swallow or complain that it feels as if food is stuck in his or her throat. Or the patient may have a diagnosis such as dementia or a stroke in which pharyngeal stage problems are common. When pharyngeal stage problems are suspected, the SLP can conduct an additional assessment procedure.

Observation of Tim's oral structures indicated good dentition, but asymmetry in both the tongue and cheeks. This was evidenced by a "droop" on the right side of his face and tongue, which could mean reduced or absent muscular movement. Food was used as a part of Tim's BCA, but he had to be constantly reminded that he needed to put the spoon in his mouth and chew and swallow. Chewing was slow and labored. He had trouble making a bolus with crackers and could not use his tongue to efficiently move the bolus to the back of his mouth. He had much better control and ease of movement with the chocolate pudding. The initiation of the swallow appeared delayed, and Tim coughed for several minutes after each of the four bites. It appeared Tim had possible pharyngeal stage deficits. Therefore, he was referred for an instrumental assessment.

Instrumental Assessment of Dysphagia

An instrumental assessment is used to get a better understanding of pharyngeal stage functioning. The most commonly used instrumental procedure is referred to as a **modified barium swallow (MBS)**. This procedure is a fluoroscopic image that is recorded on videotape. The SLP and a radiologist perform this procedure together. The patient is brought into the room where X-rays are taken. The patient sits in a special chair that can be positioned for optimal eating. The SLP places barium-coated food in the patient's mouth, and the radiologist takes a moving picture or fluoroscopy of the patient chewing and swallowing. Pharyngeal stage functioning can be visualized, and any abnormalities in structure or function can be identified on the video X-ray image. If the patient aspirates, this can also be seen on the video. Use of the MBS allows the dysphagia team to understand the cause of the dysphagia and to make recommendations for treatment. It also provides key information as to whether the patient is able to eat safely.

Another commonly used instrumental procedure is endoscopy. A flexible scope in inserted through the nose and positioned just above the epiglottis. The patient is then given food that has been mixed with dye. As the patient eats, the examiner observes the pharyngeal structures and functions through the scope. As with the MBS, endoscopy provides information about the adequacy and safety of the swallow.

Based on the results of Tim's BCA, he was referred for an MBS. He was given three consistencies of food: thin liquid barium, pudding-like barium, and a cookie coated with barium. The video study showed that Tim had a delayed swallow and weak pharyngeal constrictor muscles. The delayed swallow caused a small amount of the thin liquid to be aspirated before the swallow was initiated. Pieces of the cookie got "stuck" in his throat, and it took several extra swallows to clear all the food from the pharyngeal area. This situation was caused by the weak pharyngeal muscles.

Treatment Planning

The entire dysphagia team reviews all of the information that has been gathered about the patient and writes a treatment plan that will allow the patient to be well nourished and safe. This plan usually addresses a number of different aspects of the eating and swallowing process (Table 9-1).

Once a dysphagia treatment plan has been formulated, the team determines the procedures for carrying out the recommendations. The entire dysphagia team works together to ensure that the patient remains safe and well nourished. Dysphagia assessment and treatment are ongoing processes. Patients continually change and improve and the treatment plan needs to reflect these changes as they occur.

Tim had many of the dysphagia symptoms that are common after TBI, and his treatment plan reflected the presence of these symptoms. Tim's treatment plan contained four important elements that were directed toward his current level of swallowing: (1) *Positioning*—Tim needed to be positioned upright in his wheelchair. This aided him in the use of his weakened muscles and helped direct the food toward the esophagus and reduced the risk of aspiration. (2) *Cueing*—Tim had another person sitting with him during the meal to remind him to chew and swallow each bite of food before putting another bite in his mouth. Tim tended to stuff too much in at one time, which is a safety concern. Tim also needed to be reminded that there was food on his plate and that he needed to eat it. (3) *Bolus modifications*—the results of the dysphagia assessment showed that Tim had difficulty with thin liquids because of his delayed swallow and with foods that needed to be chewed because of his weak pharyngeal constrictor muscles. The dysphagia team recommended that Tim's diet consist of thickened liquids and foods with a pudding consistency. This allowed Tim to eat safely and obtain adequate nutrition. (4) *Swallowing strategies*—during the MBS, the team observed that it took Tim several swallows to clear the pharyngeal area of food. Based on this finding, it was recommended that after every three or four bites that Tim be directed to take two or three "dry swallows." As Tim continued to improve in both his cognitive and motor skills, the dysphagia plan was revised to meet his changing skills.

DYSPHAGIA IN CHILDREN

The focus of pediatric dysphagia treatment is different from treatment of adult dysphagia. Adult dysphagia deals with the treatment and assessment of swallowing after an injury or the onset of an illness; these patients had normal swallowing abilities that were impaired as a result of the illness or injury. In cases of pediatric dysphagia,

Table 9-1 Typical Aspects of a Treatment Plan for Dysphagia

Aspect	Questions
Positioning	What is the best position for the patient while eating?
	Does the patient need any special head or neck support?
	How long should the patient remain upright after eating?
Environmental modifications	Does the patient need a quiet room to eat in?
	What kind of reminders or cues does the patient need to put the food in his or her mouth and remember to chew and swallow?
Adaptive feeding equipment	Does the patient need a nonslip bowl, a spoon with a special handle, or a cup with a spout?
Bolus modifications	What consistency of food is easiest and safest for the patient to eat?
	Is it thin or thickened liquids or finely chopped or pudding-like food?
	Does the patient do better with hot or cold foods?
	How much food should be given for each swallow?
Swallowing techniques	Can the patient be taught any compensatory strategies to avoid aspiration?
	Does the patient need instructions for safe swallowing such as multiple swallows for each bolus or alternating liquid and solid foods?
	Can the patient's swallow be improved through the use of touch or cold? Does the application of ice and pressure to the anterior faucial pillars improve a swallow that is delayed?
	Are there interventions that can make a permanent change in the swallow over the course of time? Will facial exercises, vocal adduction exercises, breathing exercises, or pharyngeal strengthening exercises improve the dysphagia?
	Are there sensory stimulation procedures such as the use of cold or touch that will help to facilitate a swallow?
	Will any rehabilitation maneuver that aids in directing bolus flow or increasing laryngeal elevation be of benefit?

the SLP treats children who have yet to acquire normal eating skills. These children have a medical condition, genetic disorder, or illness that has been present since birth or shortly after birth and therefore prevents the development of normal swallowing skills. These etiologies affect the development of swallowing in a number of different ways. The child might have a respiratory problem that does not allow for the "suck, swallow, breath" pattern necessary for infant feeding. Or the child may have a sensory deficit such as autism that could cause rejection of some food textures. A cleft lip or palate significantly changes the anatomy and physiology necessary for feeding development.

The goal of dysphagia assessment and treatment with children is to aid in the development of skills needed to keep the child safe and well nourished. At the same time, the dysphagia team develops a plan to ensure that the child will stay well nourished while these skills are being developed. Children may be referred for a dysphagia evaluation based on a number of different referral criteria or etiologies. Following are two of the most common etiologies, prematurity and cerebral palsy, and the resultant swallowing problems.

Prematurity

The ability to suck and swallow develops prenatally. Swallowing is thought to begin somewhere between 12 and 17 weeks gestation. It is known that the fetal swallow aids in controlling the amount of amniotic fluid ingested. However, sucking is not firmly established until 30 to 34 weeks gestation. Along with the development of sucking, primitive reflexes help the newborn to establish a functional eating pattern. These reflexes also develop during the last 4 to 8 weeks of gestation. For this reason, a premature baby may not have the ability to suck milk from a nipple. Weak facial muscles and underdeveloped lungs can also contribute to this difficulty. The full-term normal infant uses a rhythmic suck–swallow–breathe pattern to take in nutrition. The premature baby may exhibit an uncoordinated suck and swallow, a weak suck, or breathing disruptions during feeding.

Cerebral Palsy

Children with cerebral palsy have a wide range of feeding problems. The type and severity of the feeding problem depend on the degree of motor deficit. There are several different kinds of cerebral palsy, and each has a different movement pattern. Typically, there is an increase in muscle tone and a decrease in the range of movement.

Cognitive deficits can also result in problems that affect all stages of the swallow. With cognitive deficits, the child may not understand what food is or that it needs to be put in the mouth to be eaten. There may be a reduction in lip closure, lingual control, or jaw control. Bolus formation is often poor, and increased time may be required for oral transit. Children with cognitive deficits may have inadequate velopharyngeal closure, which causes a delay in the pharyngeal swallow. Laryngeal elevation and pharyngeal peristalsis may also be affected by the abnormal tone and muscle strength. The child with cerebral palsy is often a slow, inefficient eater with a high risk for aspiration.

Pediatric Dysphagia Evaluation

The assessment procedures for children are similar to those for adults. The SLP reviews past medical history and current medical status, performs a NICE, and then, if warranted, proceeds to do an instrumental examination. For children, each step has a different focus or different questions to be answered. The following is a review of each of the assessment procedures with the key changes that are needed for the pediatric population.

Review of Medical and Feeding History and Current Feeding Methods

Because the focus of pediatric dysphagia is children who are having difficulty acquiring normal eating skills, it is crucial to understand any underlying medical conditions and how these conditions may contribute to current feeding problems. Therefore, to understand why a child has not developed normal eating and swallowing skills, the SLP must gather information about the child's prenatal history, birth history, early feeding problems, preferred positioning, preferred textures, types of utensils, respiratory status, use of alternative feeding methods, medications, seizures, and signs of distress during eating.

Bedside Clinical Assessment

The BCA provides information about a child's current eating status. The examination includes information about the child's level of alertness, muscle tone, movement patterns, respiratory status, and structure and function of the face and mouth. As with adults, the BCA leads to a determination of whether it is safe to use food as a part of the swallowing assessment. If food can be used, sucking or chewing is observed. The SLP looks for lip, tongue, and jaw movements, along with any changes in respiratory function. With children, the way in which the lips and tongue are used to get the food off the spoon is also noted, along with the kind of motor movement that is used for chewing. If a baby is being evaluated, the SLP assesses the rate and strength of sucking, along with the suck–swallow–breathe sequence. Any additional behaviors such as nasopharyngeal reflux, lethargy, coughing, choking, gagging, or arching of the back are noted. As with adults, if the results of the NICE indicate possible pharyngeal stage problems, then an instrumental assessment is completed.

Instrumental Assessment

Currently, the MBS procedure is used to a much greater degree than endoscopy with the pediatric population. For an MBS with children, additional procedures include (1) conducting the MBS in the child's current seating system; (2) using food textures that are similar to what the child currently eats; and (3) using the child's own utensils—bottle, special cup, spoon, and so on.

Pediatric Treatment Planning

Based on the information gained from the review of the child's medical and feeding history, NICE, and MBS, the dysphagia team formulates a treatment plan designed to address two major goals. The first goal is a way for the child to meet current nutritional needs while remaining safe so that the child can grow and remain healthy. The second goal is focused on techniques or strategies that will improve both oral-motor and pharyngeal stage functioning. This second goal is also directed toward normalizing the child's eating and swallowing skills.

SUMMARY

Swallowing includes a series of overlapping stages that prepare food and move it through the pharynx and esophagus to the stomach. Swallowing disorders frequently occur with speech disorders and fall within the professional province of the SLP. The dysphagia team uses clinical and instrumental procedures to identify the stage of swallowing affected and to develop strategies that allow the individual to maintain nutrition and hydration.

STUDY QUESTIONS

1. What are the stages of swallowing?

2. What are three disorders that cause dysphagia?

3. What is the SLP's role in assessing and treating swallowing disorders?

4. How are swallowing problems different in children compared to adults?

5. What happens when food or fluid enters the trachea?

6. Why is the assessment and treatment of dysphagia included in the scope of practice for the SLP?

7. In addition to the SLP, which other professionals typically are members of the dysphagia team?

KEY TERMS

Aspiration	Gastric tube (G-tube)	Modified barium swallow (MBS)
Bolus	Intravenous (IV)	Nasogastric tube (NG tube)
Dysphagia	Medulla	Peristalsis

REFERENCES

American Speech-Language-Hearing Association. (1987). *Ad hoc committee on dysphagia report.* Rockville, MD: Author.

American Speech-Language-Hearing Association. (2002). *Omnibus survey caseload report.* Rockville, MD: Author.

Cherney, L. (1994). *Clinical management of dysphagia in adults and children* (2nd ed.). Gaithersburg, MD: Aspen.

Martin, B., & Corlew, M. (1990). The incidence of communication disorders in dysphagic patients. *Journal of Speech and Hearing Disorders, 55,* 28–32.

Miller, R. M., & Groher, M. E. (1993). Speech-language pathology and dysphagia: A brief historical perspective. *Dysphagia, 8,* 180–184.

SUGGESTED READINGS

Arvedson, J. C., & Brodsky, L. (2002). *Pediatric swallowing and feeding* (2nd ed.). Clifton Park, NY: Thomson Delmar Learning.

Corbin-Lewis, K., Liss, J., & Sciortini, K. (2005). *Clinical anatomy and physiology of the swallow mechanism.* Baltimore: Thomson.

Crary, M., & Groher, M. (2003). *Introduction to adult swallowing disorders.* New York: Elsevier Science.

Fraker, C., & Walbert, L. (2003). *From NICU to childhood: Evaluation and treatment of pediatric swallowing disorders.* Austin, TX: Pro-Ed.

Murry, T., & Carrau, R. (2006). *Clinical management of swallowing disorders* (2nd ed.). San Diego, CA: Plural.

Rosenthal, S. R., Sheppard, J. J., & Lotze, M. (1995). *Dysphagia and the child with developmental disabilities.* San Diego, CA: Singular.

Yorkston, K., Miller, R., & Strand, E. (2004). *Management of speech and swallowing disorders in degenerative diseases* (2nd ed.). Austin, TX: Pro-Ed.

Individuals With Language Disorders

ten
chapter ten

Language Disorders in Infants, Toddlers, and Preschoolers

ELIZABETH D. PEÑA AND BARBARA L. DAVIS

LEARNING OBJECTIVES

1. To understand what a language disorder is.

2. To differentiate between language problems in the areas of language form, content, and use.

3. To become familiar with different service delivery settings.

4. To have a basic understanding of the components of an assessment for young children.

5. To compare and contrast different intervention approaches.

As noted in Chapter 1, many different kinds of children have difficulty learning language. For example, children who are born with Down syndrome (a genetic cause of mental retardation), severe hearing impairment (a sensory deficit), or fetal alcohol syndrome (difference in prenatal development caused by maternal alcohol use) are likely to have problems learning and using language. In addition, some children have problems acquiring language even though no obvious cause can be found. Such children are usually referred to as having a **developmental language disorder** or a **specific language impairment**.

Children with developmental language disorders may communicate differently from their peers. That is, their language abilities are more like the language of children who are much younger. Decisions about clinical diagnosis and appropriate intervention strategies are often based on comparisons of the child's language abilities with children of the same age and/or with children who have the same types of language difficulties. This chapter explores these issues in detail. First, we define some important terms to help you understand developmental language disorders.

BOX 10-1   Overview of CD-ROM Segments

The CD-ROM that accompanies this book contains four short video segments of two children (ages 3 and 5) with language impairment. All the segments provide examples of the kinds of language difficulties that children with language impairments experience. The first segment (Ch.10.01) shows language form errors. The second (Ch.10.02) and third (Ch.10.03) segments provide examples of content-based expressive difficulties. Finally, the fourth segment (Ch.10.04) shows a 3-year-old child with limited language output who nevertheless demonstrates appropriate social interaction (pragmatics).

Segments

Ch.10.01	The 5-year-old girl is interacting with her clinician by playing with a house and a set of figures. She is pretending to be an older boy who wants to drive. She makes tense agreement errors during this interaction.
Ch.10.02	In this video clip, you see a 3-year-old girl reading a book with the examiner. She responds to questions posed by the examiner.
Ch.10.03	This video clip shows the 5-year-old girl playing with a stuffed giraffe and a doctor's kit. She pretends to examine the giraffe. This segment shows her using nonspecific language in response to clinician questions.
Ch.10.04	In this example, the 3-year-old girl is playing with a dish and food set. She responds to contextualized requests nonverbally and uses some single-word utterances.

CHILDREN WITH DEVELOPMENTAL LANGUAGE DISORDERS

There are children who do not learn language easily or well for a variety of reasons. The next section of this chapter provides information about the nature of language disorders in children, the ways that language disorders are diagnosed, and some of the more prevalent types of language disorders.

Definition of Language Disorder

According to the American Speech-Language-Hearing Association (1993), "a language disorder is the impairment or deviant development of comprehension and/or use of a spoken, written, and/or other symbol system. The disorder may involve (1) the form of language (phonologic, morphologic, and syntactic systems), (2) the content of language (semantic system), and/or (3) the function of language in communication (pragmatic system) in any combination" (p. 1).

Consider this definition in greater detail. Speech-language pathologists (SLPs) can recognize errors in the form, content, or use of language. Form errors are reflected in ungrammatical sentences. For example, a child with language form errors might say something like, "*the block fall**ed** down*" or "*I play the truck*" (for *I am playing . . .*). Utterances with content errors do not make sense. For example, a child might say, "*the ball is **on** the table*" when it is really under the table. Finally, use errors interfere with the social appropriateness. Children with language use errors may interrupt people repeatedly, fail to contribute to conversations, or change the topic too often. Typically developing children make the kinds of errors just described, and children who come from different cultural and linguistic backgrounds sometimes produce these same kinds of errors. So, errors alone are not a definite indicator of a disorder. How does the clinician know when a language error indicates an impairment? What standard should language performance be compared to?

Parents and teachers become concerned about a child's language development when it appears that the child is not expressing him- or herself as well as other children of the same age. There are two ways to think about the concept of "same age." **Chronological age** refers to the amount of time that has elapsed since a child's birth. SLPs typically use chronological age in years and months to determine a child's age and to compare him or her to other children of the "same age." This is done by subtracting the child's date of birth (expressed in year/month/date) from the date of assessment (also expressed in year/month/date) to obtain an age that is expressed in years-months-days. Days from 16–31 are rounded up to 1 month, and days from 1–15 are rounded down to 0 month so that the chronological age is expressed in years and months. Assume, for example, that you were collecting a language sample on August 21, 2009 (2009/8/21), from a boy who was born on December 9, 2004 (2004/12/5). This child would be 4 years, 8 months, and 16 days old the day you collected his language sample. Rounding the days up, you would say this child was 4 years, 9 months old, and you would write his chronological age as 4;9 (years; months).

Developmental age refers to the typical chronological age at which a child can perform a skill in a given area, in this case, language. Clinicians determine developmental age by collecting samples of the child's language and comparing the child's content, form, and use of language to what is known about typical ranges of development. Children with language disorders nearly always present a pattern in which their developmental language age is lower than their chronological age. Recall from Chapter 2, however, that there is a great deal of individual variation in the rate of language development, making it impossible to pinpoint a specific age at which a particular aspect of language develops. Rather, SLPs usually think about ranges of development. For example, a child who is 4 years old may combine only two words together into short, incomplete sentences (e.g., "want car"). Sentences like this are typical for a child who is between 18 and 24 months old. In this example, it appears that the child's chronological age may be 2 years more than his language developmental age.

Some clinicians consider comparisons between a child's chronological age and his or her language developmental age when they diagnose language disorder. In the past, it has been common for clinicians to use a 1- or 2-year difference between a child's chronological age and language developmental age as a criterion for identifying a language disorder. There are two problems with this way of thinking. First, as noted earlier, it is nearly impossible to pinpoint a child's language developmental age. Second, a 1- or 2-year discrepancy between chronological and developmental ages in a 2-year-old child is not quite the same as a 1-year discrepancy between chronological age and developmental age in a 7-year-old child. For this reason, clinicians often base their decisions about the presence or absence of a language disorder on a variety of factors.

Some clinicians use poor performance on formal tests as an indicator of disorder. They administer language tests to compare a child's language ability to that of other children of the same chronological age and social/cultural background. The purpose of testing is to determine whether a child's test score is significantly lower than the average score for children that age. If a child scores too low on one or more language tests, it is assumed that he or she has a language disorder. This approach to diagnosis, known at the **neutralist approach**, does not account for social and cultural influences on language development or for the kinds of language expectations that exist in the child's everyday environment (Tomblin, 2006). Instead, it relies solely on comparisons between one child's performance and the average performance of other children of the same age. The word *neutralism* has been applied to this position because formal language tests are *neutral* on the importance of considering social norms and expectations in identification.

Paul (2006) defines a language disorder as "a significant deficit in learning to talk, understand, or use any aspect of language appropriately, relative to both environmental and norm-referenced expectations for children of similar developmental level" (p. 4). She goes on to suggest that clinicians should take into account how language problems affect daily interaction with others. If a child's language problems are likely to result in negative social, psychological, educational, and vocational consequences, Fey (1986) believes the child should receive language intervention. This approach to identifying children with language disorders is sometimes called the **normativist approach** because it values social norms and focuses on the functional consequences of problems with language.

A growing number of clinicians combine the neutralist and normativist approaches to identifying language disorder. Paul (2006) suggests that language impairment should be defined relative to both social expectations and performance on formal language tests. SLPs who take this perspective consider the child's test scores in light of the social norms in the environment, parental or teacher expectations, and the child's functional communication at home and at day care or preschool.

Types of Language Disorders

Language disorders are often categorized according to their cause. Nelson (2010) classifies the factors that play a role in language disorders into central processing factors, peripheral factors, and environmental and emotional factors. Central processing factors are thought to relate to the part of the brain that controls language and cognitive development. Types of disorders in this category include specific language impairment, mental retardation, central auditory processing disorder, autism, and acquired brain injury. Peripheral factors directly cause impairment in the motor or sensory systems. Peripheral factors influence how language is perceived and processed. Hearing impairment, visual impairment, deaf-blindness, and other physical impairments are examples of the types of peripheral factors that are related to language disorders. These factors may contribute to language impairment, but the presence of these factors does not always cause language impairments. Environmental and emotional factors that do not have a physical cause can influence language development. Problematic environmental and emotional factors include neglect and abuse, behavioral problems, and emotional problems. Finally, some language problems may be a result of a combination of factors. Unfortunately, mixed-factor causes often result in more severe disabilities that involve the cognitive, sensory, and motor systems.

Nelson's (2010) system for categorizing language disorders helps SLPs classify children with language impairments and suggests possible causes for the disorder. This system is not perfect, however. In most cases, clinicians can only speculate about the factor or factors that may have led to a language disorder originally. In addition, clinical categories of language disorders are not completely independent of each other. Many children with language impairments present language profiles that could fit into more than one category. For example, the language abilities of a child with mental retardation may be quite similar to the language abilities of a child who has been neglected or abused. Sometimes, the setting the child is observed in and the measures used during evaluation can influence how children with language impairment are identified. For example, children with language impairment may appear to fit a "central factor" diagnosis in a clinical setting based on formal language measures, whereas in a school setting, they may fit a "behavioral" factor diagnosis based on a combination of cognitive, language, and social-adaptive measures. The final problem with attempts to place children with language disorders into subcategories is that approaches to language intervention have little to do with subtypes of disorders. There is a danger in thinking that one intervention technique is right for one kind of syndrome or that a given child may be representative of that syndrome. Many intervention techniques work well with children whose language disorders result from quite different factors. Regardless of the cause or causes of a child's language disorder, clinicians should plan intervention that is appropriate for the child's developmental level, that matches his or her interests, and that provides the child with the kind of language needed to function better in his or her everyday environments.

Age-Related Stages

Language disorders may be characterized somewhat differently for infants and toddlers in comparison to preschoolers. Age distinctions matter because children have different communication abilities and needs as they develop. A language disorder may manifest one way at one point in time and another way at a later point.

At or near the time of birth, few overt communication behaviors can be assessed. Nonetheless, some infants are eligible for services and receive them. Clinicians who work with infants often base their decisions to provide treatment on the presence or absence of conditions such as prenatal (before birth) or perinatal (at birth) risk factors that are known to lead to language impairment and other developmental disorders.

As the infant develops during the first year of life, clinicians can attend to behavioral risk factors that are closely tied to communication. These include lack of eye contact, lack of consistent responsiveness to the environment, and slow development of speech and motor milestones (Billeaud, 1995). At present, very precise ways to identify children at risk for language impairment in the first year of life are nonexistent unless they are severely involved.

Infants' comprehension of language form, content, and use grows dramatically during the second year of life (ages 12 months to 24 months) as they begin to understand more about the environment that surrounds them and begin to exhibit language-based communication. Between the ages of 12 and 24 months, many communication, vocabulary, and speech behaviors develop, which provide more behaviors for clinicians to examine in language assessment. By the time children are 3 years old (the beginning of the preschool period), clinicians can look for a full range of language abilities (phonology, morphology, semantics, syntax, and pragmatics).

Careful description of children's language difficulties in different contexts and their level of development is necessary for identifying language disorders and planning intervention. A description of a child's language strengths and needs in the areas of language form, content, and use helps clinicians consider individual components of language as well as the ways components interact.

DISORDERS OF FORM, CONTENT, AND USE

As noted in Chapters 2 and 11 SLPs typically examine three aspects of language development: form, content, and use. **Form** refers to the structure of language including syntax, morphology, and phonology. **Content** refers to the meaning of language, known as semantics. **Use** refers to the social aspects of language, known as pragmatics.

Comprehension and **expression** are additional facets of description that are important in understanding language disorders in children. Comprehension relates to the child's understanding of the world. For an infant, comprehension may be restricted

BOX 10-2 **"I Drive the Car"**

CD-ROM segment Ch.10.01 shows a 5-year-old girl playing with cars. She is pretending she is a 15-year-old boy who is learning to drive. She makes agreement errors as she interacts with her clinician. She says, "I drive the car," using the present instead of the past tense. Next, she says, "I didn't got yours," using the past tense instead of the present tense. In addition, in this sentence, she uses the more general verb "get" instead of "drive," which is a content-based error.

to understanding that his or her mother's tone of voice changes when she wants the baby's attention. As children grow and develop, they begin to understand language at finely grained levels. For example, 2-year-old children usually understand questions such as, *What is that?* Four-year-old children can understand questions like, *What is he doing with that?*

Language also involves expression; children must learn to produce language that integrates the dimensions of form, content, and use. Infants may not be able to produce words, but they may cry in certain ways to indicate hunger or pain. Thus, different cry patterns are a form of communication that conveys meaning to familiar communication partners. As they get older, children think more complex thoughts, and they learn the words and sentence structures needed for conveying those thoughts to others.

Language Disorders Related to Form

Children with language disorders frequently have trouble with the grammatical aspects of language. The next section summarizes the kinds of problems that infants, toddlers and preschoolers can have with the various dimensions of language form.

Infants/Toddlers

The earliest forms of communication in infants include vocalizations (including crying), body movements, and gestures (such as pointing). By the end of the first year, some children may produce a few consistent forms that are recognizable to familiar partners as "first words."

Two risk factors that are predictive of later language disorders in infants and toddlers include low frequency of vocalization and lack of syllable productions in babbling (Roberts, Rescorla, Girous, & Stevens, 1998). Extensive use of gesture in the absence of vocalization is also considered an important signal of potential risk for language disorder. It is important to remember that there is a great deal of individual variability in normal development during this period, and risk factors for later communication disorders are not well established. However, infants and toddlers with overt medical conditions such as prenatal (before birth) or perinatal (at birth) infections, low birth weight, pulmonary (breathing) difficulties, intracranial hemorrhage (bleeding from the blood vessels in the brain), and other birth defects often present communication disorders later in life (Tomblin, Hardy, & Hein, 1991).

Preschool Children

During the preschool period, children exhibit rapid growth in aspects of language form (phonology, morphology, and syntax). Typical preschool-age children should be able to produce most speech sounds and use them in a variety of words. They can be understood most of the time, although some of the more difficult sounds such as /r/, /s/, and /l/ may be mispronounced, and the children may make some errors producing long words like *hippopotamus*. Preschoolers also learn inflections for nouns and verbs (for example, *-ed* and *-s*) and how to create simple and complex sentences. Review Chapter 2 for more information on typical language development.

Every child with a language disorder presents a different language profile. But some specific aspects of grammar are likely to be omitted or used incorrectly. For example, in English bound morphemes such as *-ed* and *-s* may be problematic for children with language impairments. These children are likely to omit or use the wrong "be" verb forms (e.g., *am, is, are, was, were*). Certain classes of morphemes such as articles and pronouns can also be difficult to learn. Similar to the situation with the "be" verbs, children with language disorders often omit or misuse articles and pronouns. For example, a 4-year-old might say, *Him got ball*. Finally, children with form difficulties often produce sounds and sequences of sounds incorrectly. Children may have trouble actually making all the sounds of their language, or they may be able to produce all the sounds but not use them correctly in a variety of words. Chapter 5 details ways in which preschoolers may manifest form-based articulatory and phonological disorders.

Language Disorders Related to Content

Disorders related to content during the infant/toddler phase usually include difficulties establishing consistent contact with communication partners. Additional risk factors include poor turn taking and lack of balanced initiation and response in interactions with their caregivers. Impediments to this process may be sensory (hearing or vision deficits), motor (cerebral palsy or low muscle tone), cognitive (mental retardation), or social-emotional (effects of neglect). The effect of these impediments is to render either the child or the environment unable to maintain the consistent contact necessary for the development of meaning.

Semantic knowledge and use are important aspects of language development and assessment. For children who are producing about one to two words per utterance (between the ages of 18 and 36 months), Brown (1973) suggests examining the use of relational categories. These categories account for most of what children at this stage of development are producing (see Table 10-1).

At more advanced stages of development, it is important to observe children's knowledge of different word classes. For example, preschool children should be able to respond to questions that begin with *what, where, whose, why, how many, how,* and *when*. They should have knowledge of concepts such as colors and spatial terms. They should be able to categorize objects, and they should be able to describe and understand similarities and differences among objects.

Semantic difficulties that preschool children with language impairments exhibit include restricted vocabulary size and reduced comprehension of basic concepts (spatial terms, temporal terms, deictic terms, kinship terms, color terms, etc.). They may have a limited range of semantic relations that are expressed within sentences such as

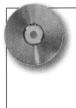

BOX 10-3   "Touch and Feel" Book

CD-ROM segment Ch.10.02 shows a 3-year-old girl looking through a "touch and feel" book with an examiner. Each page in the book has a picture of an object. The child's attention is focused on concepts such as texture, color, and functions. This child has some difficulty understanding the content of the book. Although she is able to understand language in context, she has difficulty understanding and expressing concepts such as colors, descriptions (soft/scratchy), and actions (What's he doing?).

Table 10-1   Semantic Categories

Semantic Category	Subcategories	Examples
Basic concepts	Spatial terms	up, down, in
	Temporal terms	when, before
	Deictic terms	this/that
	Kinship terms	dad, sister, aunt
	Relational terms—physical	thick/thin
	Relational terms—interrogatives	who, which, what
	Colors	blue, green, red
Semantic relations	Possessor + possession	Mom shoe
	Recurrence + X	Cracker more
	Attribute + entity	sock stink
	Nonexistence or disappearance	Bye-bye juice
	Rejection or negation	No
	Demonstrative + entity	This juice
	X + locative	Sit down
	X + dative	Ten (take this) mom
	Agent + action	Daddy eat
	Action + object	Throw ball
	Agent + object	Dog ball
Embedding and conjoining	Sequential	And then, First . . . next
	Causal	Because
	Conditional	If . . . then
	Temporal	When, before, after, then
	Disjunctive	But, or

Source: Adapted from Brown, R. (1973). *A first language: The early stages.* Cambridge, MA: Harvard University Press.

> **BOX 10-4 "Doctor, Doctor"**
>
> CD-ROM segment Ch.10.03 shows a 5-year-old girl playing with a giraffe and a doctor's kit. She pretends to examine the giraffe. The child uses nonspecific language. The toys are used as props that provide context for listener understanding. Children with content-based difficulties often use more "general" language in interaction. In one case, she says, "How about if I do this" to indicate tapping the giraffe's legs with the hammer. Later, the clinician asks the child, "Why did the giraffe say ouch?" Notice that the child acts out the response and says, "Because this was going like this." Children with language impairment often use nonspecific words in the place of specific vocabulary and explanations.
>
> A little later, the child reaches for the otoscope, and the clinician asks her what it's for. Note the amount of time that it takes the child to respond and the nonspecific response, "It's for checking something." It's important to note that previously in the interaction, the child has said she was going to check the giraffe's ears, so she has the vocabulary and knowledge of the function. However, she does not recall words at the moment they are needed to answer the question.

possession, recurrence, and location, or between clauses such as sequential, causal, and conditional. Finally, preschoolers with language impairment may have problems using a range of conjunctions (e.g., *but*, *so*).

Language Disorders Related to Use

Children with impairments in prelinguistic aspects of language use may not use their bodies for varied types of communication with those around them (**prelinguistic communication**). The most consistent manifestation of use impairments is found in children older than 6 months of age who fail to engage in intentional actions related to the world around them. These children appear to be passive observers in life rather than active participants. Later, these children may not point at objects they want, and they may use words to express a restricted range of meanings. For example, a typically developing 14-month-old child may use the word *Daddy* in a variety of contexts (indicating surprise when Daddy walks into a room, asking for help, telling who a pair of shoes belongs to, and naming a person in a picture). The same age child with a language disorder may use the word *Daddy* only when his mother points to his father and asks, "Who's that?" These differences show a restricted range of communicative functions and lack of communicative initiation.

By the time they are between 3 and 5 years old, typically developing children take turns for three to five exchanges, adjust their speech style to the listener, and make revisions during turn taking. During conversations with their peers, preschoolers are able to use phrases and sentences to both initiate and to respond in conversation. Social initiations include making requests, comments, statements, disagreements, and performatives (claims, jokes, teasing, protests). Responsive acts include responses to

> **BOX 10-5   Pragmatics**
>
> CD-ROM segment Ch.10.04 shows a 3-year-old girl interacting with the examiner while playing with a set of food and dishes. She uses a few words, typically in one-word utterances. Her low level of language output suggests difficulties in the area of expressive language. She does understand quite a bit of contextualized language and demonstrates appropriate social pragmatic responses to adult requests. In this example, she understood and responded to the request, "Would you pour me some milk?" She selected a cup, got the milk bottle, poured pretend milk, and handed it to the examiner. She then responded affirmatively to the question, "Do you want some milk?" by pouring herself pretend milk and drinking it.

requests for information, action, clarification, attention, assertives, performatives, and imitations. Additionally, preschoolers can select, introduce, maintain, and change topics quite readily (Fey, 1986).

Problems affecting the area of pragmatics may include limited verbal communication and a lack of a variety of language forms. Preschoolers may have difficulty initiating and maintaining communication. For example, they may not know how to ask for clarifications when they don't understand something, or they may not know how to restate something they have said (a conversational repair) when someone does not understand them. They may also express their meanings in appropriate ways. Most preschoolers learn their teachers' names quickly, and they know how to ask for something politely. In the preschool classroom, they might say something like, *Miss Jones, can I have some crayons?* The child with a language disorder might say something like, *Teacher, want colors.*

SERVICE DELIVERY

Language intervention is usually conducted in two types of service delivery settings: educational and medical. Educational service delivery settings are those affiliated in some way with an educational institution such as a public or private school. Medical service delivery settings are affiliated with a hospital or rehabilitation unit. In both settings, the SLP operates in concert with the family to make decisions regarding assessment and treatment of the preschooler with language disorders. There are differences in the kinds of services routinely provided in these settings. The following subsections explore the differences between the two types of service delivery settings in greater detail.

Educational Settings

Laws affect the way intervention is provided to infants and toddlers in educational settings. PL 99-457 and the Individuals with Disabilities Education Act of 2004 (IDEA) require early identification and intervention services for children from birth to 36 months of age. PL 99-457 emphasizes the provision of services designed to help families address children's special needs within the context of the family. An important part of working with infants and toddlers in educational settings is a focus on family-centered practice. **Family-centered practice** is when speech-language professionals work with families to identify, describe, and develop an appropriate intervention plan for each child. The family has the ultimate choice in the kinds of services provided and in the extent they want to participate in the process. It is important for professionals to seek the family's perspective on the child's strengths and needs. Because the emphasis is on working in the context of the family, assessment and intervention decisions should be consistent with cultural expectations. The primary concerns of the family may be different from those of professionals, but the family is allowed to make final decisions about the nature and the extent of the services provided. Thus, professionals should serve as a support and resource for family decision making.

For children birth to 3 years of age, PL 99-457 mandates service provision in the "least restrictive environment." In many states, the "least restrictive environment" is interpreted to mean the child's own home. This setting allows the family to be involved in the implementation of the treatment plan to the fullest extent possible. There are times, however, when the home may not be the best place for intervention. For example, some families may not want strangers in their home, preferring instead to take their child to a school or clinic for intervention.

IDEA Part B relates specifically to services for preschool-age children. Like PL 99-457, IDEA Part B states that parents should be part of the assessment process from the onset. Parents must be notified about any services for or evaluation of their child. They must be told about their right to view any records or reports regarding their child. Parents also have the right to seek an evaluation outside the local educational agency. Thus, the law requires that parents are integrally involved in assessment and intervention decisions.

SLPs often work collaboratively with preschool teachers and early childhood special educators to provide intervention within classrooms. The SLP may suggest ways the teacher can help the child participate in daily classroom activities. For example, a child who has difficulty with *why* questions may need to be asked simpler *what* questions during circle time, while the teacher and other children model ways of responding to *why* questions. This way, the child can participate during circle time with a high level of success.

Medical Settings

In medical settings, assessment and intervention practices are often driven by insurance company requirements. This is a consequence of the way medical services are funded in the United States right now. The active involvement of parents and families is optional based on the rules and procedures of each medical setting. The child is viewed as an individual for purposes of service reimbursement, and assessment and treatment are much more likely to be conducted in individual sessions. Clinicians who are delivering services for insurance reimbursement rarely provide intervention in the child's everyday environment. But they typically make home suggestions to increase carryover.

Reimbursement for assessment and treatment in both public and private medical settings is in a state of transition, as both government and private insurers deal with changes in Medicare, Medicaid, and managed health care. SLPs will need to remain flexible in the near term in medical service delivery settings to continue to develop and maintain best clinical practices in a changing field.

ASSESSMENT

Two important roles of SLPs are to evaluate children's language development and determine whether or not they present a language disorder. This section provides information about methods for assessing language development and diagnosing language disorders in infants, toddlers, and preschoolers.

Infants/Toddlers

Assessment of language disorder in infants and toddlers is related to the issue of prediction (Rescorla & Alley, 2001). Clinicians must collect the kinds of information about the child's language development that will help them predict which children with delays will eventually develop normally and which children will continue to show speech and language impairments. The most severely involved infants and toddlers with known etiologies for their impairment are the easiest to diagnose. Infants and toddlers with less overt developmental delays (e.g., those who may show only language impairment) are not easily diagnosed because their differences may be at the lower end of the range of normal variation for a period of time.

Often, assessment with this population is conducted simultaneously by professionals from different disciplines. In educational settings, IDEA mandates assessment teams made up of professionals from a variety of disciplines. As a result, the SLP will likely work closely with occupational therapists, physical therapists, social workers, and educational professionals. The most common model of assessment and team collaboration is termed **transdisciplinary assessment** (Kaczmarek, Pennington, & Goldstein, 2000). Transdisciplinary assessment involves collaboration and consensus building among professionals from many disciplines. One professional is usually designated as the coordinator of care to reduce the number of professionals handling the young child and to decrease the amount of intrusion into a family's life. The team is headed by different professionals depending on the most crucial problem for the child.

In medical settings, infants and toddlers are likely to be evaluated and diagnosed by a **multidisciplinary assessment** team, which usually includes a physician, an occupational therapist, a physical therapist, a social worker, and an SLP plus other medical specialists as needed. In the multidisciplinary approach, professionals conduct their own independent evaluations and then share their results in a team meeting. There is likely to be more limited exchange of information across disciplines than is typical of the transdisciplinary model. The physician, as the head of each team, has the final say over which professionals see the child and what recommendations result from the assessment process.

Test instruments and analyses are more likely to be broad-based assessments of general development than to be focused on communication or language development alone. One reason for this broad focus is the criteria for entry into educational intervention programs as well as the likelihood of multiple areas of impairment in medical settings. Although criteria vary from state to state within the United States, three types of diagnostic categories are typical: developmental delay (delay in one or more areas including motor, cognitive, sensory, social-emotional), atypical development (development in one or more of the preceding areas that is not typical of normally developing children at any stage), or medical risk factor (known risk factors for developmental delay such as severe mental retardation or cleft palate). With such broad criteria, assessment instruments are needed that qualify children for services and indicate directions for intervention in a number of areas.

Two types of tests are available for this population: **standardized assessment** instruments and **criterion-referenced assessment** instruments. Standardized tests compare the child to other children the same chronological age in a given area (e.g., motor development). An example of a standardized test is the Battelle Developmental Inventory, Second Edition (BDI-2) (Newborg, 2007). The BDI-2 is a test that can be used to obtain developmental age scores for personal-social skills, adaptive behaviors, motor skills, communication, and cognition.

Criterion-referenced tests outline patterns of strength and areas that need intervention within a single child (e.g., child is not sitting up at 15 months, needs help with muscle strength). The Rosetti Infant Toddler Language Scale (Rosetti, 2006) is a criterion-referenced scale that is often used to plan intervention rather than to compare toddlers to others their age. It has items in the areas of interaction-attachment, pragmatics, gesture, play, language comprehension, and language expression. Most instruments for prelinguistic children include a direct child response format (ask questions and wait for responses), an observational format (watch the child play), and a parent report format (ask the parent questions) to provide as many ways as possible for the clinician to explore the child's skills. In addition, informal observation and sampling are important because the infant or toddler may not be able to cooperate with a test procedure because of age or extreme disability.

Preschool Children

Preschool children who are suspected of having language impairment should undergo a complete language evaluation. Generally, assessment questions take two forms: "Does this child have language impairment?" and "What should be done about it?" Most of the time, the clinician should answer both questions with an assessment of language abilities related to expectations for the child's chronological age. The first question is one of identification. The child is compared to typically developing peers to find out whether language development is significantly delayed in comparison to children who are the same chronological age. This comparison can answer whether the child's language is impaired. Next, the clinician analyzes the child's language to determine the child's level of language development. Intervention often focuses on language skills that are lacking in the child with a language disorder but that usually appear in younger, typically developing children who are functioning at the same language level. In other words, the clinician looks for aspects of language that make the child with a language disorder different from most children.

A combination of assessment tools and analyses is appropriate for understanding the difference between the child's developmental and chronological age levels. These include use of standardized testing, criterion-referenced testing, and **interactive assessment**.

As noted in the previous section, SLPs can use standardized assessment to determine how a child compares to peers. Some of the tests used for this age and purpose include the Preschool Language Scale-4 (PLS-4; Zimmerman, Steiner, & Pond, 2002), Clinical Evaluation of Language Fundamentals-Preschool-2 (CELF-P:2; Wiig, Secord, & Semel, 2005), and Test of Language Development-4 Primary (TOLD-P:4; Newcomer & Hammill, 2008). These tests evaluate many areas of language form and content and provide a score of general language performance that clinicians can use to compare the child to same-age peers. The kinds of items that appear on these tests include asking the child to point to colored blocks in response to an examiner's question (as on the PLS-4), questions about a story (as on the CELF-P:2), and sentences the child is asked to repeat (as on the TOLD-P:4). Some tests are specific to one area of language. For example, the Expressive One-Word Picture Vocabulary Test-2000 (Brownell, 2000) provides information about expressive vocabulary by asking the child to name pictures presented on test plates. It is important to note that many of the tests used to assess language ability do not do a good job of distinguishing between children with typical development and those with language impairment (Spaulding, Plante, & Farinella, 2006). Thus, it is critical that in selecting tests clinicians use those that have the best classification accuracy.

Criterion-referenced approaches to assessment are used to help clinicians develop better descriptions of performance and to plan intervention. Examples of criterion-referenced procedures include checklists of language behaviors, inventories, and language sampling. For example, language sampling provides useful information about a child's level of syntactic or grammatical performance. The examiner records by video or audiotape a play session or a conversation with the child. These sessions usually last about 20 minutes. The conversation is transcribed (written out), and the clinician analyzes and codes at least 50 sequential utterances. Clinicians usually determine the mean length of utterance, which is the average number of morphemes in each utterance. They also look for the types of syntactic structures that the child uses, and they assess the types of meanings that the child expresses. These measures are compared to what is known about language development to determine where the child is in the language development process. Incorrect forms or missing forms may become targets for intervention, depending on when they are expected to develop.

For vocabulary development, a standardized test may tell whether the child is performing below the expected chronological age level. However, it does not tell what kinds of words or word classes the child is having difficulty with. Further observation of vocabulary knowledge and use using structured probes may provide this information. For example, clinicians can devise a list of question types, prepositions, or attributes (color, size, shape) that the child may need for preschool success. Then, they can systematically test these through play to see what the child can express or understand. One example of such a probe would be to devise a "hiding game." With a puppet or stuffed animal, the clinician hides a ball in various places (in, under, on top) and the child helps the puppet find the ball. The clinician may ask the child to help the puppet find the ball that is under the bed to test comprehension of spatial prepositions or to tell the puppet where the ball is to test expression of spatial terms.

Pragmatics or use is best assessed through observation of communication interactions. Again, the clinician may have a predetermined checklist of pragmatic behaviors to use in observing a child's communication. One possibility is to examine children's interactions with peers during a specific time period using Fey's (1986) model of assertiveness and responsiveness (see Figure 10-1). Here, the clinician writes down what the child says and does to initiate conversation (assertive acts) and to respond to others' initiations (responsive acts) during a predetermined length of time (for example, 10 minutes). The clinician tallies assertive versus responsive acts. Also, the clinician may note the percentage of communicative acts that were verbal or nonverbal and whether they were appropriate or inappropriate. The summary provides a picture of the types of interaction the child prefers and how the child performs these acts.

Nonbiased Assessment

SLPs should make sure their assessment is culturally and linguistically appropriate. This is especially important for infants, toddlers, and preschoolers. Not all children learn English as a first (or second) language. The developmental course of other languages is not necessarily like that of English. In addition, not all families share the same set of interaction styles or beliefs about the nature and role of children in the family and in the community. The possibility of a mismatch between parental and SLP expectations and beliefs makes it important for clinicians to understand variation in language learning and in socialization practices (refer to Chapter 3 for more information on these topics).

Historically, children from non-English-speaking backgrounds have been assessed in English. This practice may lead to misdiagnosis. Think about how well you would do on an intelligence test administered in Russian. Assuming you don't speak or understand Russian, you probably would not appear to be very smart, would you? Unfortunately, assessments conducted in children's second language can lead to misdiagnoses such as language impairment or mental retardation. Even though it seems obvious that children cannot be assessed in a language that is not their own, problems continue to persist. Some of these problems occur because the process of learning a second language or dialect variations is not well understood. Other problems may occur because interaction styles reflective of different cultures do not match mainstream expectations for test-taking behavior. For example, in some cultures, parents emphasize single-word labels during interactions with their children. These children are well prepared for taking a single-word expressive vocabulary test that requires a naming response. In other cultures, parents may not label objects for their children as often. A single-word expressive vocabulary test

Transcription/Description of Communicative Act	Assertive	Responsive

Figure 10-1 Observation of child interaction.

would be an unusual experience for these children. It is likely that their performance would be a reflection of their lack of experience with this type of task rather than language impairment.

Testing the Limits

Interactive assessment of form, content, and use allows SLPs to test beyond the limits of the behaviors that the child displays in nonteaching (e.g., testing) situations. In interactive assessment, the clinician evaluates how easily or well a child learns something that is specifically taught. It is like turning the teaching part of the child's intervention into assessment. This type of assessment helps rule out whether poor test performance is a result of little or limited exposure to the types of questions being asked or of not understanding the task itself. For children from culturally and linguistically diverse backgrounds, this step is particularly important. Many times, these children are misdiagnosed because they may not know the rules of testing language. They may be in the process of learning English as a second language. Furthermore, interactive assessment helps to guide intervention. There are differences between children who quickly and easily learn something new and those for whom new learning is difficult.

Interactive assessment is guided by several principles. First, there is intent to purposefully teach new information or new strategies (based on standardized and nonstandardized procedures). Second, the examiner observes what the child does as a result of the teaching. Third, this information helps the examiner to make a judgment about how much change the child is able to make in a short period given adult support.

The general procedure for utilizing interactive assessment is to examine the results of standardized or criterion-referenced assessment to determine where the child may be having difficulty. Typically, the clinician then targets one or two specific areas in a short intervention. The intervention is guided by principles of mediated learning that focus on helping children understand the goal of teaching, helping them hypothesize, and helping them develop strategies that will lead to success in the identified area of weakness. For example, if a child has trouble with vocabulary, the examiner would help him or her understand that the goal of the task is to think about names for things. The examiner might also help the child talk about hypothetical situations such as not having specific names for things and to think of different ways that vocabulary is used.

After a short mediation (typically two 20- to 30-minute sessions), the child is retested on what was taught to assess what changes occurred with teaching. The clinician also observes the approach and strategies the child uses in completing the test task. For example, if the focus was on vocabulary because the child scored low on an expressive vocabulary test, the clinician might see whether the child was able to respond to more items. The clinician may also see whether the error types differed from pre- to posttest. Children may make more attempts at naming or may move from using descriptions at the time of the pretest to using more nouns at the time of the posttest. Children who are able to make great changes after a very short period of teaching may have had limited experience with the task and may not need intervention. Children who make moderate or few changes from pre- to posttest and who demonstrate difficulty learning during the teaching sessions may require therapy. It is likely that those children who made moderate changes would make more rapid progress in therapy than children who made almost no change.

INTERVENTION

According to Fey (1986), intervention approaches with young children who have language impairment generally fall along a continuum of clinician-centered approaches to child-centered approaches. **Clinician-centered approaches** are those in which the clinician controls the intervention context, goals, and materials. **Child-centered approaches** often use less structured settings and stimulate language development indirectly in concert with the family.

Clinician-centered approaches are based on behavioral principles of learning in which the stimulus (clinician input) is designed to produce a correct response (child output). When the child produces the desired response, the clinician systematically provides reinforcement to increase the likelihood that the correct response will occur again. Advantages of this approach are that the clinician can provide lots of practice and the child receives immediate feedback. On the other hand, these approaches are often criticized for being too dissimilar to the situations in which language is actually used. Unfortunately, the unnaturalness of this kind of intervention reduces the likelihood that children will use the forms they learn in everyday conversations and interactions.

Child-centered approaches focus on facilitating language through more indirect means. The clinician is there to facilitate language through play or a whole language approach, but does not direct the activity. Similarly, family-centered approaches, especially in the case of early intervention, focus on the family as the primary unit of intervention. So, child-centered therapy looks much like play. However, the key is to have a clinician who is maximally responsive to the child and responds in ways that are known to facilitate language development. Often clinicians will provide input at a higher rate than what children otherwise receive. Also, rather than focusing on specific language structures (i.e., auxiliary verbs), the clinician focuses on overall communication. The role of the clinician is to respond to communication attempts consistently and to provide linguistic models for the child to learn. Facilitative techniques include self-talk and parallel talk by the clinician in which running commentaries about the clinician's actions (self-talk) or the child's actions (parallel talk) are provided. Imitating the child may increase the probability that the child will, in turn, imitate the imitation. The clinician can expand a child's sentence to provide a more complete or complex model for the child, increasing the possibility that the child will realize the relationship between the meanings he or she wanted to express and the language forms that can express those meanings. Extensions provide additional content to what the child says. Again, this technique increases the possibility that children will use longer utterances.

A third intervention approach is somewhat in the middle of the two endpoints of the continuum that we have presented. This is referred to as a **hybrid approach**.

Hybrid approaches focus on one or two specific language goals. The clinician selects the activities and materials rather than following the child's lead and responds to the child's communication to model and highlight the specific forms targeted for intervention. One example of a hybrid approach is *focused stimulation*, in which the clinician designs the materials and activities in such a way that the child is likely to produce utterances for the targeted language form. Furthermore, the clinician provides lots of models within this context without requiring the child to produce the form. This technique helps children to improve comprehension as well as **production** skills.

Several language stimulation techniques have been shown to be helpful for children with language impairment. On the more clinician-centered side are techniques such as drill and drill-play. More child-centered techniques include indirect stimulation and whole language approaches. Table 10-2 provides some examples of these language stimulation techniques.

Regardless of which type of approach SLPs use, they need to think about the following parameters to select appropriate intervention targets:

Prior knowledge: Clinicians need to think carefully about the child's level of conceptual and linguistic development. Selected language goals need to be slightly more advanced than the abilities the child has and those that are likely to occur next in development.

Information processing: Clinicians need to take maximum advantage of the child's information processing system. For maximum attention, memory, and perception, they should provide slow-paced input, stress important words, give repeated examples, and vary the examples given.

Motivation: Clinicians should think about what the child finds interesting. Play-based intervention that takes the child's interests, needs, and cultural values into consideration should be incorporated into the intervention plan.

SUMMARY

Working with young children with language impairment is one of the many roles of an SLP. The SLP needs to know the laws and the professional guidelines that govern intervention with infants, toddlers, and preschoolers. The SLP works to improve the language of young children either directly through the assessment and intervention process or indirectly by working with families and others who interact with the child, such as parents and teachers. It is important that SLPs who work with young children have an understanding of normal as well as disordered language development and have a wide range of approaches for identification and intervention with this population. In this chapter, we have given you a broad overview of language impairments and some of the options clinicians have for working with this population.

Table 10-2 Language Stimulation Techniques

Stimulation Technique	Focus	Example
Drill	Clinician-centered	Phonology—contrastive drills. The clinician models word pairs that differ by one (target) phoneme, and the child repeats the pairs, for example, *cap/tap* (for targeting /k/.
Drill play	Clinician-centered	Syntax—sentence completion tasks given in a play situation. For example, when children produce the syntactic target in response to picture cards, they can move forward on a game board.
Self-talk	Child-centered	Clinicians talk about what they themselves are doing, seeing, and feeling as they play with children in an unstructured setting. This technique is especially appropriate for children whose language is emerging.
Parallel talk	Child-centered	Clinicians talk about what children are doing or looking at as they play in an unstructured setting. Again, this technique is appropriate with children who are beginning to use language to communicate.
Expansion	Child-centered	Clinicians repeat the child's utterance, adding grammatical and/or semantic information to make it complete. For example, the child might say, "Daddy peeling orange," and the clinician then says, "Daddy *is* peeling *an* orange."
Extension	Child-centered	Clinicians add information to what the child has said. For example, if the child says, "Daddy orange," the clinician might add, "Daddy peels the orange."
Recast	Child-centered	This is similar to expansions, but here the clinician changes the voice of the original statement. In the preceding example, where the child says, "Daddy orange," the clinician might recast the utterance as a question, "Is Daddy peeling the orange?"
Build-ups and breakdowns	Child-centered	The clinician expands the child's utterance (build-up), and then breaks it down into its components, and then builds it up again. Continuing with the previous example of the child saying, "Daddy orange," the clinician might then say, "Daddy is peeling the orange. Daddy is peeling. Peel the orange, Daddy. Daddy is peeling the orange."

BOX 10-6   Personal Story

Many clinicians (or future clinicians as the case may be) who are reading this chapter may not realize the importance of the distinctions between the different service delivery settings described here. Casey, an SLP, gained a full appreciation for these differences while working as an SLP in a developmental day care in Casper, Wyoming. Prior to working in Wyoming, she had only experienced a multidisciplinary model of service delivery. SLPs go in, do their own assessment, write their own report, make their own recommendations, and provide their prescribed intervention.

She became aware of the benefits of transdisciplinary assessment through her association with a young man whom we call Christopher. Christopher was 2 years old. He had been developing typically until he was found to have a fast-growing tumor in his spine (neuroblastoma). After the removal of the tumor, he was left with multiple problems including an inability to eat, walk, talk, and visually track objects or people. Needless to say, Casey's team of occupational therapists (who work with small motor movements like feeding), physical therapists (who work with large motor movements like walking), and SLPs (who work with feeding, speech, and language) was called to complete an evaluation. They worked under an educational and transdisciplinary model.

The team conducted the assessment plan over the course of a few days, and Christopher's parents were wholly integrated members of that team. They wrote one comprehensive report and made their recommendations as a unified team. The intervention was conducted in the same manner, with all professionals and family members working toward common goals. Although they provided fairly intensive, daily services to Christopher, they sent only one professional out per day (or two at the same time who worked together), armed with common goals constructed by all of their team members. Their intrusion into the lives of the family was minimal and Christopher's gains were good. He regained most of his skills with regard to eating, walking, and talking over the course of the following year.

Casey's old notion of a medical, multidisciplinary model would have involved separate assessments (by all team members), separate reports, separate intervention plans, and individually scheduled visits with each of the members of the team. One can only imagine how difficult it would have been for the family had they had to schedule three visits minimum (occupational, physical, and speech therapy) per day, 5 days per week to work with a severely involved 2-year-old while at the same time juggling naptime, playtime, doctor visits, and other family responsibilities.

STUDY QUESTIONS

1. What is a language disorder?

2. Define chronological age and developmental age.

3. Name and give an example of the three components of language.

4. What are similarities and differences in working with children 0–3 years old and 3–5 years old?

5. Why is the development of language use important?

6. How do you think language form and language content interact with language use?

7. How does the setting in which SLPs work with children affect service delivery?

8. What kinds of assessments are appropriate for young children?

9. What do different types of assessment contribute to the total picture of the child?

10. What are advantages and disadvantages of child-centered, clinician-centered, and hybrid intervention approaches?

KEY TERMS

Child-centered approaches
Chronological age
Clinician-centered approaches
Comprehension
Content
Criterion-referenced assessment
Developmental age
Developmental language disorder

Expression
Family-centered practice
Form
Hybrid approaches
Interactive assessment
Multidisciplinary assessment
Neutralist approach

Normativist approach
Prelinguistic communication
Production
Specific language impairment
Standardized assessment
Transdisciplinary assessment
Use

REFERENCES

American Speech-Language-Hearing Association. (1993). *Definitions of Communication Disorders and Variations* [Relevant Paper]. Available from www.asha.org/policy

Billeaud, F. (1995). *Communication disorder in infants and toddlers: Assessment and intervention.* Boston: Andover Medical Publishers.

Brown, R. (1973). *A first language: The early stages.* Cambridge, MA: Harvard University Press.

Brownell, R. (2000). *Expressive One Word Picture Vocabulary Test—2000 Edition.* Novato, CA: Academic Therapy Publications.

Fey, M. (1986). *Language intervention with young children.* Austin, TX: Pro-Ed.

Kaczmarek, L., Pennington, R., & Goldstein, H. (2000). Transdisciplinary consultation: A center-based team functioning model. *Education & Treatment of Children, 23*(1), 156–172.

Nelson, N. W. (2010). *Language and literacy disorders: Infancy through adolescence*. New York: Allyn & Bacon.

Newborg, F. (2007). *Batelle Developmental Inventory, Second Edition*. Rolling Meadows, IL: Riverside Publishing.

Newcomer, P., & Hammill, D. (2008). *Test of Oral Language Development: Primary—4th Edition*. Austin, TX: Pro-Ed.

Paul, R. (2006). *Language disorders from infancy through adolescence: Assessment and intervention*. St. Louis, MO: Mosby.

Rescorla, L., & Alley, A. (2001). Validation of the Language Development Survey (LDS): A parent report tool for identifying language delay in toddlers. *Journal of Speech, Language, and Hearing Research, 44*(2), 434–445.

Roberts, J., Rescorla, L., Girous, J., & Stevens, L. (1998). Phonological skills of children with specific expressive language impairment (SLI-E): Outcomes at age 3. *Journal of Speech, Language, and Hearing Research, 41*, 374–384.

Rosetti, L. (2006). *Rosetti Infant Toddler Language Scale*. East Moline, IL: Lingui Systems.

Spaulding, T. J., Plante, E., & Farinella, K. A. (2006). Eligibility criteria for language impairment: Is the low end of normal always appropriate? *Language, Speech, and Hearing Services in Schools, 37*(1), 61–72.

Tomblin, B., Hardy, J. C., & Hein, H. (1991). Predicting poor communication status in risk factors present at birth. *Journal of Speech and Hearing Research, 34*, 1096–1105.

Tomblin, J. B. (2006). A normativist account of language-based learning disability. *Learning Disabilities Research & Practice, 21*(1), 8–18.

Wiig, E., Secord, W., & Semel, E. (2005). *Clinical Evaluation of Language Fundamentals—Preschool, Second Edition*. San Antonio, TX: Psychological Corporation.

Zimmerman, I., Steiner, V., & Pond, R. (2002). *Preschool Language Scale-4*. San Antonio, TX: Psychological Corporation.

SUGGESTED READINGS

Leonard, L. B. (1998). *Children with specific language impairment*. Cambridge, MA: MIT Press.

McCauley, R. J. (2001). *Assessment of language disorders in children*. Mahwah, NJ: Erlbaum.

McCauley, R. J., & Fey, M. E. (Eds.). (2006). *Treatment of language disorders in children*. Baltimore, MD: Brookes.

Owens, R. E. (2004). *Language disorders: A functional approach to assessment and intervention* (4th ed.). Boston: Allyn & Bacon.

Polloway, E. A., Smith, T. E. C., & Miller, L. (2004). *Language instruction for students with disabilities*. Denver, CO: Love Publishing.

eleven

Language Disorders in School-Age Children

RONALD B. GILLAM AND DOUGLAS B. PETERSEN

LEARNING OBJECTIVES

1. To understand the nature and consequences of language disorders in school-age children.

2. To differentiate between language disorder, learning disability, and dyslexia.

3. To learn aspects of language development that are especially difficult for school-age children with language disorders in the primary and secondary grades.

4. To know the laws that directly affect the way services are delivered to school-age children with language disorders.

5. To learn about assessment procedures that are commonly used to evaluate language disorders in students in the primary and secondary grades.

6. To learn about typical intervention procedures that are used by speech-language pathologists who treat school-age children with language disorders.

Approximately 7% of all school-age children have unusual difficulties learning and using language, and more than 1 million children receive language intervention services in public schools each year (U.S. Department of Education, 2005). Many more children receive treatment for **language disorders** in hospitals, rehabilitation agencies, and private clinics. Clearly, language intervention comprises a large proportion of the health and education services that are provided to children with disabilities.

Some children are relatively poor language learners. There are numerous causes of language disorders in school-age children including intellectual and cognitive impairments, problems processing information (deficits in attention, perception, and memory), hearing loss, emotional disorders, and neglect. Recall that in most cases of language disorders, the cause or causes of the child's language-learning difficulties are not known.

BOX 11-1   Overview of the CD-ROM Segments

The CD-ROM that accompanies this text contains four video segments that accompany this chapter. The first segment shows an 8-year-old girl who has been diagnosed as having specific language impairment, central auditory processing disorder, and learning disabilities. This segment was included to demonstrate some of the language difficulties that these children present. The second and third segments demonstrate formal tests of receptive and expressive language. The fourth segment shows part of a language intervention session with an 11-year-old boy with autism.

Segments

Ch.11.01	The clinician is collecting a language sample from Jennifer, age 8. Jennifer tells the clinician about an incident that happened with her bird. Jennifer's language includes lots of mazes (false starts, repetitions, and revisions). Notice that the mazes occur when she is unsure of the correct grammatical structure to use and when she is constructing longer, more complex sentences.
Ch.11.02	The clinician is administering the Grammatic Understanding subtest of the Test of Language Development—Primary: 3rd Edition (TOLD-P:3) to Jennifer. This is a test of receptive language. Jennifer points to one of four pictures on a page that the clinician names.
Ch.11.03	The clinician is administering the Grammatic Completion subtest of the TOLD-P:3 to Jennifer. This is a test of grammatical morphology. The clinician says part of a sentence. Jennifer provides the last word, which must contain a certain grammatical marker (plural, past tense, present progressive, etc.) to be correct.
Ch. 11.04	Trey, an 11-year-old boy with autism, is participating in a language intervention activity with his clinician. This activity was designed to help Trey improve his problem solving and his explanatory language.

A variety of causes of language disorders can have the same effects on language development. Regardless of the cause (traumatic brain injury, autism, auditory processing deficits, etc.), many children with language disorders present similar clusters of problems. Frequently, these children do not attend well to what their parents and teachers say, do not mentally process and represent multiple pieces of language information at once, do not readily relate new information to what they already know, and/or do not retain new information in a manner that permits easy retrieval. These kinds of problems interfere with children's ability to take maximum advantage of the language-learning opportunities that exist in primary and secondary school classrooms. That is why children with language disorders usually need specialized assistance beyond the education that is routinely provided by classroom teachers.

This chapter provides information about language disorders in school-age children. The school-age years are divided into two periods, the primary grades (K–5) and the secondary grades (6–12). The first section of this chapter explains the laws that affect public education and describes the contexts in which language intervention is delivered in school settings. The second section of the chapter concerns issues related to delivering services to school-age children with language disorders. It reviews critical aspects of language development and language disorders during the primary grades (K–5) and the secondary grades (6–12) and summarizes basic assessment and intervention principles that relate to these areas of language development.

SERVICES FOR SCHOOL-AGE CHILDREN

A number of laws affect the way language intervention services are provided to pre-schoolers. There are also laws that affect the assessment and treatment of language disorders in school-age children. In 1973, the U.S. Congress passed a law, commonly referred to simply as **Section 504**, that prohibited any agency receiving federal funding from discriminating against individuals with disabilities. The term *discrimination* has been interpreted very broadly with respect to educational opportunities. Basically, a child is the subject of discrimination if, as a result of a disability, he or she cannot benefit from the same kinds of educational experiences that are routinely available for nondisabled students. As a result of Section 504, all public schools are required by law to ensure that, to the fullest extent possible, children with disabilities can profit from the instruction that is offered in classrooms. This is done by providing appropriate accommodations to the curriculum and/or modifying the way the curriculum is taught. Children with language disorders fall under the umbrella of Section 504 protection.

The requirements of Section 504 have been specified in greater detail over the years, and Congress has passed a number of bills that provide federal funding for special education. **Public Law 94-142, the Education of All Handicapped Children Act of 1975**, guaranteed a free appropriate public education in the least restrictive environment to all children with disabilities.

Those three concepts, *free public education, appropriate public education, and least restrictive environment*, may appear to be fairly simple ideas when considered individually, yet when those ideas are combined, and applied collectively as in PL

94-142, they emerge as an intricate construct of checks and balances that place the primary focus on children's individual educational needs.

For example, if the idea of least restrictive environment was taken out of context, it could be interpreted to mean that all children, regardless of disability, should be placed in the general education classroom during the entire school day. Yet, consider when the idea of least restrictive environment is combined with the idea of appropriate education; the individual child's needs are brought to the forefront because it is no longer simply a question of which setting is the least restrictive, it is also a question of which setting is the most appropriate. For certain children, it could be that the most appropriate public education in the least restrictive environment is in a special education classroom for part of the day.

The idea of a free public education is equally important to consider in the proper context. A free public education could simply mean that all children must receive a public education free of charge. Although this is correct (all children must receive a free public education), greater implications emerge when the ideas of a free public education and an appropriate public education are combined. Once again, the individual child's needs are brought forward. For example, some children require assistive technology devices and other special needs items that can be quite expensive, yet necessary, for an appropriate education to take place. PL 94-142 acknowledges that the expenses related to providing for the special needs of children with disabilities are the responsibility of the public.

There was a time when children with severe cognitive disabilities, cerebral palsy, deafness, blindness, and other impairments were sent to special schools. Many times, these children were not allowed to attend the schools in their neighborhood. In some states, parents were told that if they wanted their children to receive treatment, they had to send them away from home to live in residential institutions. This was unfair to parents and children. In essence, it amounted to discrimination against children with disabilities. The requirement in PL 94-142 that services must be provided in the least restrictive environment has resulted in an increase in the number of special education services that are provided in neighborhood schools and in regular classroom settings. As a result, there are far fewer residential schools for children with disabilities. Children are sent to institutions like a state residential school for the deaf and blind only when their parents and school district representatives agree it is the most appropriate educational placement.

To make important decisions regarding what constitutes a free and appropriate public education in the least restrictive environment for each individual child with a disability, an **individualized education program (IEP)** is created. An IEP is drafted and implemented by a team of people who have the child's best interests at heart. Recent changes to the law reduced the stipulations concerning who must attend an IEP team meeting; nevertheless, the child's parents, the general education teacher, a local education authority and those professionals, such as special education teachers, psychologists, speech-language pathologists (SLPs), audiologists, and occupational therapists who have an interest in helping that child, should be participants.

In 1990, the name of the Education of All Handicapped Children Act was changed to the **Individuals With Disabilities Education Act (IDEA)**. Some of the key provisions of this act are listed in Table 11-1. As part of the budget process each year,

Congress must reauthorize the funding mechanisms that make it possible for school districts to provide a free appropriate public education in the least restrictive environment for all children.

Table 11-1 Important Requirements of the Individuals With Disabilities Education Act (IDEA)

Parent Notification	In most cases, parent consent is required before children can be referred for special testing and again before they can be tested.
Comprehensive Evaluation	Children must receive a full and individual evaluation by a team of professionals to determine whether they have disability. This evaluation must be conducted in the child's native language unless it is clearly not feasible to do so.
Determination of Disability	Following their assessment, professionals must meet with the child's parents to report their results and to determine whether the child has a disability. A *disability* is defined as a child with mental retardation, hearing impairments (including deafness), speech or language impairments, visual impairments (including blindness), serious emotional disturbance, orthopedic impairments, autism, traumatic brain injury, other health impairments, specific learning disabilities, deaf-blindness, or multiple disabilities. For children between the ages of 3 and 9 years, a disability can also mean a child who is "experiencing developmental delays, as defined by the State and as measured by appropriate diagnostic instruments and procedures, in one or more of the following areas: Physical development, cognitive development, communication development, social or emotional development or adaptive development."
Individualized Education Program (IEP)	If it is determined that a child has a disability, school personnel meet with the parents to develop an individualized education program (IEP). This program is a written statement that specifies the child's strengths and weaknesses, the child's levels of educational performance, the measurable goals that the child needs to meet to profit from instruction, the type of services the child will receive, and the amount of time each week that services will be provided.
Review of Placement and Services	Each year, members of the IEP team and the child's parents meet in person, if possible, to hold an IEP meeting to review the child's progress, to determine whether the child is still eligible for special education services, and to create a new IEP (if needed).
Due Process	Parents have the right to review all records related to their child's education, to have their child evaluated by an independent professional, and to request a hearing if they are not satisfied with the type or amount of services recommended for their child.

Parents can request a hearing with a state-appointed officer when they believe the school district has not met the requirements of IDEA. Either side (parents or school districts) can appeal a hearing decision to a higher court. Students in communication sciences and disorders need to understand the requirements of IDEA so that they can be certain they always provide services to children in a manner that is consistent with the laws that regulate special education and related services in the schools.

IDEA has been revised many times since 1975. Congress passed the most recent amendments in December 2004, with final regulations published in August 2006 (U.S. Department of Education, 2006). Some of the latest amendments reduced the amount of evaluations, meetings, and paperwork required of SLPs who work in public schools. For example, it is no longer required to conduct an evaluation every 3 years when a child's parents and the school agree that a reevaluation is not necessary to determine eligibility for special education. Also, when changes to a child's IEP are needed, a recent IDEA amendment allows the parent and the school to agree to forgo a meeting and develop a written document to change the current IEP. Furthermore, changes in the law allow IEP team members to be excused from attendance if their area is not being discussed. These changes in the law could help reduce the number of meetings that an SLP is required to attend throughout the school year. Recent changes in IDEA could also reduce paperwork demands. For example, although it is still required that each IEP include a statement of measurable annual goals, including academic and functional goals, the previous regulations requiring that each IEP contain benchmarks or short-term objectives for each of the annual goals have been removed.

Note that in the examples provided, the changes to IDEA do not necessarily eliminate the option to perform a 3-year evaluation, hold additional IEP team meetings, or write short-term IEP objectives. The new changes simply do away with the legal mandate to do so.

The **No Child Left Behind Act (NCLB)** of 2001 is the reauthorization of the Elementary and Secondary Education Act, first enacted in 1965. Some key provisions of this act are listed in Table 11-2. NCLB is an ambitious congressional act that is based on stronger accountability for academic achievement, more freedom for states and communities, research-based education methods, and more choices for parents. The act states that all schools must make adequate yearly progress in raising the percentage of students who are proficient in math and reading. Student progress must be assessed every year in grades 3 through 8, and at least once in high school. Most children who are receiving special education services, including speech and language services, are not exempt from the requirements outlined by NCLB.

NCLB was based on an idea that most educators consider commendable: to promote high standards and accountability for the learning of all children, regardless of their background or ability. Nevertheless, some professionals feel that NCLB places too much emphasis on standardized testing and promotes the practice of "teaching to the test." Other professionals disagree with the punitive measures directed toward schools that repeatedly do not demonstrate adequate yearly progress. Some people feel that NCLB was written without carefully considering the needs of students with disabilities.

Table 11-2 Important Terms for No Child Left Behind (NCLB) 2001

Accountability	No Child Left Behind holds schools and school districts accountable for results. Schools are responsible for making sure children are learning.
School District Report Cards	No Child Left Behind gives parents report cards so that they can see which schools in their district are succeeding and why.
Scientifically Based Research	No Child Left Behind focuses on teaching methods that have been supported by research to be effective.
Reading First	Reading First is the part of No Child Left Behind that is dedicated to ensuring that all children learn to read on grade level by the third grade. Reading First provides money to states and many school districts to support high-quality reading programs based on scientific research.
Title I	This is the part of No Child Left Behind that supports programs in schools and school districts to improve the learning of children from low-income families. The U.S. Department of Education provides Title I funds to states to give to school districts based on the number of children from low-income families in each district.
State Assessments	This refers to the tests developed by each state that students will take every year in grades 3–8 and at least once in high school. Using these tests, the state will be able to compare schools to each other and know which ones need extra help to improve.
Adequate Yearly Progress (AYP)	This is the term No Child Left Behind uses to explain that a particular school has met state reading and math goals.
School in Need of Improvement	This is the term No Child Left Behind uses to refer to schools receiving Title I funds that have not met state reading and math goals (AYP) for at least 2 years. If a school is labeled a "school in need of improvement," it receives extra help to improve and students have the option to transfer to another public school, including a public charter school. Also, students may be eligible to receive free tutoring and extra help with schoolwork.
Supplemental Educational Services (SES)	This is the term No Child Left Behind uses to refer to the tutoring and extra help with schoolwork in subjects such as reading and math that children from low-income families may be eligible to receive. This help is provided free of charge and generally takes place outside the regular school day, such as after school or during the summer.
Highly Qualified Teacher (HQT)	This is the term No Child Left Behind uses for a teacher who proves that he or she knows the subjects he or she is teaching, has a college degree, and is state-certified. No Child Left Behind requires that students be taught by a Highly Qualified Teacher in core academic subjects.

IDEA and NCLB must be reauthorized by Congress periodically. To help continually improve legislation and retain the advances that have been made in special education and related services to children with disabilities, including children with language disorders, it is important for students and professionals in communication sciences and disorders to stay informed about congressional actions related to these laws. Most SLPs enter the profession because they are advocates for children with disabilities. They want to provide the best possible services to these children and want these children to receive as much help as they need to succeed socially, academically, and vocationally. With that goal in mind, many professionals in communication sciences and disorders strongly support increased funding for special education programs across the nation.

LANGUAGE DISORDERS

Many preschool-age children have significant limitations in their ability to learn and use language. These children's development in areas of language form (morphology and syntax), content (size of the lexicon and semantic relations), and/or use (pragmatics and socialization) lags behind that of their same-age peers. Some of these children benefit from early intervention and have language growth spurts that enable them to develop language skills that appear to be similar to their age peers by the time they are 5 years old (Paul, Hernandez, Taylor, & Johnson, 1996). However, these same late-talking children who seem to catch up by age 5 often continue to have lower language and reading skills into their teenage years (Rescorla, 2002, 2005). Those children whose language disorders are more severe and who do not seem to improve by an early age frequently have significant difficulties with social and academic language during the elementary school years (Aram & Hall, 1989; Paul, Murray, Clancy, & Andrews, 1997). Often, these same children continue to exhibit social, academic, and vocational difficulties well into the secondary grades (Bishop, 1997; Stothard, Snowling, Bishop, Chipchase, & Kaplan, 1998) and even into adulthood (Records, Tomblin, & Buckwalter, 1995). For this reason, professionals need to be diligent in their efforts to identify children with language disorders as early as possible and to provide them with the kinds of intervention they need to succeed.

Language Disorder, Learning Disability, or Dyslexia?

Reading and writing are language-based skills. When children enter kindergarten, they usually have a great deal of knowledge about the vocabulary, grammar, and use of their language. This knowledge is based on their experiences with listening to and speaking the language that surrounds them. To learn how to read and write, children must organize their knowledge of language on a new level. They need to figure out how to use sequences of letters to represent the phonemes, words, sentences, and stories that have been part of their oral language for some time. To read, children must decode sequences of letters into language. To write, they must encode their language into sequences of letters. It only makes sense that children who have difficulty comprehending and producing spoken language are at a significant disadvantage when they begin to learn how to read and write. Therefore, it should not be surprising that most children with language disorders have significant difficulties with the development of literacy.

Children with learning disabilities and children with dyslexia have difficulties learning how to read and write. Recent research shows that children with language disorders have the same kinds of problems. One question that naturally arises with school-age children is, "What is the difference between a language disorder, a learning disability, and dyslexia?"

Children with language disorders have difficulty with the comprehension and/or the expression of language form, content, or use, and these problems place them at risk for social, educational, and vocational difficulties. Students with learning disabilities sometimes have difficulties learning and using language as well. According to the Individuals with Disabilities Education Act (2004), a "**specific learning disability** is a disorder in one or more of the basic psychological processes involved in understanding or in using language, spoken or written, which may manifest itself in the imperfect ability to listen, think, speak, read, write, spell, or do mathematical calculations. (section 602, paragraph 30)"

Some professionals believe that learning disabilities in the areas of speaking and listening are, in fact, language disorders. Reading and writing are language-based skills. Therefore, difficulties learning to read, write, and spell are often symptoms of language disorders.

Many researchers believe **dyslexia** is a neurologically based, phonological processing disorder that interferes with single-word decoding (Lyon, 1995). According to Catts and Kamhi (1999), dyslexia is one type of a developmental language disorder in which the child's specific difficulties are in the area of phonological processing skills that relate to reading. That is, students with dyslexia have specific problems learning and using sound–symbol relationships (phonics) during reading. This negatively affects their ability to "sound-out" words.

What is the difference between a language disorder, a specific learning disability, and dyslexia? According to one perspective, there is no difference. They are all manifestations of language-learning difficulties. However, theory and practice are two different things. Children with similar symptoms are often labeled differently because professionals from various disciplines use different procedures to diagnose language disorders, specific learning disabilities, and dyslexia.

Children are diagnosed as language disordered when they have difficulties with language form, content, and use that are unexpected given their chronological age. That is, they are significantly poorer at comprehending or producing language than are other children their same age. Clinicians make this determination by comparing children's performance on standardized tests to the norms for children who are their same age. They also make this determination by analyzing the level of language and the patterns of form, content, and use errors in conversational and narrative language samples. Comparing a child's language abilities to the abilities of typically achieving children the same age is referred to as **chronological age referencing**. That is, the expected language ability for a particular age is the reference on which a determination of a language disorder is based.

Up until the most recent IDEA reauthorization, a specific learning disability was diagnosed by law as a severe discrepancy between a child's intellectual quotient (IQ) and his or her academic achievement. IDEA 2004 changed the way in which specific learning disabilities are determined. The current version of IDEA states that school districts are no longer required to take into account a severe discrepancy between ability (IQ) and achievement when determining whether a child has a specific learning disability. Many people and organizations advocated for this change in the law. They expressed concerns that under the discrepancy model, many children had deficits in academic achievement for as long as 3 or 4 years before they demonstrated a "severe discrepancy." Another concern was that children with high IQs could qualify for special assistance with relatively mild academic problems, whereas children with lower-level IQs had to demonstrate much more severe academic problems to qualify for services. For example, a child with an IQ score of 100 (right at the average) and a standard score of 85 on a test of reading could be identified as having a **learning disability** in the area of reading because there was a significant discrepancy between his or her standard scores on an IQ test and his or her standard scores on a reading test. Consider a child who is the same age and has a lower standard score (75) on a reading test. If the second child earns a standard score of 87 on an IQ test, this second child would not be labeled as learning disabled and would not qualify for special education services because he or she did not present a significant discrepancy between ability and achievement. Thus, the problem with **discrepancy modeling** is that two children with similar difficulties with reading and with similar needs for extra assistance did not always receive the same help.

The language in IDEA 2004 does not specifically state that a school district cannot use a discrepancy model to diagnose a specific learning disability. It simply states that it is no longer required by law to do so, and that a state may prohibit the use of a discrepancy model to diagnose a specific learning impairment if it so desires. This update to IDEA permits individual states to begin to use other methods for diagnosing specific learning disabilities. IDEA 2004 suggests that school districts can use a process that determines whether a child responds to scientific, research-based intervention as part of the evaluation procedures for determining a specific learning disability. There is congressional support for models that focus on assessment, are related to instruction, and promote intervention for identified children.

Response to intervention (RTI) is an example of an alternate method that can be used to identify children with learning disabilities. RTI is based on changes in instruction to find what works best for the individual child. An important element of an RTI model is the potential for early intervention when children first present with academic difficulties. Once a child is recognized as having academic difficulty, additional instruction can be implemented until that child "responds," improving his or her skills. Often a tiered approach is suggested in which a child moves to increasingly more intensive levels, or "tiers," of instruction until his or her response to that intervention is acceptable.

RTI should be considered only one component of the process to identify children in need of special education and related services. Determining why a child has not responded to scientific, research-based interventions requires a comprehensive evaluation. IDEA 2004 states that an evaluation must include a variety of assessment tools and strategies and cannot rely on any single procedure, such as RTI, as the sole criterion for determining eligibility for special education and related services.

The line separating a language impairment and a specific learning disability in the areas of listening, speaking, reading, writing, and spelling will likely become even less clear than before. Because SLPs can and should have a significant role to play in a RTI model, or in any model used to diagnose a specific learning disability, it will be important for SLPs to monitor and help shape these new methods.

Dyslexia is diagnosed by examining children's reading ability. As noted earlier in the chapter, dyslexia has come to mean a difficulty decoding print caused by phonological processing (phonological awareness) problems. Most professionals test for dyslexia by administering reading tests and tests of phonological processing skills like the ability to blend sounds together (b – o – t = boat) to make words or the ability to listen to a word and then make a new word by removing the first or last sound (say *boat* without the *t*).

Some children who have difficulties in the areas of speaking, listening, reading, writing, and spelling happen to have characteristics of a specific learning disability and have phonological processing problems that adversely affect their reading. These children could be labeled as having a language disorder, a learning disability, or dyslexia. The important message is that language disorders; learning disabilities in speaking, listening, reading, writing, and spelling; and dyslexia are all language-based problems. Because these terms have similar diagnostic criteria, children with quite similar language abilities and disabilities can sometimes be classified with different labels.

CRITICAL AREAS OF LANGUAGE DEVELOPMENT DURING THE SCHOOL-AGE YEARS

Recall from Chapter 2 that many aspects of language form, content, and use continue to develop during the school-age years. For the purposes of this chapter, we focus on three critical aspects of language development during the primary grades (complex sentences, narration, and literacy) and three different aspects of development during the secondary grades (subject-specific vocabulary, expository texts, and metacognitive strategies). Although there are many types of language disorders and many different kinds of language needs, these are the skills most often assessed and treated during the school-age years.

Primary Grades (K–5)

SPLs often assess complex sentence production, narrative abilities, and literacy abilities in primary-grade children. Frequently, these same skills are targeted in language intervention.

Complex Sentences

Most children use more complex sentences and a greater variety of complex sentence forms during the school-age years (see Table 11-3 for a list of different types of complex sentences). As children have more complex things to talk about, they need to have a command of various kinds of complex language forms that can express their ideas. Children experiment with the kinds of syntactic devices that are required for "literate" language, and they discover when and how to use these complex structures. Unfortunately, complex sentences pose unusual difficulties for many children with language disorders, and these difficulties are especially evident when children are reading and writing (Gillam & Carlile, 1997; Gillam & Johnston, 1992).

Often, children with language disorders use more mazes when they are producing complex sentences. A **maze** is a repetition, a false start, or a reformulation of a sentence. For example, in the CD-ROM video segment Ch.11.01, Jennifer says, "But one time, when I had a b-, when uh, I uh, when last Christmas, I, uh uh, my aunt Mary Ann, my aunt, she gave me a bird, and her, and I called him Tweetie Bird." What Jennifer is trying to say is, *Last Christmas my aunt Mary Ann gave me a bird named Tweetie.* Jennifer has difficulties with pronouns and with adverbial phrases, and these difficulties get in the way of her ability to formulate and organize what she wants to say about her bird. These are not unusual problems for many school-age children with language disorders.

Narration

Narration (storytelling) is a critical aspect of language development during the school-age years. Children socialize by telling each other stories about their lives, they use stories as mental tools for remembering events, and they learn to read and write stories.

Table 11-3 Examples of Complex Sentences

Sentence Type	Example
Simple sentence	I *saw* the girl.
Compound sentence (and, but, so, or)	I *saw* the girl, and I *said*, "Hello." I *saw* the girl, but she didn't *see* me.
Complex Sentences	
Adverbial clauses	If you *see* the girl, *call* me. I'll *call* her because she *is* my friend.
Relative clauses	
Subjective	The girl who *had* brown eyes was *walking* with my sister.
Objective	My sister was *walking* with the girl who *had* brown eyes.
Infinitive (with second subject stated)	I *want* you to *play* with me.
Clausal complements	I *saw* the elephant *run* away. I *heard* the band *playing* its new song.
Multiple embedded clauses	He *said*, I *hope* you *remember* who you are *supposed* to talk to because I'm *going* to be mad if you *say* this to the wrong person.

Note: Main verbs are italicized.

Children's narratives become longer and more complex during the primary grades as they learn how to create more elaborate episodes (see Chapter 2). They also develop the ability to weave multiple episodes into their stories.

If children with language disorders have trouble creating complex sentences, it should not be surprising that they also have trouble combining groups of sentences into stories. Studies of the narrative abilities of children with language disorders have shown they routinely tell shorter stories that contain fewer story grammar elements and that are less coherent than the stories of typically developing children. As you might imagine, difficulties with narration interfere with socialization and with the development of literacy.

Literacy

Learning how to read is probably the most important achievement during the primary grade years. Children are taught how to decode words in kindergarten and first grade. Instruction in second grade is usually designed to make decoding skills more automatic. Beginning in third grade, the primary emphasis of instruction changes to the ability to use reading as a tool for learning. As noted earlier, reading and writing are language tasks, and many school-age children with language disorders have literacy-learning problems.

There are various models of reading acquisition. However, the **simple view of reading** (Gough & Tunmer, 1986) is excellent in providing a fairly straightforward outline of the relationship between language and literacy. The simple view of reading suggests that reading is composed of two components: language comprehension and word recognition.

Children who have difficulty with language comprehension are likely to have problems understanding both verbal language and written language. The relationship between language and reading comprehension can be viewed in the reverse manner as well. That is, children who have a deficit in reading comprehension will likely have difficulty with language comprehension (Catts, Adlof, & Weismer, 2006). Children with reading comprehension difficulty are sometimes able to decode and recognize words well, but they are unable to understand those words' individual or collective meaning.

On the other hand, there are those children who have reasonably good language comprehension, but poor word recognition. **Word recognition** has two important subskills: the development of **mental graphemic representations (MGRs)**, and word **decoding**.

MGRs (also referred to as visual or mental orthographic images) allow readers to identify words almost instantaneously without the need to decode or "sound them out." Fluent readers use MGRs most of the time when reading. Only when a new or uncommon word is presented will a fluent reader need to use decoding. Using MGRs is often referred to as "sight word reading," although the phrase *sight word* is not an entirely accurate description of the process. Some evidence suggests that words are not simply remembered and then recalled through a visual process. It has been shown that the complexity of the sounds in words make a difference in how easily a word can be remembered and recalled (Apel, Wolter, & Masterson, 2006).

Although being able to rapidly identify words is an extremely important reading skill, the ability to decode words is equally important. Recall that children begin to think about their own language at about the time they enter kindergarten. This ability is called metalinguistic awareness. Decoding, or the ability to "break the code" of letter–sound combinations, requires one aspect of metalinguistic awareness called phonological awareness. Phonological awareness is the ability to identify the phoneme structure of words. For example, if a child can recognize that the word *bat* rhymes with the word *cat*, or if a child can tell you that the word *light* starts with the sound /l/, then he or she is demonstrating phonological awareness.

Phonological awareness skills are required to decode words. If a child is not "aware" of the individual sounds in a word, then he or she will not be able to extract those sounds from their corresponding letter or combination of letters. For example, the word *bat* has three distinct phonemes /b/, /æ/, and /t/, and is commonly written with three letters, *b*, *a*, and *t*. Without the awareness of those individual sounds, decoding could not take place. Phonological awareness has been shown to be extremely important in the development of reading, especially for the word learning skill of decoding. Unfortunately, many children with language disorders have difficulties with phonological awareness (Gillon, 2005).

Because children who have language impairments tend to also have difficulty with reading comprehension and word recognition skills, including phonological awareness, SLPs can have an important role to play in the identification and remediation of reading difficulties. SLPs have a knowledge base related to receptive and expressive language and phonological awareness. They are in a unique position to help teachers, parents, and students understand how oral language abilities are inextricably tied to the development of literacy.

Secondary Grades (6–12)

When SLPs assess and/or treat language disorders in children who are in the secondary grades, they often focus on vocabulary that is associated with specific subject areas (e.g., geometry, world history or biology), comprehension and production of expository texts (discourse for teaching or explaining something), and/or metacognitive strategies for learning.

Subject-Specific Vocabulary

As mentioned in Chapter 2, children's vocabularies expand dramatically during the school-age years. Much of this expansion relates to the acquisition of subject-specific vocabulary in subject areas such as mathematics, social studies, and the sciences. Many students with language disorders have difficulty understanding and remembering subject-specific vocabulary, and this difficulty contributes to school failure. Therefore, SLPs who work with adolescents with language disorders often help these children acquire the vocabulary they need to succeed in their courses.

Expository Texts

Adolescents become adept at the rhetorical conventions of argument and persuasion. These skills require them to present information about persons, facts, and dates and to provide specific details, generalizations, and conclusions. Children encounter these same forms of discourse, called **expository texts**, in their academic textbooks. Students with language disorders frequently have difficulties understanding the expository texts they must read for their courses (Gillam & St. Clair, 2007). They may not understand cause-and-effect relationships that are expressed in their science or history textbooks. They also have difficulties creating the kinds of expository texts that are needed to complete assignments for class such as book reports, essays, and term papers. These difficulties can contribute to school failure.

Metacognitive Strategies

Adolescents learn to employ strategies for learning school subjects. Throughout the elementary school years, teachers support students as they learn the fundamentals of reading, writing, and mathematical computation. During the middle and high school years, there is a greater expectation for independence in academic learning. To be academically successful, adolescents must know how to acquire, store, recall, and use knowledge from assignments they complete outside of class.

Metacognitive strategies are effortful actions that students use to accomplish specific learning goals. For example, students may reread passages they do not understand completely, take extra notes, memorize their notes by saying them out loud, or create their own practice tests. Adolescents with language disorders often demonstrate inefficiency or even reluctance in applying these kinds of effortful learning strategies.

ASSESSMENT

IDEA requires clinicians to follow a sequence of steps when they conduct language assessments with school-age children. When classroom teachers have concerns about a child's language ability, they must do their best to help the child in the classroom using scientific, research-based intervention methods before they refer the child for special education testing. Table 11-4 lists a number of strategies that teachers can use to facilitate language development in the classroom.

If a classroom teacher tries these facilitative strategies with little success, he or she can refer the child for a speech and language assessment. Before any testing can begin, the child's parents should be informed of the reasons why the child was referred and the tests that will be administered. Under most circumstances, the actual assessment can begin only after the child's parents give their permission for testing.

The assessment practices for school-age children are much like the language assessment practices that were discussed in Chapter 10. As is the case with preschoolers, the assessment of school-age children is usually conducted by a multidisciplinary assessment team. Language assessment usually includes a review of the child's records, observation of the child in the classroom setting, administration of one or two standardized tests, and the collection and analysis of language samples.

Most SLPs who work in school settings give one of three standardized tests: TOLD-P:3 (Newcomer & Hammill, 1997; there is also a version of this test for adolescents), the Clinical Evaluation of Language Fundamentals: 4th Edition (Semel, Wiig, & Secord, 2004), or the Comprehensive Assessment of Spoken Language (Carrow-Woolfolk, 2004). SLPs usually evaluate language comprehension and language expression. The CD-ROM that accompanies this book contains examples of two subtests from the TOLD-P:3 that are used for assessing comprehension and production (CD-ROM segments Ch.11.02 and Ch.11.03).

One of the most critical aspects of a speech and language evaluation is the language sample. When SLPs assess a school-age child, they usually converse with the child for about 20 minutes, and then they have the child tell a story. One common procedure for collecting a narrative sample is to ask children to narrate a wordless picture book like Mayer's (1969) *Frog, Where Are You?* The child tells a story that corresponds to a series of pictures. This sampling procedure is useful for eliciting complex sentences and literate language forms from children.

The CD-ROM video segment Ch.11.01 shows part of a language sample that was collected from Jennifer, an 8-year-old girl with specific language impairment. Video

Table 11-4 Alternative Strategies That May Be Used by Classroom Teachers and Speech-Language Pathologists in Classroom Settings

Strategies

1. Simplify teacher questions.
2. Shorten teacher directions.
3. Require the child to restate teacher directions.
4. Give the child extra time to organize thoughts.
5. Give cues to assist the child in word retrieval.
6. Explain questions and instructions in greater detail.
7. Repeat the child's statements, adding grammatical markers to make them complete.
8. Ask questions that encourage the child to explain his or her answers in more detail.
9. Explain concepts in greater detail.
10. Respond positively to any verbal output from the child.
11. Provide a "buddy" to assist the child when he or she is confused.
12. Show the child how to ask for assistance and/or clarification.
13. Provide minilessons on using descriptive language.
14. Ask questions that encourage the child to make connections between new and previously taught information.
15. Teach the child to make semantic maps of stories and expository texts he or she reads.
16. Use pictures and objects while you are giving directions or explaining concepts.

segment Ch.02.01 (contained on CD-ROM Volume 1) shows five children who are narrating *Frog, Where Are You?* Clinicians record the samples of conversation and narration they elicit from children and write down everything the child says. This written record is called a **transcript**. A transcript of a conversation is provided in Box 11-2 titled "Mazes and Complex Sentences." The transcript of the narration is provided in Chapter 2 in Box 2-4, "Speech Sound Acquisition." Clinicians can tell where children are in the language development process by analyzing the length and types of their utterances. Clinicians also look for patterns of language form, content, and use errors.

BOX 11-2   Mazes and Complex Sentences

Play CD-ROM segment Ch.11.02 on Volume 2 of the CD-ROM set. Jennifer is talking to the clinician, who is a certified and licensed SLP. Can you identify how many complex sentences there are? Note the number of mazes in her language and where they occur in her sentences. The mazes are clues to aspects of language that are difficult for her. Mazes are noted in parentheses in the transcript.

Conversation: "Bird"

Context: Jennifer is telling the examiner about her pet bird.
Note: The angle brackets (< >) indicate overlap between speakers. The *x* indicates an unintelligible word.

J: Jennifer   **E:** Examiner

J: (But one time, when I had a b-) (when uh) (I uh) (when) last Christmas (x uh uh) aunt Mary Ann) my aunt, she gave me a bird (and her) and I called him Tweetie Bird.
E: A real bird?
J: Uh-huh.
E: She gave you a real bird?
J: Yeah.
J: And uh and one time, Tweetie pooped on my head by accident.
J: <Poop!>
E: <Oh, not> really.
J: Oh, yes he did.
E: How did that happen?
J: Because, when he was climbing up here, he pooped by accident.
E: You would let him climb on you?
J: Yeah, and he climbed right up here, then climbed right up here, then he pooped.
E: Oh, my goodness.
E: But you don't think he really meant to do it.
J: M-m.
E: So, sometimes you would let him go out of his cage?
J: No, (I let x) (I) I x x x.

J: (Uh) one time (when I was) (when I) (when I was uh) when I was playing, I stepped on Tweetie by accident, like this.

J: Then, he said, "Tweet tweet tweet tweet tweet tweet."

J: Then we had to take him to the vet.

E: Is that really true that you <stepped on> him?

J: <Uh-huh>

J: M-hm.

J: (It was very acci-) it was a accident.

J: Then I said, "I hope Tweetie doesn't die."

J: And Mom said, "(I hope he wasn't) (I hope he didn't) I hope he doesn't."

E: What happened when you took him to the vet?

J: (Oh we uh) I took Tweetie (and, and) and then I took Tweetie out, then the man said, "Well, that's a fine-looking bird."

J: "Maybe someday you will be a doctor (uh) when you grow up."

J: And I, and Mom laughed.

E: She did?

J: Uh-huh.

E: Yeah.

J: My sister cried when she wanted a turn.

E: Do you think you would like to be a veterinarian when you grow up?

J: No, I would like to be a artist from Walt Disney.

Assessment practices with adolescents are similar. In their language evaluations of adolescents, most clinicians administer at least one standardized test and collect a language sample. Formal tests usually provide a gross estimate of general language functioning in comparison to other children who are the same age as the child who is being assessed. Informal assessments are usually more informative for evaluating the adolescent's content-specific vocabulary knowledge, use of expository texts, and meta-cognitive strategies.

In addition to testing and language sampling, SLPs often include an interactive assessment procedure in evaluations of adolescents. In the interactive assessment, the clinician attempts to teach the child a history or science lesson. For example, we recently taught one student about the Santa Fe Expedition. We read a passage from a textbook aloud, asked the student to summarize it aloud, and then conversed with the student about what we just read and how she might go about studying this information on her own. After we asked a few questions about the content of the material that was read, we reread the passage and asked the child to summarize it again. We evaluated the amount of content-specific vocabulary that the student used, the amount of change in the child's ability to elaborate on details during her summary, and the child's ability to plan an effective study strategy.

BOX 11-3   Standardized Testing

The CD-ROM contains two segments that show standardized testing. In segment Ch.11.02, an SLP is administering the Grammatic Understanding subtest of the TOLD-P:3 to an 8-year-old girl. The task requires the child to listen to the sentence that LaVae says and then point to the picture on the page that best represents the sentence. This is a test of the ability to comprehend and remember sentences (an aspect of language form).

Segment Ch.11.03 shows the same SLP administering the Grammatic Completion subtest of the TOLD-P:3. In this task, the SLP says a sentence or two but leaves off the last word. This is called a *cloze* task. For example, she says, "Carla has a dress. Denise has a dress. They have two _____." If the child knows the plural morpheme -*s*, she should answer, "dresses." This task assesses language production (expressive language).

INTERVENTION

Over the years, clinicians have used a variety of procedures to promote language development in children with language disorders. Recall from Chapter 10 that some of the primary types of facilitative interactions with preschoolers include imitation, modeling, expansion, focused stimulation (including milieu teaching), and growth-relevant recasts. These types of facilitative interactions can be used to teach different kinds of intervention targets to school-age children as well. However, SLPs use two types of language intervention quite often with children in the primary and secondary grades. These intervention procedures are called **literature-based language intervention** and **classroom collaboration**. The following sections discuss some general principles of language intervention with school-age children and then describe literature-based language intervention and classroom collaboration.

General Principles of Language Intervention With School-Age Children

Language intervention with school-age children can be conducted individually or in groups. In school settings, most language intervention is provided in groups. There are theoretical and practical reasons for intervening in the context of groups. Theoretically, there may be a benefit to socially mediated peer interactions. On a practical level, groups are scheduled simply to accommodate the SLP's need to see a greater number of children.

The clinician's primary job is to influence language learning through social interaction. The idea is that children who experience cognitive and linguistic activities in social situations will come to internalize them gradually over time. First, the child and the clinician work together, with the clinician doing most of the work and serving as a model. As the child acquires some degree of skill, the clinician gives the child more responsibility for the communication that takes place in the activity. Gradually, the child takes more of the initiative, and the adult serves primarily to provide support and help when the child experiences problems. Eventually, the child internalizes the language that is necessary to complete the activity successfully and becomes capable of performing the activities independently. An example of a clinician and child participating in intervention activities is shown in Box 11-4.

Gillam and van Kleeck (1996) suggest that intervention should primarily focus on social-interactive and academic uses of language in pragmatically relevant situations. Many intervention activities benefit both memory and language. New clinicians should keep the following language intervention principles in mind as they plan and conduct activities.

Promote Attention

Individuals with various kinds of language disorders evidence difficulties with attention. Learners process information more quickly after they have activated relevant information in long-term memory. Second, language learning is enhanced when learners selectively attend to the most critical information. Clinicians can mediate preparatory attention in adolescents by explaining what they plan to work on and why it is important. Clinicians can mediate selective attention by making the intervention models as clear as possible and by limiting distractions. For example, Ellis Weismer and Hesketh (1998) report that children learned to produce novel words that clinicians had emphatically stressed better than they learned novel words that had been produced with regular stress. These authors conclude that the emphatic stress helped direct the children's selective attention to new information to be learned.

Speak Clearly and Slowly

Speech perception and speed of cognitive processing contribute to learning language. Some children with developmental language disorders have difficulties perceiving and understanding rapidly produced speech. As noted by Ellis Weismer (1996), when clinicians slow their rates of speech, they provide learners with more time for processing, encoding, storage, and retrieval.

Plan Activities Around Topics or Concepts That Are Familiar to the Learner

Greater prior knowledge enables learners to attend more carefully to new information, which leads to better language learning. Clinicians who want to teach new language

---

BOX 11-4 Language Intervention

CD-ROM segment Ch.11.04 shows an SLP conducting a language intervention lesson with an 11-year-old boy named Trey. Trey has been diagnosed with autism. The clinician and Trey are working on an activity that has been designed to promote problem solving and explanatory language. What types of language facilitation techniques does the clinician use to assist Trey when he encounters difficulty?

forms or new communicative functions should make optimal use of the learner's prior knowledge. For example, an 8-year-old boy with a language impairment might be very interested in the World Wrestling Entertainment, and he might know a great deal about the wrestlers. If he had trouble with subject–verb agreement, it would make sense for the SLP to use growth-relevant recasts while talking to this child about wrestling and to work on writing and revising sentences contained in stories or reports on wrestling events.

Help Learners Organize New Knowledge

Learners can remember much more information when they have organized their knowledge meaningfully. For example, people struggle to recall 20 randomly presented letters, but they can easily remember 60 or 80 letters when the letters are part of words that comprise sentences. Following the same logic, it makes sense to help learners organize new knowledge in ways that facilitate recall. Practice with paraphrasing sentences and paragraphs from expository texts can help learners in the elementary grades use their own prior knowledge, vocabulary, and language structures to organize new information. Adolescents can be taught learning strategies that help them organize and recall information contained in their textbooks (Gillam, 2007).

Provide Learners With Retention Cues

Clinicians need to build bridges between what they are teaching and learners' knowledge and expectations. Learners can internalize clinician questions, summaries, drawings, and pictures as recall cues. Recall cues provided by clinicians, parents, or teachers can be powerful. Children who are given retention cues during language intervention activities learn more than children who do not receive extra cues.

These are some general suggestions for conducting language intervention activities with school-age children. The next sections explain two specific language intervention approaches that SLPs use often with children in the primary and secondary grades.

Literature-Based Language Intervention

Many clinicians use book discussions as the primary context for intervention. This type of intervention has been shown to be helpful for spoken language, listening, reading, and writing (Gillam, 1995; Gillam, McFadden, & van Kleeck, 1995). In this approach, activities that facilitate semantics, syntax, morphology, narration, and phonological awareness are centered around a common theme that is introduced in a story. Activities usually include prereading discussions about concepts that are contained in the books, reading and rereading the story on a number of occasions, retelling the story, and conducting various language activities, called minilessons, that are related to the story that was read, writing parallel stories, and discussing related books. Clinicians who believe that children need to learn language within natural contexts tend to use facilitative interactions (focused stimulation, modeling, recasting, and others listed in Chapter 10) as part of all their interactions with children.

Classroom Collaboration

Many SLPs who work in public school settings are beginning to conduct language intervention in the regular classroom. Usually, clinicians try to integrate their language-learning goals (complex sentence usage, narrative abilities, phonological awareness, vocabulary, expository texts, learning strategies, etc.) into the curriculum. They do this to make language intervention more functional for children. Sometimes, SLPs and classroom teachers work together to plan and carry out language-learning activities with the whole class. For example, some SLPs conduct minilessons on creating narratives with the whole class. The SLP will display an overhead that contains a story like, "Once there was a whale. He swimmed. Then he got sick. Then he got better." The SLP and the class might work together to make this kind of story more complex and complete. Children give suggestions for changes, and the SLP writes them on the overhead. Then, the class votes on the changes they like best, and they construct new sentences with the SLP's help. The SLP may repeat this overhead editing process two or three times until the class has a story they are all proud of.

Some SLPs work with small groups of students in the classroom. For example, van Kleeck, Gillam, and McFadden (1998) describe a language intervention procedure in which they conducted phonological awareness activities with small groups of prekindergarten and kindergarten children as part of their center time. Children worked on rhyming and phoneme awareness activities in their "sound center" three times each week for 10-minute periods. The whole class rotated through the sound center on the same schedule that they rotated through other centers that were available in the classroom. At the end of the year, these children were better at phonological awareness activities than a comparison group of first-graders who had been in these same classrooms 1 or 2 years before.

Finally, SLPs often consult with teachers about language intervention activities that can be conducted in the classroom. They might suggest language intervention procedures that the teacher can carry out as part of the regular classroom day. The teacher is responsible for actually conducting the activities. Classroom teachers have many responsibilities that they need to worry about. Asking them to act as a "speech and language clinician" in addition to their other duties is asking a lot. For this reason, collaborative teaching or small group activities within classrooms are usually preferred over consultation approaches.

SUMMARY

This chapter discusses language disorders and language intervention with school-age children. IDEA requires states to provide these children with a free, appropriate public education in the least restrictive environment. Parents must be notified whenever children are to be tested for a language disorder, and they should be part of the decision-making team after testing.

Children with language disorders who are in the primary grades often have difficulties with understanding and producing complex sentences, with narrative development, and with the phonological awareness abilities that support literacy development. Children with language disorders who are in the secondary grades often have difficulties with content-specific vocabulary, expository texts, and metacognitive learning strategies.

SLPs assess these language abilities with the use of standardized tests and informal assessment procedures such as language sample analysis, narrative analysis, and interactive learning assessment practices. In interventions with school-age children, they use many of the same language-facilitation techniques that were explained in Chapter 10. Clinicians who work with school-age children also use literature-based intervention procedures and classroom collaboration.

BOX 11-5   Personal Story

I (RBG) worked as a public school speech-language pathologist in Douglas, Wyoming. During my first year on the job, one child on my caseload, a kindergartner named Jay, had a profound impact on my approach to therapy. Jay was one of the most severely speech and language impaired children I have ever worked with. He only produced 10 consonants and 7 vowels correctly and he omitted the final sounds from most words when spoke. He also spoke in very short, incomplete sentences. So, Jay might come up to another child in his class and say something like, "I wat mu la ni." for "I watched a movie last night." Many children chose not to play or socialize with Jay because they couldn't understand what he said.

In graduate school, I had been taught to use a pretty structured approach to speech and language therapy. I often showed the children pictures and made them practice saying individual speech sounds or syllables or short sentence patterns such as, "The boy is running. The boy is playing. The boy is jumping. The boy is riding."

One day, Jay's teacher came to watch one of his therapy sessions. She indicated to me that I was working on skills and activities that would not help him very much in the classroom. I decided to spend a morning observing Jay in her room. As a result, I changed the way I approached Jay's therapy. We worked on such things as giving "show-and-tell" presentations, on talking to other children during play, on asking questions, and on listening to stories, answering questions about them, and retelling them. Jay's speech and language skills improved considerably, and he was able to interact more successfully in his classroom. Based on the success I had with Jay, I changed nearly all of my intervention so that we worked on activities that were directly related to the way that the children used language in their daily lives.

STUDY QUESTIONS

1. What aspects of language development are especially difficult for school-age children with language disorders in the primary and secondary grades?

2. What is the difference between a learning disability, a language disorder, and dyslexia?

3. Describe what a maze is.

4. What is the difference between Section 504 and IDEA?

5. What is an IEP?

6. What is RTI?

7. What procedures are commonly used to assess language disorders in school-age children?

KEY TERMS

Chronological age referencing
Classroom collaboration
Decoding
Discrepancy modeling
Dyslexia
Expository texts
Individualized education program (IEP)
Individuals with Disabilities Education Act (IDEA)

Language disorder
Learning disability
Literature-based language intervention
Maze
Mental graphemic representations (MGRs)
Metacognitive strategies
No Child Left Behind Act (NCLB)

Public Law 94-142, the Education of All Handicapped Children Act of 1975
Response to intervention (RTI)
Section 504
Simple view of reading
Specific learning disability
Transcript
Word recognition

REFERENCES

Apel, K., Wolter, J. A., & Masterson, J. J. (2006). Effects of phonotactic and orthotactic probabilities during fast mapping on 5-year-olds' learning to spell. *Developmental Neuropsychology, 29*(1), 21–42.

Aram, D. M., & Hall, N. E. (1989). Longitudinal follow-up of children with preschool communication disorders: Treatment implications. *School Psychology Review, 18*(4), 487–501.

Bishop, D. V. M. (1997). *Uncommon understanding: Development and disorders of language comprehension in children*. Hove, England: Psychology Press/Erlbaum (UK), Taylor & Francis.

Carrow-Woolfolk, E. (2004). *Comprehensive assessment of spoken language*. Circle Pines, MN: American Guidance Service.

Catts, H. W., Adlof, S. M., & Weismer, W. E. (2006). Language deficits in poor comprehenders: A case for the simple view of reading. *Journal of Speech, Language, and Hearing Research, 49*, 278–293.

Catts, H. W., & Kamhi, A. G. (1999). *Language and reading disabilities*. Needham Heights, MA: Allyn & Bacon.

Ellis Weismer, S. (1996). Capacity limitations in working memory: The impact on lexical and morphological learning by children with language impairment. *Topics in Language Disorders, 17*(1), 33–44.

Ellis Weismer, S., & Hesketh, L. (1998). The impact of emphatic stress on novel word learning by children with specific language impairment. *Journal of Speech, Language, and Hearing Research, 41*, 1444–1458.

Gillam, R. B. (1995). Whole language principles at work in language intervention. In D. Tibbits (Ed.), *Language intervention: Beyond the primary grades* (pp. 219–256). Austin, TX: Pro-Ed.

Gillam, R. B., & Carlile, R. M. (1997). Oral reading and story retelling of students with specific language impairment. *Language, Speech, and Hearing Services in Schools, 28*, 30–42.

Gillam, R. B., & Johnston, J. R. (1992). Spoken and written language relationships in language/learning-impaired and normally achieving school-age children. *Journal of Speech and Hearing Research, 35*(6), 1303–1315.

Gillam, R. B., McFadden, T., & van Kleeck, A. (1995). Improving the narrative abilities of children with language disorders: Whole language and language skills approaches. In M. Fey, J. Windsor, & J. Reichle (Eds.), *Communication intervention for school-age children* (pp. 145–182). Baltimore, MD: Brookes.

Gillam, R. B., & van Kleeck, A. (1996). Phonological awareness training and short-term working memory: Clinical implications. *Topics in Language Disorders, 17*(1), 72–81.

Gillam, S. L. (2007). Understanding and remediating text comprehension deficits in school-age children. In A. Kamhi, J. Masterson, & K. Apel (Eds.), *Clinical decision making in developmental language disorders* (pp. 267–284). Baltimore, MD: Brookes.

Gillam, S. L., & St. Clair, K. (2007). Comprehension of expository text: Insights gained from think-aloud data. Manuscript in preparation.

Gillon, G. (2005). The efficacy of phonological awareness intervention for children with spoken language impairment. *Language, Speech, and Hearing Services in Schools, 31*, 126–141.

Gough, P. B., & Tunmer, W. E. (1986). Decoding, reading and reading disability. *Remedial and Special Education, 7*(1), 6–10.

Individuals with Disabilities Education Act of 2004, P.L. 108-446. (2004). Title I, Part A, Section 602 Definitions. U.S. Government Clearing House.

Lyon, R. (1995). Toward a definition of dyslexia. *Annals of Dyslexia, 4*, 3–30.

Mayer, M. (1969). *Frog, where are you?* New York: Penguin Books.

Newcomer, P. L., & Hammill, D. D. (1997). *Test of Language Development—Primary* (3rd ed.). Austin, TX: Pro-Ed.

Paul, R., Hernandez, R., Taylor, L., & Johnson, K. (1996). Narrative development in late talkers: Early school age. *Journal of Speech and Hearing Research, 39*, 1295–1303.

Paul, R., Murray, C., Clancy, K., & Andrews, D. (1997). Reading and metaphonological outcomes in late talkers. *Journal of Speech, Language, and Hearing Research, 40*, 1037–1047.

Records, N. L., Tomblin, J. B., & Buckwalter, P. R. (1995). Auditory verbal learning and memory in young adults with specific language impairment. *Clinical Neuropsychologist, 9*, 187–193.

Rescorla, L. (2002). Language and reading outcomes to age 9 in late-talking toddlers. *Journal of Speech, Language, and Hearing Research, 45*, 360–371.

Rescorla, L. (2005). Language and reading outcomes of late-talking toddlers at age 13. *Journal of Speech, Language, and Hearing Research, 48*, 1–14.

Semel, E., Wiig, E., & Secord, W. (1996). *Clinical evaluation of language fundamentals* (3rd ed.). San Antonio, TX: Psychological Corporation.

Stothard, S. E., Snowling, M. J., Bishop, D. V. M., Chipchase, B. B., & Kaplan, C. A. (1998). Language-impaired preschoolers: A follow-up into adolescence. *Journal of Speech, Language, and Hearing Research, 41*, 407–418.

U.S. Department of Education. (2005). *Twenty-Sixth Annual (2004) Report to Congress on the Implementation of the Individuals with Disabilities Education Act.* (Publication No. ED01CO0082/0008). Washington, DC: U.S. Government Printing Office.

U.S. Department of Education. (2006). *Federal Register. Assistance to states for the education of children with disabilities and preschool grants for children with disabilities; Final rule.* Washington, DC: U.S. Government Printing Office.

van Kleeck, A., Gillam, R., & McFadden, T. U. (1998). A study of classroom-based phonological awareness training for preschoolers with speech and/or language disorders. *American Journal of Speech-Language Pathology, 7*, 66–77.

SUGGESTED READINGS

Butler, K. G., & Silliman, E. R. (2002). *Speaking, reading, and writing in children with language learning disabilities: New paradigms in research and practice.* Mahwah, NJ: Erlbaum.

Catts, H. W., & Kamhi, A. G. (Eds.). (2005). *Language and reading disabilities* (2nd ed.). Needham Heights, MA: Allyn & Bacon.

Falk-Ross, F. (2002). *Classroom-based language and literacy intervention: A programs and case studies approach.* Boston: Allyn & Bacon.

Johnston, J. (2006). *Thinking about child language.* Eau Claire, WI: Thinking Publications.

Kamhi, A., Masterson, J., & Apel, K. (2007). *Clinical decision making in developmental language disorders.* Baltimore, MD: Brookes.

Leonard, L. B. (1998). *Children with specific language impairment.* Cambridge, MA: MIT Press.

Naremore, R. C., Densmore, A. E., & Harman, D. R. (1995). *Language intervention with school-age children: Conversation, narrative, and text.* San Diego, CA: Singular Publishing.

Nippold, M. A. (1998). *Later language development: The school-age and adolescent years* (2nd edition). Austin, TX: Pro-Ed.

Silliman, E. R., & Wilkinson, L. C. (Eds.), (2004). *Language and literacy learning in schools.* New York: Guilford.

Ukrainetz, T. A. (2006). *Contextualized language intervention: Scaffolding PreK–12 literacy achievement.* Eau Claire, WI: Thinking Publications.

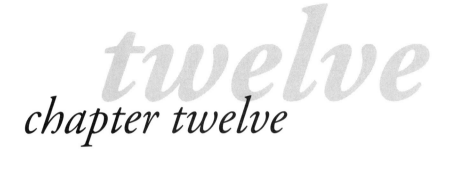

chapter twelve

Acquired Neurogenic Language Disorders

THOMAS P. MARQUARDT AND SWATHI KIRAN

LEARNING OBJECTIVES

1. To learn the primary causes of brain damage that result in communication disorders in adults.

2. To learn why the site of brain damage influences the type of language disorder.

3. To understand the components of language that can be impaired.

4. To understand the different types of aphasia based on their characteristics.

5. To learn the different treatment options for adults with language disorders.

The disorders considered in this chapter are called *neurogenic* because they involve impairment of the nervous system. Damage to the nervous system results in different types of language disorders depending on the site and extent of the lesion and the underlying cause. The disorders are termed *acquired* because they result from brain injury that disrupts the planning, formulation, and execution of language.

Although this chapter focuses primarily on neurogenic language disorders, it is important to note that injury to the nervous system frequently affects every aspect of the individual's life. The combined impact of paralysis of one side of the body, vision problems, and communication difficulties make everyday activities difficult and frustrating. A communication disorder is only one consequence of damage to the nervous system that the individual must face. This chapter discusses the causes of brain injury, the consequences of the damage, and the role of the speech-language pathologist (SLP) in helping the individual regain success in everyday communication situations.

CAUSES OF BRAIN DAMAGE

Four primary causes of brain damage can affect communication: stroke, head injury, infections and tumors, and progressive degeneration of the central nervous system. The effects of these disease processes on communication depend on whether the left, right, or both sides of the brain are involved.

The most frequent cause of brain damage is a **cerebrovascular accident (CVA)**, or stroke. Strokes can result from an **embolus**, a moving clot from another part of body that lodges in the artery, or a **thrombosis**, which occurs when an artery has gradually filled in with plaque. Both types of stroke result in the closing of an artery to the brain, which leads to the deprivation of oxygen (**anoxia**) to an area of the brain, with subsequent death of the tissue (**infarct**). A stroke may be preceded by a **transient ischemic attack**, a temporary closing of the artery with symptoms that disappear within 24 hours. **Hemorrhages** are another type of stroke that involves bleeding in the brain. A common cause of a hemorrhage is a ruptured **aneurysm**, a weakening in the artery that bulges and eventually breaks, interrupting blood flow to tissues fed by the artery.

The prevalence and morbidity vary for each of the etiologies of stroke. Thromboses occur more frequently than do hemorrhages, but individuals with thrombosis are more likely to survive the stroke. Strokes occur most often in older adults because the blood vessels of the brain become blocked and brittle as a result of arteriosclerosis.

The effects of a stroke are immediate. The individual may lose consciousness, have difficulty speaking, and be paralyzed on the side of the body opposite the hemisphere of the brain that was damaged. Typically, these effects are most prominent during the first 3 to 5 days after the stroke and are related to swelling of brain tissue (**edema**) and reductions in blood flow. After this period, there is a recovery of function (**spontaneous recovery**) associated with a reduction in edema, a return to more normal blood flow, and a reorganization of nervous system processes. Recovery generally is better if the brain damage is small and the stroke occurs at a young age.

A second type of brain damage is caused by trauma to the head. In penetrating injuries, a foreign object enters the skull and causes focal damage along the route the object travels. Symptoms vary depending on the part of the brain that has been damaged. In closed head injury, most often caused by motor vehicle accidents or falls, the brain is twisted and forced against the interior of the skull. Damage may include bruises on the surface of the cortex (**contusions**), tearing of structures and blood vessels (**lacerations**), and damage to nerve cells in the connecting fibers of the brain (**diffuse axonal injury**). Coupled with this damage may be hemorrhages within the brain (**intracerebral**) or within tissue coverings of the brain (**meninges**) that form **hematomas** (areas of encapsulated blood).

Head injuries can range from mild to severe depending on the force of the impact and the amount of brain tissue affected. Missile wounds, such as gunshots, may affect a very specific area of the brain. Damage sustained in a motorcycle accident will generally affect many different parts. The greater the severity and extent of the injury, the more that motoric, cognitive, and communication skills will be affected. In severe head injury the individual may be comatose and not remember the incident at all when he or she recovers. The length of time the person is in a coma varies but is usually longer when the brain trauma is more severe.

Additional causes of damage to the nervous system are space-occupying growths within the skull and infections. **Neoplasms** (new growths) and tumors, which can be malignant or benign, can occur within the interior of the brain or on the surface within the tissue coverings. These growths take up space and, depending on their type, cause destruction of brain tissue and increased pressure in the skull. Brain tumors can be slow or fast growing. Slow-growing tumors have a better prognosis. When their primary effect is to take up space, the symptoms reported are dizziness, headache, memory deficits, and generalized sensory and/or motor problems. Infections, when treatable with antibiotics, may produce temporary effects, but also may produce permanent damage because they destroy areas of brain tissue.

A final cause of brain damage is progressive deterioration of brain functions, often caused by a gradual loss of brain cells resulting in brain atrophy. For example, Alzheimer's disease, which makes up 70% of the cases of **dementia**, results from degeneration of neurons, the accumulation of amyloid plaques, and tangles (twisted stands of proteins) formed inside brain cells. A similar disorder, Pick's disease, results from deposition of Pick's bodies (rounded microscopic structures) within neurons. Huntington's disease and Parkinson's disease are characterized by degenerative changes in subcortical structures such as the basal ganglia. Progressive and ultimately global deterioration of cells leads to impaired cognitive, communicative, and motor functioning impairments.

APHASIA

Aphasia is a language disorder caused by left hemisphere damage, typically resulting from a stroke. Auditory comprehension, verbal expression, and reading and writing deficits are common characteristics of the disorder. Phonology, syntax, semantics, and pragmatics can all be affected. Typically, some aspects of language are more or less impaired than others.

Patterns of Communication Performance in Aphasia

The Boston Diagnostic Aphasia Examination (Goodglass, Kaplan, & Barresi, 2001) is used to identify patterns of impairment for this classification system. This test includes items such as picture naming, sentence repetition, yes/no questions, rhythm, writing, and repetitive movements of the speech production structures at maximum rates. Performance on the test items reflects an individual's abilities in four primary language areas: naming, fluency, auditory comprehension, and repetition. Clinicians use the patterns of strengths and weaknesses in these areas of communication to classify the type of aphasia.

Naming

Naming is the process of knowing and retrieving the label for an object, picture, or concept. If someone were to ask you, "What are you reading?" the ability to respond "A *book*" involves a complex process in which you must identify and say the label for the object you are holding. First, you access the conceptual store that identifies the item as something with a cover, lots of pages, and that you read. Next, you identify a semantic label that best fits the concept you established, in this case "book." In the third step, you develop a phonological form for the label, for example, b-oo-k. Finally, your brain programs the speech movements needed to say the word.

Naming deficits can result from a problem at any stage of the process. Individuals with naming problems have difficulty naming a concept and will instead say the wrong name, say a word that is phonologically or semantically similar, use a nonsense word,

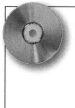

BOX 12-1   A Woman With Aphasia

A woman with aphasia is shown on Volume 2 of the CD-ROM. Included are a brain scan (segment Ch.12.01) and segments that show her talking (Ch.12.02 and Ch.12.03), following instructions (Ch.12.04), and repeating phrases (Ch.12.05 and Ch.12.06). These tasks allow the clinician to classify the patient into one of the types of aphasia.

BOX 12-2   Word-Finding Problems

CD-ROM segment Ch.12.01 is a computerized tomography (CT) scan showing a lesion to the left frontal area of the brain.

In segment Ch.12.02, Mrs. L. is describing moving to Arizona. Word-finding problems are evident, but she uses compensatory strategies including describing the location of the city, gesturing, and shifting some of the communicative burden to the listener. Notice that Mrs. L's speech is nonfluent but not agrammatic. She uses fully grammatical sentences, but they are produced slowly and with some struggle.

or avoid giving a name. **Neologisms** are new words such as the use of *gabot* for *table*. When a nonsense word of this type is produced, the individual may have no awareness that it is not meaningful to the listener. Selection of an alternate for an intended word in a category, such as *lion* for *tiger*, is an example of a **verbal paraphasia**; substitution of one or more sounds in the phonological realization of the word (*gable* for *cable*) or transpositions of sound elements are called **literal paraphasias**, both of which are relatively common in aphasia. At times, the individual uses strategies to locate and produce the word (**circumlocution**). The individual describes the characteristics of the item, how it is used, and in what circumstances, but cannot name it.

Although the errors provide information on the type of naming problem, at times the individual may indicate that he does not know the name of the item. In this case, failure to name does not provide information on why the task cannot be carried out. It could be a result of a failure in recognizing the item, difficulty retrieving the label, or an inability to access the motor program for the word's production.

Clinicians use various tasks to assess naming. For example, the clinician may show the individual a picture of a chair, cactus, or spoon and ask him or her to name the item. The clinician might also ask the individual to name all the jungle animals he or she can think of and words beginning with the letter *s*. The kinds of errors made on the tasks allow the clinician to determine the severity of the naming impairment and make predictions about the stage(s) in the process that have been affected by the brain damage. Naming is a complex process that may have more than a single level at which it is impaired. Naming deficits are a universally expected feature of aphasia regardless of the lesion site. Because damage to the right hemisphere and progressive global deterioration of the brain also may cause naming problems, the deficit is an indicator of a neurogenic communication disorder rather than a specific type of aphasia.

Fluency

In fluent speech, syllables are produced rhythmically, and speakers use pitch and stress variations that are appropriate to the intended meaning of the utterance. In aphasia, patients with fluent speech present with an overall ease of speaking, normal length and rate, and adequate melody. In contrast, nonfluent speech is characterized by effort, a slow rate, and abnormal pauses. Typically, fluent speech is observed in patients with posterior lesions, and nonfluent speech is characteristic of patients with anterior lesions. Clinicians listen for unusual patterns of rhythm, rate, ease of production,

BOX 12-3   Word Retrieval

In segment Ch.12.03, Mrs. L is trying to say the word *Missouri*. She retrieves the name of *Kansas City*, but she begins saying the word *Arizona*. This is an example of a perseverative response because she has just finished talking about that state. She realizes the error and chooses the strategy of orally spelling the word until the clinician produces the word *Missouri* for her.

and intonation (variations in pitch and stress) as individuals engage in conversation, describe pictures, give directions, and tell stories.

Auditory Comprehension

Auditory comprehension is the ability to understand spoken language, that is, words, commands, questions, or groups of utterances. Auditory comprehension is a complex process that involves being able to segment the sounds heard into meaningful phonemes, understanding the meaning of the words within the sentence, and retaining the message in memory long enough to understand it and formulate a response. The ability to understand language interacts with the ability to discriminate between words and to remember instructions. Some patients are able to participate in casual conversations by giving appropriate replies but fail standardized tests. Other patients demonstrate severe limitations in comprehending single words.

Clinicians assess auditory comprehension by asking questions, making statements, or giving commands, to which the individual must respond. Responses can be nonverbal to ensure that the individual is not limited by an inability to produce language. The clinician may ask the individual with aphasia to point to the door or ceiling, to follow complex instructions such as placing a pencil between a cup and a spoon, and to respond to questions such as "Does a stone float?"

Repetition

Repetition of words and phrases assesses the integrity of connecting pathways between Wernicke's area of the temporal lobe and Broca's area of the frontal lobe. When asked to repeat a phrase, the individual must hear the phrase (Wernicke's area) and then organize the output for repetition (Broca's area). Damage to Broca's area or Wernicke's area affects spontaneous production as well as repetition. However, when the major pathway (the arcuate fasciculus) between the two areas has been damaged, individuals

---

BOX 12-4   Simple and Complex Commands

CD-ROM segment Ch.12.04 demonstrates Mrs. L's ability to perform simple and complex commands without error.

BOX 12-5   Repetition of Short Phrases

In CD-ROM segment Ch.12.05, Mrs. L repeats short phrases with only minor articulation errors.

Notice in CD-ROM segment Ch.12.06 that Mrs. L has difficulty with longer and more unusual phrases. There also is evidence of a verbal paraphasic response with a self-correction.

usually exhibit a marked difficulty repeating words and phrases but minimal problems with auditory comprehension or fluency. The ability to repeat may be entirely lost and replaced with paraphasias and omissions.

Sentence Formulation and Production

The process of formulating and producing a sentence is complex and involves several stages. For example, to say the sentence "The chef is baking a cake," an individual first must access the conceptual store to plan the message, then select nouns and verbs (*bake, chef, cake*) along with other plausible entries (*cook, make, pie*). The verb chosen (*bake*) assigns functional roles to the nouns (e.g., who is doing what to whom). The individual arranges the sentence in grammatical order by inserting appropriate grammatical markers (e.g., *is, are, the*). Impairments in sentence production vary from omission of verbs, incorrect ordering of words (e.g., *chef cake baking*), or omission of function words such as articles, prepositions, and conjunctions (e.g., *chef is bake cake*). These errors in sentence production are called agrammatism.

Classification of Aphasia

The categories of naming, fluency, auditory comprehension, and repetition provide a method for describing the symptoms of aphasia. The classification of aphasia type can be based on differences in relative impairment of naming, fluency, auditory comprehension, and repetition. The next section reviews the different types of aphasia. The system for classifying aphasia does not work for every case. A significant portion of the aphasic population (approximately 25%) cannot be reliably assigned to a specific category because their disorder includes patterns that are indicative of more than one type of aphasia. Descriptions of the different types of aphasia are listed in Table 12-1.

Broca's Aphasia

Damage to Broca's area on the posterior inferior frontal lobe (see Figure 12-1) causes a type of aphasia that is marked by difficulty with fluency. The lesion most frequently involves the lateral aspect of the frontal lobe, including the insula, in addition to Broca's area. Broca's aphasia is characterized by nonfluent, effortful speech and **agrammatism**. Oral expression is slow with very short sentences (3–4 words in length) that contain mostly content words (nouns and verbs). Function words such as articles, prepositions, and conjunctions are frequently omitted. The speaker's prosody is usually quite flat, meaning there is little change in stress or rate. In response to a question about what happened to cause his aphasia, a 42-year-old man responded "Shot in head. Communicate hard. Me zero talk." This type of agrammatic verbal expression is also observed in phrase repetition and in writing. Patients are usually aware of their struggle to produce speech, and they make repeated efforts to correct their errors. Auditory comprehension is relatively intact, although not entirely spared. When they are asked to follow directions that require comprehension of function words ("Put the ball *under* the box") or grammatically complex sentences ("Point to the boy who is pushing the girl"), comprehension errors are more frequent.

Table 12-1 Classification of Aphasia

	Broca	Wernicke	Global	Conduction	Anomia	Transcortical Motor	Transcortical Sensory
Speech	Nonfluent	Fluent (paraphasic)	Nonfluent	Fluent	Fluent (pauses)	Nonfluent	Fluent (echolalic)
Naming	Impaired	Paraphasic (mix up sounds in words)	Impaired	Variable	Impaired	Impaired	Impaired
Comprehension	Impaired for complex items	Impaired	Impaired	Intact	Intact	Intact	Impaired
Repetition	Impaired	Impaired	Impaired	Impaired	Intact	Intact	Intact
Reading	May be impaired	Impaired	Impaired	May be intact	Intact	May be intact	Impaired
Writing	Impaired	Impaired	Impaired	May be intact	Intact	Impaired	Impaired
Location of lesion	Broca's area	Wernicke's area	Perisylvian region	Left superior temporal region or inferior parietal lobule	Diffuse/focal	Sparing Broca's area	Sparing Wernicke's area

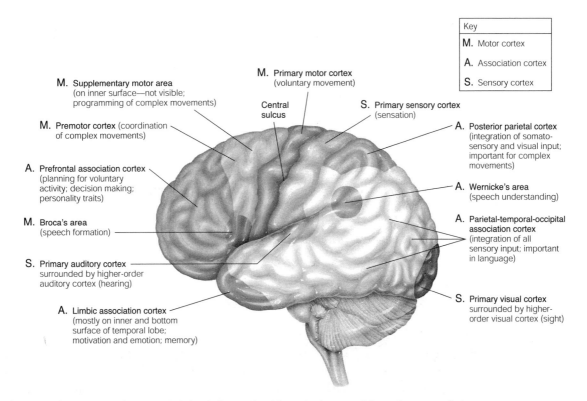

Figure 12-1 Lateral aspect of the left cerebral hemisphere, with major speech-language areas labaeled. BA = Broca's area, WA = Wernicke's area, AG = angular gyrus, SMG = supramarginal gyrus, SMA = supplementary motor area, and OM = orofacial motor cortex. *Source:* Chiras, D. D. (2008) *Human Biology* (6th ed., p. 200). Jones and Bartlett.

Wernicke's Aphasia

Damage to Wernicke's area and tissue surrounding the superior posterior temporal lobe causes a type of aphasia that is marked by deficits in auditory comprehension and fluent oral expression. Individuals with Wernicke's aphasia have marked difficulty in comprehending language, spoken or written. Sometimes the deficit in auditory comprehension is so severe that patients cannot even identify single words. Speech output has normal intonation and stress. However, speech production is filled with verbal paraphasias (mixing up sounds in words) and neologisms (making up new words). This kind of speech may seem "empty" because of the lack of intelligible content words. Some patients are not aware their speech is not understandable, and they show little obvious concern about their problems with communication. The use of meaningless neologisms may be so frequent that speech sounds like jargon (these sequences of phonemes that sound like words were discussed in Chapter 2). For this reason, the individual is described as having **jargon aphasia**. In addition to problems with speech, reading and writing abilities are significantly affected. Repetition is impaired, and writing mirrors oral expression with the production of neologisms and paraphasias.

Conduction Aphasia

Recall from Chapter 4 that there is a group of fibers (the arcuate fasciculus) that connects Broca's area to Wernicke's area and the supramarginal gyrus. Damage to this pathway results in a type of aphasia in which there is an impaired ability to "conduct" information from one part of the nervous system to another. This disconnection results in an inability to repeat what was heard because the auditory input cannot be transmitted to the area of the brain where speech output is organized. Individuals with conduction aphasia have marked problems with repeating phrases in the context of normal auditory comprehension. Their oral expression is fluent, but it often includes frequent literal paraphasias (transpositions of sounds) because of a deficit in the person's ability to select and order phonological elements of words. The literal paraphasias, such as *cake* for *take*, appear in their speech and in their writing. These patients often try to correct their phonemic errors by saying the word repeatedly.

Anomic Aphasia

Anomia literally translated means "without words." The primary deficit of patients with anomic aphasia is a marked difficulty in retrieving the names of objects, pictures, or concepts. Auditory comprehension, verbal expression, and repetition are otherwise relatively unimpaired. Their connected speech is characterized by a marked absence of nouns. Patients produce paraphasias and circumlocutions in an attempt to convey meaningful information. The site of lesion cannot be reliably inferred from these behaviors, although most physicians and clinicians suspect that the patient has suffered a posterior lesion in the temporal-parietal area. In some cases, lesions elsewhere in the left hemisphere have resulted in similar symptoms.

Transcortical Aphasia

Widespread "watershed" lesions of the frontal and temporal-parietal areas interrupt the ability to process sensory information and to program sequential skilled movements. Generally, there is widespread damage to these areas of association cortex. Wernicke's area, the arcuate fasciculus, and Broca's area are usually left intact. Transcortical aphasias are found most often in older individuals because the nervous system damage that causes this type of aphasia results from a gradual deterioration of the blood supply at the periphery of the major arteries to the brain.

There are two types of transcortical aphasia. When the damage involves the frontal lobe, a type of aphasia termed "transcortical motor" results. Patients with this type of aphasia often have good auditory comprehension and repetition, but they have significant difficulty initiating speech production. When you ask a patient with transcortical motor aphasia a question, you will likely get a grammatically complete response. However, the response will be nonfluent. Even though this type of patient responds to questions, he or she is not assertive. That is, the patient does not ask many questions and does not add information to a conversation unless specifically asked.

When the damage involves areas of the posterior part of the brain around Wernicke's area, a type of aphasia termed "transcortical sensory" results. Patients with transcortical sensory aphasia have severe deficits in auditory comprehension. However, their speech is usually fluent, and they can repeat words and sentences that are spoken to them. This combination of good repetition ability and poor comprehension results in an unusual pattern of behavior. These patients are able to repeat commands verbally, but they are unable to understand or carry them out.

Global Aphasia

When the damage to the left hemisphere is extensive enough to involve a wide area of the lateral aspect, all parts of language processing are severely impaired. Patients with global aphasia have nonfluent verbal expression, poor auditory comprehension, and difficulty repeating words and sentences. In the most severe form of global aphasia, the patient's lexicon (his or her bank of available vocabulary items) is reduced to a few words that are used repeatedly to respond to questions. These patients cannot even follow one-stage commands or repeat single words. Their speech output may be accompanied by gestures that are not meaningfully employed for communication.

ASSESSMENT AND DIAGNOSIS OF APHASIA

Immediately following brain injury, when language ability is most impaired and variable, the SLP observes and interacts with the patient to determine the level of impairment in verbal expression, auditory comprehension, repeating, reading, and naming. This assessment is usually conducted while the patient is recovering in the hospital. When conducting the assessment, the SLP usually employs informal tasks to evaluate language skill, such as engaging the patient in conversation, asking the patient to name items located in the hospital room, and asking the patient to follow simple commands.

During the first few weeks following brain injury, there is a period referred to as "spontaneous recovery." This is a period of significant changes that occur from day to day as the nervous system recovers and reorganizes from reduced responsiveness of distant neurons, abnormal release of neurotransmitters, and reduced blood flow to the brain. These early changes are followed by a rewiring of synapses associated with the physiological recovery process. Communication during this period is variable and is affected by fatigue, medical complications, and medications. The SLP's role is to make a preliminary determination of the type and extent of aphasia and to serve as a resource for the patient and the family. Of particular importance at this point is the provision of information to the patient and family about the effects of stroke and the development of a functional communication system for the patient.

The SLP may administer a more formal assessment that includes an aphasia test battery when the patient becomes more stable. The Boston Diagnostic Aphasia Examination (Goodglass et al., 2001), the Porch Index of Communicative Ability (Porch, 1967), and the Western Aphasia Battery (Kertesz, 1982) are three examples of comprehensive aphasia batteries. Each test contains tasks that assess reading, writing, auditory comprehension, naming, and other language abilities. Following the broad assessment of language function, the SLP may conduct more specific evaluations of naming, semantic processing, sentence production, reading, and writing. Results from these assessment tasks are placed in the context of other information about the patient's medical, educational, and family history to arrive at a differential diagnosis, that is, a labeling of the language deficit pattern. The diagnosis is valuable to the extent that there are treatment programs proven to be most effective for particular disorders.

The SLP also assesses functional communication skills or the ability to communicate meaning in familiar contexts regardless of the quality of the spoken language. It has been long observed that individuals with aphasia communicate more effectively than one might expect given their poor performance on formal language tests. Aphasics often use compensatory skills such as gesturing, intonation, facial expression, and writing to supplement residual verbal expression and to facilitate communication success. Functional measures such as the Functional Communication Profile (Sarno, 1969) and assessments based on role-playing as in the Communicative Abilities in Daily Living test (Holland, 1980) are often used to estimate the individual's ability to communicate in everyday situations.

Motoric, visual, and cognitive deficits commonly associated with aphasia may complicate the assessment process (see Figure 12-2). When there is damage to the frontal lobe, a **hemiplegia** (muscle weakness or paralysis) is often observed on the side of the body opposite from the side of the brain damage. A motoric impairment may make it difficult for a patient to follow commands. Vision may also be affected because of interruption in the visual pathways between the optic chiasm and the visual processing areas of the occipital lobe. An example of a visual problem that accompanies some aphasias is **homonymous hemianopsia**, which is a loss of one half of the visual field on the side opposite the brain hemisphere that was damaged. A homonymous hemianopsia may make it difficult for a patient to see objects to name them or point to them, or it may impair reading. Cognitive deficits such as a decreased ability to remember or maintain attention can co-occur with aphasia. The ability to follow commands, answer questions, and repeat phrases are all dependent on the ability to attend to and remember what was heard. A clinician conducting a speech and language assessment must also be aware of how the patient's response is influenced by these nonlinguistic variables.

Case Study: Mrs. L

Mrs. L, age 68 years, incurred a left hemisphere CVA when she was 65 years old. A CT scan revealed a subcortical lesion involving the left middle cerebral artery in the basal ganglia. As a result of the stroke, Mrs. L had a nonfluent aphasia, minimal

BOX 12-6 Patterns of Performance

Review the brain scan and CD-ROM segments of Ms. L again. Note that her diagnosis is based on the pattern of communication abilities/disabilities.

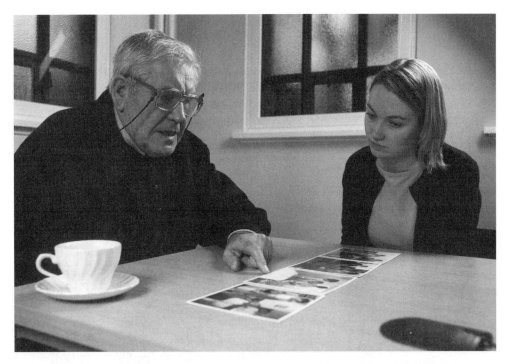

Figure 12-2   Patient with aphasia responding to pictures. *Source:* © Colin Cuthbert/SPL/Photo Researchers, Inc.

comprehension deficits, and a right hemiparesis. Results from the Boston Diagnostic Aphasia Examination 3 years postonset of brain damage showed mild to moderate problems in auditory comprehension and repetition and in reading and writing skills. Mrs. L's word finding and articulation were the most impaired areas of communication. An SLP administered a measure of functional communication, the Communicative Abilities in Daily Living (Holland, 1980). This test revealed minimally reduced functional communication abilities with mild difficulty with memory, word finding, and interpreting nonliteral situations and incongruous language.

Based on the assessment, Mrs. L was diagnosed as having mild Broca's aphasia. Her auditory comprehension was minimally impaired, but her speech production was nonfluent, with word-finding problems and difficulty on more demanding repetition tasks. Mrs. L had an excellent recovery, which was anticipated because she was highly motivated, the lesion was small, and therapy for this type of aphasia is usually quite effective.

THE TREATMENT OF APHASIA

Assessment provides the basis for treatment by identifying the type and severity of aphasia and a general picture of the communication tasks the patient can perform. SLPs may provide aphasia treatment in individual or group therapy sessions. The initial goal is to provide the patient with a reliable communication system. Just like language intervention with young children, intervention with adults who have aphasia must begin at the level of communication ability of the person. In the case of severe aphasia, intervention activities may target the production of single words or the use of some gestures. In the case of less severe aphasia, intervention activities may target oral expression abilities, reading, and/or writing. There are two primary goals in therapy: maximizing language abilities and developing compensatory communication strategies.

Specific Treatment Approaches for Aphasia

Treatment for aphasia may produce significant improvement in language functioning for an extended period after brain injury and have important effects on quality of life. A primary communication problem for many individuals with aphasia is naming. The SLP can facilitate word retrieval by using tasks that improve conceptual retrieval of the word (e.g., apple: *red, fruit, has seeds*), matching the picture of an apple to a word, choosing related words (e.g., *apple-orange*), or sorting pictures. The SLP also can work on improving access to words by employing tasks such as phonological rhyming (e.g., *berry-merry*), phonemic cueing (e.g., *tuh* for *table*), and matching pictures to sounds (Raymer, Thompson, Jacobs, & LeGrand, 1993). When individuals with aphasia have a mild language deficit or can retrieve words but cannot formulate grammatical sentences, focusing on verb access and assembling nouns and verbs together using picture cues may promote sentence production. Similarly, reading and writing deficits can be addressed by focusing on word retrieval using semantic tasks or tasks that involve the relearning of spelling to sound correspondence rules (e.g., RABBIT: /r//a//b//b//i//t/; Kiran, Thompson, & Hashimoto, 2001). Treatment items that are personally relevant have a higher probability of affecting everyday communication. It also is important for SLPs to promote any form of communication output for individuals with aphasia, whether it is oral, written, or gestural.

For example, Ms. CA was a country singer from Virginia. She and her husband had produced several successful music records and traveled across the country to give live performances. At age 55, Ms. CA suffered a stroke in the left hemisphere and was diagnosed with conduction aphasia. She received extensive therapy, but 8 months later continued to have significant communication problems.

Ms. CA subsequently was involved in experimental therapy. Because one of her main communication problems was finding the right word (word retrieval problems), she was provided with treatment to improve her naming skills. Upon completion of treatment, she reported that her ability to name objects had improved but that she was disappointed that she still could not sing her old songs. She was then involved in a treatment program to improve the ability to produce sentences, and she made significant gains. Over the course of the treatment program, her language abilities improved from a diagnosis of moderately severe aphasia to only mild aphasia 2 years later. Ms. CA had also begun practicing songs again, and although she was not sure whether she would ever return to giving live performances, she sang for small audiences in her hometown.

Improving communication skills can also be addressed in group therapy. Group sessions are often used for practicing communication skills in a nonthreatening and supportive environment. When three or four individuals with aphasia meet together with an SLP, they have an opportunity to use their own regained communication skills and to observe the kinds of communication strategies that other members of the group use. The group chooses topics for discussion, such as the best sites to visit in the city, how I met my spouse, hobbies, and places traveled to on vacations. Although an SLP leads the group, the focus is on helping individuals with aphasia to communicate with each other, demonstrating communication strategies in a supportive environment.

Family Participation in Therapy

Group therapy can also be an opportunity for individuals and their families to engage in open discussion of the consequences of stroke and positive strategies for dealing with everyday problems they encounter. Meetings of this type are helpful because aphasia affects the family as well as the patient, and there are important changes in family responsibilities and interactions. Waisanen (1998), in interviews with wives of stroke patients about changes in their lives, reported the following comments:

> "I have to do everything that (my husband) used to do, because he really can't do much of anything around the house."

> "He's like three different people, like three personalities. He's his old self, he is childish, and at times he even acts retarded. But these things pass, and they're not him. Basically he's his sweet gentle self."

> "My circle of friends are the same, his are not. I learned early on that the men drop off. They don't come to see him; they don't check on him. I think they don't want to put themselves in his place."

There is a reorganizational change that takes place in the family. Family members may experience feelings of loss, anger, and grief as the patient and family recover from the changes caused by the stroke. Spouses who have not worked outside the home may become the primary wage earners. Some old friendships wither, and new ones are made as the patient and family change to meet the challenges brought about by brain injury. One aspect of therapy directed by the clinician is to assist the family in developing new ways to communicate effectively and devising strategies for improving the patient's ability to communicate meaningfully.

RIGHT HEMISPHERE COMMUNICATION DEFICITS

Aphasia, as discussed, results from neurological damage to the left hemisphere of the brain. The left hemisphere is generally considered to house the neuroanatomic structures associated with the form and content of language. Damage to the right hemisphere also affects the communication process in aspects related to language use rather than form or content. Aspects of communication dependent on the functioning of the right hemisphere can be broadly considered within the following areas, which are addressed in detail: affective processing, comprehension of indirect meanings, and the structuring of conversational and narrative discourse.

An important aspect of communication is the ability to interpret the emotion that overlays the spoken word. Emotion is generally conveyed through facial expressions and changes in intonation. Patients with right hemisphere damage often have difficulty conveying emotion through facial expression and prosody. Sometimes they exhibit a reduced sensitivity to displays of emotion in others as well. An individual with right hemisphere damage will fail to understand the angry tone behind a statement such as, "Thanks for forgetting to pick me up after work," and interpret it based on the words as a genuine expression of gratitude. An inability to interpret the underlying emotion can result in misinterpretation of the message.

The right hemisphere seems to be involved in the ability to produce the "big picture" from the details. Individuals with right hemisphere damage often see the details but are unable to understand the broader meaning they represent. They also have difficulty interpreting nonliteral meanings of phrases. They understand the individual meanings of the words but cannot put them together to grasp the figurative meaning. They have difficulty interpreting metaphors and analogies such as "The man is a knight in shining armor" and "He is big as a house." This kind of figurative language is usually interpreted in concrete terms. Coupled with the inability to use abstract interpretations of figurative language is a lack of appreciation of humor. This happens because humor is based on ambiguity and incongruities that do not make sense if they are interpreted literally.

Discourse in a communication context is difficult for the individual with right hemisphere brain damage. Narration and conversation discourse are marked by an overabundance of detailed information, with some of the information not directly relevant to the topic. Some individuals with right hemisphere damage begin to talk too much, even though they may have been somewhat reticent prior to experiencing a brain lesion. This results in inefficient communication, and the listener must infer how all the extra information that is provided relates to the topic of discussion. For example, Mr. P, a 72-year-old retired businessman with a history of right hemisphere brain damage, was asked to tell about what happened at the time of the stroke. He indicated that he was playing golf and noticed a tingling in his left leg. He then proceeded to describe the rules of golf, the best golf courses in Texas and Colorado, the brand names of golf equipment, and the merits of playing golf. He only returned to the topic of what happened at the time of the stroke after prompting from the examiner.

Stories told by these individuals often are poorly organized, making it difficult for listeners to tell exactly who did what to whom. Individual elements of a story may be described, but the description includes both important and unimportant information. These individuals suffer from an inability to isolate the most important facts, to integrate this information, and to interpret the main theme or underlying cause of events.

In conversations, individuals with right hemisphere damage demonstrate an inability to maintain the topic. Conversational interactions are complicated by deficits in turn taking and by the patient's assumption that the listener has more shared knowledge about people, ideas, and events than the listener really does. When asked to provide information, patients often give listeners facts not related to the topic at hand. Sometimes, they continue talking in a rambling fashion.

Assessment for right hemisphere disorders focuses on the expected areas of deficit. Typically, SLPs administer a collection of tasks that focus on prosody, inference, discourse comprehension, and production. They also use conversation and narrative tasks to assess aspects of language pragmatics that are expected to be impaired. As with individuals with aphasia, treatment is geared toward developing compensatory strategies for problems the individual may be experiencing. Rather than focusing on basic language production issues, treatment goals for individuals with right hemisphere lesions usually focus on attention, memory, story interpretation, and the ability to make inferences.

Brain Trauma

As discussed earlier, brain trauma involves neurological damage caused by injury to the head. The trauma usually results in damage to multiple areas in the brain, as well as the connecting fibers within the brain. Because brain trauma tends to be diffuse, multiple motor, speech, language, and cognitive functions may be impaired. Some patients may exhibit symptoms characteristic of aphasia if language areas in the left hemisphere are damaged. However, the majority of the characteristics of communication disorders resulting from brain trauma are most often associated with disrupted cognitive processes.

The effect of brain trauma on cognitive processes varies as a result of the extent and severity of injury. Immediately after the trauma, there is a period of "black-out" that may last just seconds but that can extend as long as months. When the individual regains consciousness, typically he or she experiences a loss of memory about the accident. The effect of traumatic brain damage is usually disrupted orientation, attention, memory, visual processing, and executive function that become more apparent as the patient recovers.

Various scales such as the Levels of Cognitive Functioning Scale (Hagan, 1984) have been developed to monitor the behavioral changes associated with recovery from traumatic brain injury. They are not objective tests. Rather, they are measures of tested or observed behavior that can be employed to monitor improved performance as the brain recovers. Initially, individuals who have experienced brain injury will open their eyes but will be severely confused (they know who they are, but they are confused about where they are) and restless. This stage is followed by improved orientation and a reduction in confusion, but severe problems in attention, memory, and problem solving continue. Over time, these problems resolve, but even with rehabilitation, there are often lasting problems.

The course of these predictable changes is dependent primarily on the severity of the brain trauma. In mild brain trauma, cognitive processing deficits may be noticeable only when the individual must perform in a complex situational environment, such as dealing with a computer crisis that arises at work. In severe trauma, recovery may be limited to the development of some self-help skills with required supervision in everyday situations. Individuals with traumatic brain injury exhibit a wide range of communication and cognitive deficits. The language/communication deficits include problems in word finding, formulating grammatical sentences, spelling, reading, and writing. They also have difficulty taking turns and staying on topic during conversations, and in understanding facial expressions, body language, and humor/sarcasm. The deficits in communication are intricately linked to cognitive problems such as maintaining attention and in reasoning, problem solving, and judgment. Brain trauma also makes it difficult for these individuals to plan, set goals, and evaluate their own performance.

Researchers have shown that in many cases, increasing the dependence on attention or memory leads to increased difficulty with comprehension. For example, adolescent boys with brain trauma were able to correctly determine whether two complex sentences had the same meaning, but only if they compared two sentences (Turkstra & Holland, 1998). If they compared three sentences, the memory demands were too high, and they answered incorrectly. Cognitive processing deficits may lead to poor comprehension of written and auditorially presented information.

Dementia

Recall that dementia is characterized by deterioration of cognitive and language abilities resulting from progressive degeneration of the brain caused by Alzheimer's disease, multiple strokes, Parkinson's disease, and so on. Symptoms vary depending on the underlying disease process, but in general the disorder is marked by memory problems, changes in personality, orientation problems, and episodes of confusion. The most prominent of these deficits is in memory. Initially patients have difficulty retaining information (i.e., working memory) and may misplace valuable objects (i.e., episodic memory). As the disease progresses, memory for words and their meanings is also impaired (semantic memory). Ultimately, long-term memory for people, faces, and past events is impaired.

The communication problems that are identified in individuals with dementia vary with the progression of the disease. Bayles (1986) observed that individuals in the early stages of dementia experience word omissions and trouble thinking of the correct word. They also have a reduced ability to comprehend new information, and they tend to drift from the topic. However, their grammar is generally intact. By the middle stages of the disease, vocabulary is noticeably diminished and they have difficulty comprehending grammatically complex sentences. In conversation, individuals with dementia may express ideas with little sensitivity to the communication partner. They may also fail to correct errors. By the late stages of the disease, severe anomia (inability to recall words) and jargon can be observed along with sentence fragments. These individuals produce few complex sentences, and their conversation is marked by meaningless content, repetition of words, and little meaningful use of language. By this stage, patients may be dependent on assistance for most self-help skills, and they may need continuous monitoring and support.

There are few test batteries for communication problems associated with dementia. The Arizona Battery for Communication Disorders in Dementia (Bayles & Tomoeda, 1993) includes a number of assessment tasks that are sensitive to deficits in dementia. Included are tasks such as naming, pantomime expression, oral description of objects, and oral and written discourse. The test battery includes normative data for normal older individuals and individuals with dementia.

Unfortunately, direct therapy for patients with dementia typically is not helpful. However, Bourgeois (1991), in a review of reports from fields such as psychology, nursing, and communication sciences and disorders, concluded that there are some positive outcomes from programs for dementia that focus on changing the communication environment, counseling caregivers, and providing group therapy.

SUMMARY

There are many variations in the kinds of communication disorders that result from brain injury. Where the injury occurred, how much of the brain is damaged, and the cause of the problem all influence the type of communication disorder that results. Communication disorders may involve all aspects of language (such as in aphasia), or they may be limited primarily to activities such as an inability to interpret the emotion of the speaker or take turns in a conversation (as frequently happens following right hemisphere damage). The role of the SLP is to identify the type and severity of communication deficits and to implement a plan of remediation to address these problems.

STUDY QUESTIONS

1. What are three types of brain damage that cause aphasia?

2. What are the primary differences between Broca's and Wernicke's aphasia?

3. What are three deficits associated with damage to the right hemisphere?

4. How are the cognitive deficits in dementia different from those found in brain trauma?

5. What are the expected emotional responses of the family to a family member who has had a stroke?

6. What types of errors do patients with naming impairments demonstrate?

7. What are some of the physiological processes that occur in recovery from brain damage?

8. What are the similarities and differences between conduction aphasia and anomic aphasia?

9. What are the different types of memory problems observed in individuals with dementia?

KEY TERMS

Agrammatism	Edema	Lacerations
Aneurysm	Embolus	Literal paraphasia
Anoxia	Hematoma	Meninges
Aphasia	Hemiplegia	Neologism
Cerebrovascular accident (CVA)	Hemorrhage	Neoplasm (tumor)
Circumlocution	Homonymous hemianopsia	Spontaneous recovery
Contusions	Infarct	Thrombosis
Dementia	Intracerebral	Transient ischemic attack
Diffuse axonal injury	Jargon aphasia	Verbal paraphasia

REFERENCES

Bayles, K. (1986). Management of neurogenic communication disorders associated with dementia. In R. Chapey (Ed.), *Language intervention strategies in adult aphasia* (2nd ed.). Baltimore, MD: Williams & Wilkins.

Bayles, K., & Tomoeda, C. (1993). *The Arizona Battery for Communication Disorders* (ABCD). Phoenix: Canyonland Publishing.

Bourgeois, M. (1991). Communication treatment for adults with dementia. *Journal of Speech and Hearing Research, 14,* 831–844.

Brookshire, R. (1998). *Introduction to neurogenic communication disorders* (5th ed.). St. Louis, MO: Mosby.

Goodglass, H., Kaplan, E., & Barresi, B. (2001). *The assessment of aphasia and related disorders* (3rd ed.). Philadelphia: Lippincott, Williams & Wilkins.

Hagan, C. (1984). Language disorders in head trauma. In A. Holland (Ed.), *Language disorders in adults: Recent advances* (pp. 245–282). San Diego, CA: College-Hill Press.

Holland, A. (1980). *Communicative Abilities in Daily Living.* Baltimore, MD: University Park Press.

Kertesz, A. (1982). *Western Aphasia Battery.* New York: Grune & Stratton.

Kiran, S., Thompson, C., & Hashimoto, N. (2001). Effect of training grapheme to phoneme conversation in patients with severe oral reading and naming deficits: A model based approach. *Aphasiology, 15,* 855–876.

Porch, B. (1967). *The Porch Index of Communicative Ability.* Palo Alto, CA: Consulting Psychologists Press.

Raymer, A., Thompson, C., Jacobs, B., & LeGrand, H. (1993). Phonological treatment of naming deficits in aphasia: Model based generalization analysis. *Aphasiology, 7,* 27–53.

Sarno, M. T. (1969). *Functional Communication Profile.* New York: University Medical Center.

Turkstra, L. S., & Holland, A. L. (1998). Assessment of syntax after adolescent brain injury: Effects of memory on test performance. *Journal of Speech, Language, and Hearing Research, 41,* 137–149.

Waisanen, S. (1998). Adjusting to life with aphasia: The partner's perspective. Unpublished manuscript, University of Texas, Austin.

SUGGESTED READINGS

Bayles, K. (1982). Language function in senile dementia. *Brain and Language, 16,* 265–280.

Coelho, C. (1997). Cognitive-communicative disorders following traumatic brain injury. In C. Ferrand & R. Bloom (Eds.), *Introduction to organic and neurogenic disorders of communication* (pp. 110–133). Boston: Allyn & Bacon.

Damasio, A. (1992). Aphasia. *New England Journal of Medicine, 326,* 531–539.

Maher, L. M., & Raymer, A. M. (2004). Management of anomia. *Topics in Stroke Rehabilitation,* 11, 10–21.

Myers, P. (1997). Right hemisphere syndrome. In L. LaPointe (Ed.), *Aphasia and related language disorders* (2nd ed., pp. 201–225). New York: Thieme.

Pulvermuller, F., Neininger, B., Elbert, T., Mohr, B., Rockstroh, B., Koebbel, P., et alw. (2001). Constraint-induced therapy of chronic aphasia after stroke. *Stroke,* 32, 1621–1626.

Raymer, A. M. (2001). Acquired language disorders. *Topics in Language Disorders,* 21, 42–59.

Yaair, R., & Corey-Bloom, J. (2007). Alzheimer's disease. *Seminars in Neurology,* 27, 32–41.

Hearing and Hearing Disorders

chapter thirteen

Hearing Science

CRAIG A. CHAMPLIN

LEARNING OBJECTIVES

1. To learn how sound is generated.

2. To understand how sound travels through a medium.

3. To learn the names of important structures in the auditory system.

4. To understand how different parts of the auditory system work.

Simply defined, hearing is the sense of perceiving sound. Closer examination reveals that hearing is the result of a complicated series of events. First, an object or sound source must be set into motion. A back-and-forth movement called vibration is then transferred from the source to the surrounding medium, which is usually air. When the air particles closest to the source begin to vibrate, the sound travels away from the source in all directions via a domino-like effect. Eventually, the sound reaches the listener, who is equipped with an exquisite apparatus that catches sounds as they fly through the air. Ear structures channel the sounds deeper inside the head, where the vibrations are converted to neural impulses. The impulses travel to the brain, and sound is perceived.

This chapter discusses the generation and propagation of sound. It also names important structures of the ear and auditory nervous system and describes their function. The information that is provided in this chapter is necessary for understanding much of the rest of the book. Dr. Martin considers the measurement of hearing in Chapter 14. Chapter 15 (Audiologic Rehabilitation) and Chapter 16 (The Habilitation of Children With Severe to Profound Hearing Loss) concern ways professionals can assist individuals who do not hear well. Chapter 4 (Speech Science) discusses issues related to hearing and the hearing mechanism.

FUNDAMENTALS OF SOUND

The physical bases of sound include measurements of frequency, intensity, and phase. The psychological or perceptual measures are pitch, loudness, and timbre.

Generating Sound

As mentioned previously, sound needs to be generated before it can be heard. To be a sound source, an object must have mass and elasticity. **Mass** is defined as the amount of matter present in a given object. All objects have mass. **Elasticity** refers to an object's ability to return to its original shape after being deformed (e.g., compressed or stretched). The more elastic the object, the more likely it will be a good sound source.

Perhaps a practical example can help to illustrate the process of **sound generation**. In Figure 13-1, a guitar string has been tightly stretched between two posts. The string is at rest. This position is indicated by the solid line labeled A. The string can be deformed by pulling it upward, away from its resting position. This is position B in the figure and is shown by the long dashed line. When the string is released from position B, it is drawn downward, toward its resting position. The elastic force attempts to restore the string to its original shape. However, the string does not suddenly stop once it reaches its resting position. Because the moving string has mass and thus inertia, momentum drives it, causing it to overshoot the target. As the string continues to move away from its resting position, the elastic force steadily builds. At some point, the elastic force exceeds the opposing force of momentum and the string stops, albeit briefly. This position is indicated in the figure by the short dashed line, which is labeled C. Elasticity pulls the string toward its resting position, but again it fails to stop as momentum pushes the string past its mark. As before, the elastic force increases in

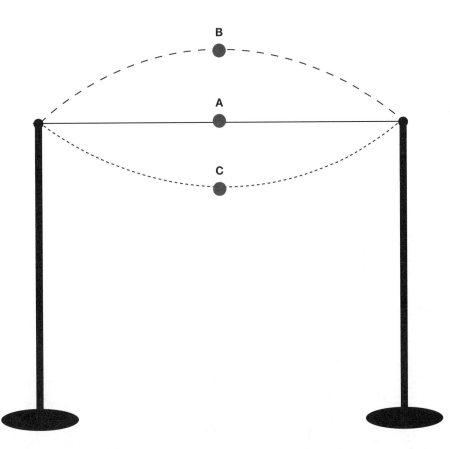

Figure 13-1 Drawing of a guitar string at three different positions during vibration. Position A indicates the resting position. Position B corresponds to the maximum positive amplitude. Position C indicates the maximum negative amplitude.

strength until it overcomes the force of momentum. Again, the string reverses its direction of travel and moves back the other way. This up-and-down motion continues until the force of friction eventually overpowers the forces of elasticity and momentum to halt the vibration.

Measuring Sound

In the previous example, the string generated vibrations, which created sound. To understand sound better, it may be instructive to consider what properties of vibration can be quantified or measured. When the string vibrates, it moves up and down. If you were to make a drawing of the string's movement over time, it would look like Figure 13-2. This graph is known as a **waveform**. The *x*-axis (horizontal line) of the graph represents the passage of time (in seconds). It shows when the vibration starts (where time equals zero) and when the vibrations stops, 3.25 seconds later in this case. The *y*-axis (vertical line) shows the distance from the resting position (in millimeters). A positive number indicates upward displacement, and a negative number indicates downward

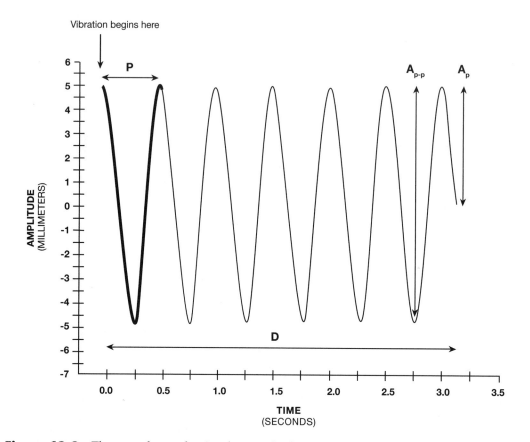

Figure 13-2 The waveform of a simple sound. The period (P), duration (D), peak amplitude (A_p) and peak-to-peak amplitude (A_{p-p}) are marked. The bold line shows one cycle of vibration.

displacement. The horizontal line (where displacement equals zero) denotes the resting position.

Recall that plucking the guitar string generated sound. The string was pulled away from its resting position, and then quickly released. For this purpose, the sound began immediately following the release of the string. On the waveform graph, this point corresponds to time of 0 seconds and a displacement of +5 millimeters. The string moves downward initially, shooting past the resting position. At a displacement of −5 millimeters, the string stops briefly before reversing its direction. The string next moves upward, zipping past the resting position, but then it slows and finally stops again when it reaches a displacement of +5 millimeters. The process begins to repeat itself—the string moves down, and then up, and then down again, and then up again, and so on.

In science, descriptions of objects and actions must be as specific as possible. Making quantitative measurements is one way to provide accurate descriptions. The waveform is useful because it allows all the characteristics of a simple sound, for example, the vibration of the guitar string, to be quantified. The four quantities that are considered are frequency, amplitude, duration, and starting phase.

Frequency refers to the number of cycles of vibration that occur in 1 second. The unit of measurement is Hertz, abbreviated Hz. The frequency of a sound is not directly available from the waveform; it must be derived from another measurement called the **period**. However, before discussing the period, you must understand what a cycle of vibration is. Examining the waveform reveals that vibration is repetitive or cyclical. A cycle of vibration is the series of unique movements an object makes. In the working example, the guitar string moves downward, and then upward. This sequence of movements corresponds to one cycle of vibration. The bold line segment in Figure 13-2 indicates a cycle. The period, abbreviated *P*, is the amount of time needed for one cycle of vibration. As shown in Figure 13-2, *P* equals 0.5 second (500 milliseconds) because that is how long it takes the string to complete one cycle of vibration.

Once the period is known, the frequency of vibration can be calculated using the formula $f = 1 / p$, where *f* represents the frequency and *p* represents the period. In the example waveform, *P* equals 0.5 second. Dividing this number into 1 yields a frequency of 2 Hz. This number means the guitar string vibrates at the rate of 2 cycles per second. It is worth noting that the frequency and period are inversely related—as *P* increases, *f* decreases and vice versa. This can be proved by inserting different values for P into the formula. In practical terms, if a sound source vibrates slowly (i.e., the period is long), it produces a low-frequency sound. Conversely, if the source vibrates rapidly (i.e., the period is short), it generates a high-frequency sound. Remember that because the *x*-axis of the waveform is time, it does not tell about frequency directly; this information must be derived by measuring the period, which is a time-based quantity.

In the waveform graph in Figure 13-2, note that the *y*-axis reveals how far away the string is from its resting position. Acoustically speaking, this measure of distance is known as the amplitude of vibration, or simply **amplitude**. The maximum displacement in the positive or negative direction is called the peak amplitude. In Figure 13-2, the peak amplitude is indicated by A_p. Sometimes, the peak amplitude can be difficult to gauge, especially if the resting position cannot be determined precisely. A solution to this problem is to measure the distance from the maximum positive peak to the

BOX 13-1   Demonstration of Sound Frequency

CD-ROM Segment Ch.13.01 contains three waveforms that are displayed successively on the screen. The sounds can be heard if the computer is equipped with headphones or a speaker. Use the Pause button on the player to freeze the image. The first wave has a frequency of 200 Hz (period = 0.005 second), the second wave has a frequency of 400 Hz (period = 0.0025 second), and the third wave has a frequency of 800 Hz (period = 0.00125 second). Note that as the frequency increases, the number of cycles visible on the screen increases, too. Conversely, as the frequency increases, the period (e.g., the distance between successive peaks in the waveform) decreases, or gets shorter.

BOX 13-2   **Demonstration of Sound Amplitude**

CD-ROM Segment Ch.13.02 presents three waveforms displayed successively on the screen. The sounds can be heard if the computer is equipped with headphones or a speaker. Use the Pause button on the player to freeze the image. Each waveform has a frequency of 400 Hz. The first wave has peak-to-peak amplitude of 6 cm, the second wave has peak-to-peak amplitude of 3 cm, and the third wave has peak-to-peak amplitude of 1.5 cm.

maximum negative peak. This measurement is called the peak-to-peak amplitude and is shown in Figure 13-2 as $A_{p\text{-}p}$.

One feature of everyday sounds is the tremendous variability in amplitude. By comparison, the amplitude of a loud sound may be 10,000,000,000 times greater than that of a soft sound. Writing numbers like this is cumbersome and may lead to inaccuracy. Consequently, the decibel, abbreviated dB, was invented. The dB is based on a logarithmic scale, rather than a linear one. Without getting into the details, a logarithmic scale is useful when working with very large (or very small) numbers. The dB, then, provides an efficient way of expressing amplitude. To get a better feel for the dB, the softest sound you can hear is about 0 dB, while the loudest sound you can tolerate is around 120 dB. Conversational speech presented at a comfortable loudness level is between 65 and 75 dB.

The duration of vibration means how long the sound lasts. In other words, the duration corresponds to the span of time marked when the source starts moving and when it stops. The duration is abbreviated *D*, and, as shown in Figure 13-2, *D* equals 3.25 seconds.

The **starting phase** of vibration describes the position of the sound source when the vibration begins. For example, the guitar string can be pulled up and then released, or it could be pulled down and then let it go. These two positions are not the same. The starting phase, as measured in degrees (0–360), quantifies the position of the sound source just before it begins to vibrate.

Simple and Complex Sounds

The four quantities just discussed—period (the inverse of frequency), amplitude, duration, and starting phase—characterize **simple sounds**. A sound is considered simple if it vibrates at a single frequency. A pure tone is an example of a simple sound. Simple sounds rarely occur in the everyday world. In fact, virtually all sounds people hear are complex sounds.

Complex sounds are vibrations that contain two or more frequencies. In a way, simple sounds are building blocks. By adding simple sounds together, extremely complex sounds such as speech or music can be created. A music synthesizer is an electronic device capable of generating *any* sound by combining simple tones.

BOX 13-3   **Demonstration of Simple and Complex Sounds**

CD-ROM Segment Ch.13.03 presents two waveforms displayed successively on the screen. Use the Pause button on the player to freeze the image. The first wave is a simple sound, a 200-Hz tone. The second wave is a complex sound, which was synthesized by adding together three equal-amplitude tones (200-, 400-, and 600-Hz).

The waveform provides a useful way of depicting simple sounds. However, the waveform of a complex sound is not particularly revealing because the specific details (e.g., the period) are obscured. An alternative method for representing complex sounds is to plot the **spectrum**. The graph has as its coordinates frequency on the *x*-axis and either peak amplitude or starting phase on the *y*-axis. The amplitude spectrum is used more often in sound applications, so the focus is on it rather than the phase spectrum.

The top two panels in Figure 13-3 show the waveform (left) and amplitude spectrum (right) of a simple sound. The single vertical line indicates that only one frequency is present. The height of the line corresponds to the peak amplitude. For comparison purposes, the waveform and amplitude spectrum of the spoken word *big* are shown in the bottom left and right panels, respectively.

It is difficult to identify the period(s) in the waveform; thus, the frequency composition of this complex sound cannot be determined using this graph. In contrast, the amplitude spectrum reveals the frequency and peak amplitude of each component. Because complex sounds are so common, the amplitude spectrum is widely used for the purpose of visualization.

Sound Propagation

In the guitar string example, plucking the string caused it to vibrate. If this were done in a vacuum like outer space, the string would eventually stop moving, and nothing more would happen. On Earth, however, air surrounds the string. When the string vibrates in this environment, it bumps into the small particles called molecules that make up air. The string pushes and pulls on the neighboring air molecules, which causes them to vibrate, too. Air molecules closest to the sound source are affected first. Then, via a chain reaction, sound energy rapidly moves away from the source in all directions. This process is known as **sound propagation**. Although the speed of sound in air is influenced by several factors including temperature and humidity, 350 meters per second is a reasonable estimate of how fast sound travels. All sounds travel at the same speed.

Farther away from the sound source, the amplitude of the vibrating air molecules decreases progressively. Sound energy is lost because of friction produced by the molecules crashing into one another. At a sufficient distance from the source, the sound's impact on air molecules is minimal, if any. This is why you are not able to eavesdrop on a conversation occurring on the other side of the room.

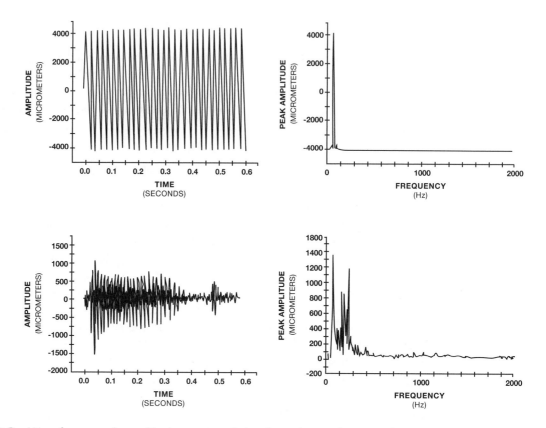

Figure 13-3 Waveforms and amplitude spectra of simple and complex sounds. The upper, left panel shows the waveform of a 50-Hz tone, while the upper, right panel is the amplitude spectrum of the tone. The lower-left panel shows the waveform of the spoken word big; the lower, right panel is the amplitude spectrum of the word.

This first part of the chapter discusses how sound is generated and how it is propagated through a medium. Listeners strive to perceive sound. The next section discusses how the structures of the ear enable hearing.

THE AUDITORY SYSTEM: STRUCTURE AND FUNCTION

Vertebrates, such as mammals (including humans), are the only animals that have an auditory system per se. One anatomic characteristic shared by all vertebrates is bilateral symmetry, which means having similar structures on both sides of the body. The auditory system of vertebrates, then, includes a pair of ears. A diagram of the ear is shown in Figure 13-4, which illustrates the structures of the outer, middle, and inner ears. This cross-sectional view is of the right ear.

The auditory system consists of two parts: the ear (the outer, middle, and inner ear), and the auditory nervous system (neural pathways, associated nuclei, and the brain). This part of the chapter names the significant structures of the auditory system

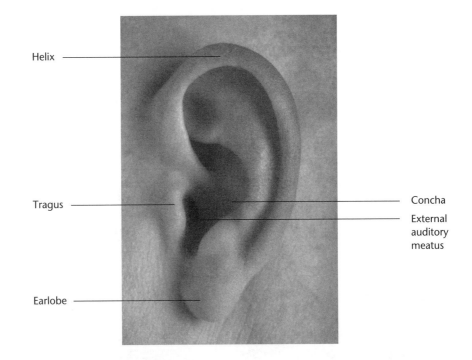

Helix

Tragus

Concha

External
auditory
meatus

Earlobe

Figure 13-4 Coronal section of the ear, including the outer, middle, and inner ears. *Source:* Chiras, D. D. (2008). *Human Biology* (6th ed., p. 226). Sudbury, MA: Jones and Bartlett.

and then briefly describes the function of each one. Because sound arrives first at the outer ear, the discussion begins there.

The Outer Ear

The outer ear consists of the **pinna** and **external auditory meatus (EAM)**. The pinna is the visible flap of skin attached to the head. Because the pinna is made of cartilage, it is quite pliable. The primary function of the pinna is to funnel sounds into the EAM. This process is facilitated by the pinna's shape (i.e., the various ridges and hollows) and its slightly forward-facing orientation. The EAM is essentially a tube that is closed at one end. In the male adult, the EAM is about 2.5 cm in length and 1.0 cm in diameter. The skin that lines the EAM contains oil glands that secrete a sticky, yellow or brown substance known as **cerumen** (earwax).

The cerumen and the tiny hairs that are also present in the EAM help protect the delicate middle ear by trapping the small debris that may enter the canal. The outer one third of the EAM is surrounded by cartilage. The inner two thirds of the canal are supported by the **temporal bone**, which is one of the bones of the skull. The skin becomes more sensitive farther inward along the EAM. In fact, tactile stimulation in this area may trigger a cough reflex. The potential for evoking this reflex, with its rapid head movement and accompanying risk of injury, is one reason to avoid using small objects to clean the EAM.

BOX 13-4   Anatomy of the Pinna

CD-ROM Segment Ch.13.04 is a photograph of the right pinna of an adult male. The important structures are labeled.

Besides their protective function, the pinna and EAM have the capacity to selectively boost or amplify sounds. Conceptually, each of these structures partially encloses a small volume of air, as an empty soda bottle does. Air can vibrate; however, it tends to vibrate at some frequencies better than others depending on the amount (volume) of air that is present. This acoustical phenomenon is known as **resonance**. To demonstrate resonance, blow across empty bottles of different sizes, and listen to the pitch of the sound that is produced. The pockets of air trapped in the pinna and EAM resonate. In the human adult, the resonant frequencies associated with these structures range from 2000 to 5000 Hz. Although the boost provided by resonance is not large (maximum effect = 10–15 dB), sounds passing through the outer ear are influenced by its resonance characteristics.

THE MIDDLE EAR

Opposite the pinna, at the other end of the EAM, the **tympanic membrane (TM)** forms the boundary between the outer and middle ears. Sound traveling down the EAM strikes the TM and causes it to vibrate just like the head of a drum, hence the common name "eardrum." The circular TM is stretched across the EAM, forming an airtight seal between the outside world and the middle-ear cavity. The area of the TM is approximately 80 mm². However, the surface of the TM is not uniformly taut. A small region (about 25% of the total) at the top of the TM is relatively loose, which may help reduce risk of rupture of this membrane.

Attached to the center of the TM is the malleus. The **malleus** is one of three bones that make up the **ossicular chain**. The ossicles are the smallest bones in the human body. The other ossicles are the **incus**, which is connected to the malleus, and the **stapes**, which is attached to the incus. The TM in children is nearly transparent, so it is possible to see the ossicles by illuminating the EAM with a special ear light called an otoscope. The TM appears cone-shaped because the ossicular chain tends to pull it inward. Therefore, shining an otoscope on the TM produces the characteristic "cone of light" on the lower, back portion of the TM's surface.

Located on the floor of the middle-ear cavity is a passageway called the **Eustachian tube (ET)** . The ET connects the middle ear to the back of the throat. Normally, the ET is closed. When the air pressure in the middle ear is less than the air pressure surrounding the body (such as at the higher altitudes reached in an airplane), the ET rapidly opens, allowing air from the mouth to pass into the middle ear. This action equalizes the air pressure in the middle ear. People know their ET is working properly when they feel their ears "pop." Yawning, swallowing, and chewing are normal activities that help the ET to pop open.

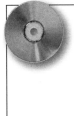

BOX 13-5   Anatomy of the Tympanic Membrane

The left panel of CD-ROM segment Ch.13.05 shows a photograph of the right tympanic membrane of an adult male. The head of the malleus can be seen on the other side of the tympanic membrane. The right panel shows the same view, except the malleus is outlined.

BOX 13-6   Anatomy of the Tympanic Membrane and the Ossicles

The left panel of CD-ROM Segment Ch.13.06 presents a model of the tympanic membrane and the three ossicles. The key structures are labeled. In the right panel, the model can be rotated, which permits viewing from various orientations. *Note*: There is no sound associated with this image.

The ossicles are suspended in the middle-ear cavity by a set of ligaments. Additionally, the **tensor tympani** and **stapedius muscles** are attached to the malleus and stapes, respectively. (The function of these muscles is considered shortly.) The ossicles provide a pathway for sound to travel from the outer to the inner ear. The vibration's journey, however, is not an easy one because the inner ear is filled with fluid. Sound energy does not transfer easily from one medium to another. When airborne sound waves encounter fluid, nearly all (approximately 99.9%) of the energy is reflected; very little (0.1%) energy is transmitted. This opposition to energy transfer is known as impedance. The ossicles exist to help overcome the effect of impedance, thus permitting more sound energy to be transmitted from the outer to the inner ear. The difference in the area of the TM compared to the stapes footplate is the primary method for **impedance matching**. The area of the TM is about 18 times larger than that of the footplate. This means that vibrations striking the TM are increased 18 times by the time they reach the much smaller footplate. The ossicles act as tiny levers, which also boost the sound amplitude. This effect is small relative to the area difference. Without impedance matching, the sound level reaching the inner ear would be reduced and hearing capacity greatly diminished.

An important role of the middle ear is overcoming the impedance mismatch between air and fluid. In certain circumstances, however, high impedance (i.e., low energy transfer) is desirable. Intense sounds are capable of producing excessive motion in the ear. Such movement is potentially harmful to the fragile sensory cells in the inner ear. To help reduce the risk of damage, a reactive mechanism has developed in mammals. The so-called **acoustic reflex** involves the tiny tensor tympani and stapedius muscles mentioned previously. Recall that the tensor tympani and stapedius muscles are attached to the ossicles. These muscles, especially the stapedius, contract reflexively when the ear is stimulated with sounds exceeding 80 dB or so. The contraction results in an overall stiffening of the ossicular chain, which increases the acoustic impedance of the ear. By increasing the acoustic impedance, the delicate structures of the inner ear are afforded some protection against intense sounds.

The Inner Ear

Like the middle ear, the inner ear resides in a hollowed out portion of the temporal bone. Actually, the inner ear consists of a series of interconnected cavities (**labyrinth**) known as the bony or **osseous labyrinth**. The osseous labyrinth is filled with fluid called **perilymph**, which is essentially saline or salt water. Floating in the perilymph is a sack known as the membranous labyrinth. The flexibility of the **membranous labyrinth** enables it to conform to the tortuous shape of the osseous labyrinth. The fluid inside the membranous labyrinth is **endolymph**. The chemical content of endolymph makes it somewhat different from perilymph.

The inner ear houses structures used for hearing and balance. The osseous and membranous labyrinths are divided into three distinct areas: the cochlea, vestibule, and semicircular canals. The cochlea contains the hearing organ, while the vestibule and semicircular canals hold the organs of balance. Because this chapter is devoted to sound and hearing, it focuses on the structures in the cochlea.

The **cochlea** is a coiled tube. There are approximately 2.5 turns in the coil of the human cochlea. The membranous labyrinth actually partitions the cochlea into three smaller tubes. The upper and lower tubes are called scala vestibuli and scala tympani, respectively. They both contain perilymph. The middle tube is called scala media; it is filled with endolymph.

The entrance to the inner ear from the middle ear is provided by the **oval window**. The stapes footplate is positioned in the oval window, which opens into scala vestibuli. Another opening into the cochlea is called the **round window**. Located on the wall of the middle-ear cavity just below the oval window, the round window leads to scala tympani. The round window is covered with a thin membrane to prevent perilymph from leaking into the middle-ear cavity. A cross-sectional view of the cochlea is shown in Figure 13-5.

When viewed in cross section, scala media is not round, but triangular. A thin layer of cells known as **Reissner's membrane** forms the top (hypotenuse) of the triangle. Reissner's membrane separates scala vestibuli from scala media. The side of the triangle consists of a collection of vessels called the **stria vascularis**, which supplies blood to the cochlea. The bottom (base) of the triangle is formed by the basilar membrane. This membrane divides scala tympani from scala media.

BOX 13-7   Inside the Cochlea

CD-ROM segment Ch.13.07 shows the cochlea as if it were cut in half. In this view, the cochlea is coiled such that the apical end is at the top of the picture. *Source:* Webster, D. B. (1995). *Neuroscience of Communication* (p. 235). San Diego, CA: Singular Publishing Group.

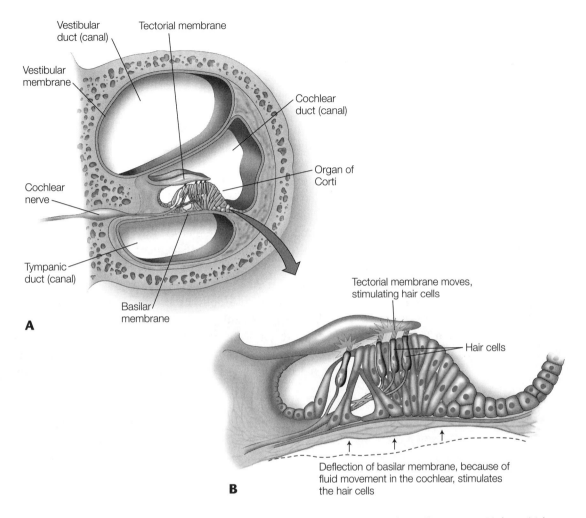

Figure 13-5 Cross-sectional view of the cochlea. *Source:* Chiras, D. D. (2008). *Human Biology* (6th ed., p. 227). Sudbury, MA: Jones and Bartlett.

The **basilar membrane** is a thin ribbon of tissue. One edge is attached to a lip of bone called the osseous spiral lamina, and the other edge supported by the spiral ligament. The basilar membrane differs from an actual ribbon in that the width and thickness are not uniform throughout its length. The end closest to the oval window, referred to as the base, is narrow and thin, which gives the basilar membrane a stiff consistency. The opposite end of the basilar membrane, called the apex, is wide and thick. The basilar membrane there is relatively flaccid. Moreover, the stiffness of the basilar membrane changes progressively from one end of the cochlea to the other. This stiffness gradient turns out to play an important role in the process of hearing.

Sound waves impinging on the TM cause it to vibrate. These vibrations are conducted to the cochlea via the ossicular chain. The stapes moves in (or out of) the oval window. The footplate pushes (or pulls) on the perilymph in the scala vestibuli, which, in turn, pushes (or pulls) the membranous labyrinth downward (or upward). The motion of the membranous labyrinth affects the perilymph in the scala tympani. The round-window membrane bulges outward (or inward) to counteract the pressure changes generated at the oval window by the stapes. The main point is that many structures in the cochlea, including the basilar membrane, are set into motion when the ear is stimulated by sound.

Recall that the basilar membrane is stiff at one end and loose at the other. One consequence of this mechanical variation is that the entire basilar membrane does not move in unison. Rather, the basal end (the one near the oval window) begins moving first, and the up-down action is transmitted down the basilar membrane toward the apex. This pattern of vibration is called the **traveling wave**. The amplitude of the traveling wave changes as it moves from base to apex. That is, the amplitude increases, reaches a maximum at a particular location on the basilar membrane, and then decreases. The place of maximal displacement is determined by the frequency of the sound. Because the basilar membrane is stiffest at the base, it vibrates best (i.e., with greatest amplitude) when stimulated by a high-frequency sound. The apex is less stiff, and thus the greatest amplitude of vibration is brought about by a low-frequency sound. Like a piano, the basilar membrane is laid systematically according to frequency, with the high-frequency "notes" at the basal end and the low-frequency "notes" at the apical end. The arrangement where each frequency is related to a particular place along the basilar membrane is known as **tonotopic organization**.

The intensity of the sound also affects the amplitude of the traveling wave. Low-intensity sounds produce a small traveling wave. Conversely, high-intensity sounds generate a traveling wave of greater amplitude. Frequency and intensity are primary characteristics of sound. The cochlea, specifically the traveling wave, provides a mechanism for sensing these two properties. Frequency content is conveyed by the location of the peak(s) in the traveling wave, while the amplitude of the peak(s) provides information about the sound's intensity.

The cochlea performs another function that is essential to hearing. For the brain to perceive sound, the vibrations must be converted from mechanical (or movement-based) energy to electrical energy. The general process of converting energy from one form to another is known as **transduction**. In the ear, transduction is accomplished by the hair cells. The **hair cells** rest on top of the basilar membrane, arranged in four rows that extend from the base of the cochlea to its apex. There actually are two types of hair cells. The three rows of outer hair cells lie closer to the stria vascularis than does the single row of inner hair cells. Several small cilia (hair-like structures) project from the top of each hair cell; hence the name. A gelatinous substance called the **tectorial membrane** arches over the tops of the inner hair cells and rests on the cilia of the outer hair cells. The tectorial membrane runs parallel to the basilar membrane. One edge is attached to the spiral limbus, which is on the opposite side of the scala media from the stria vascularis. The structures named in this paragraph are collectively known as the **organ of Corti**.

BOX 13-8   **Organ of Corti**

CD-ROM segment Ch.13.08 is a radial section through the organ of Corti. The entire organ of Corti moves up and down in response to sound stimulation. In conjunction with this motion, the tiny cilia located on the top of each hair are bent back and forth. *Source:* Webster, D. B. (1995). *Neuroscience of Communication* (p. 239). San Diego, CA: Singular Publishing Group.

The organ of Corti moves up and down when stimulated. The basilar membrane is securely attached to the osseous spiral lamina, but less securely to the spiral ligament. Further, the tectorial membrane is only anchored on one side, to the spiral ligament. Because of this arrangement, as the organ of Corti moves, it tends to pivot much like a hinge. Recall that the bottoms of the hair cells are rooted in the basilar membrane, while their tips are embedded in the tectorial membrane. Consequently, when the organ of Corti begins to move in response to sound, the cilia are forced to bend. The up-down motion of the organ of Corti is translated directly into back-and-forth movement of the cilia. This form of movement by the hair cells is called "shearing" and is crucial to the transduction process.

As stated previously, hair cells perform transduction. More specifically, the mechanical energy of vibration is converted to electrical energy. To understand how the hair cell accomplishes this, a brief discussion of electricity is necessary. An ion is a small (subatomic) particle that carries an electrical charge. Certain kinds of ions are positively charged while others are negatively charged. As the saying goes, "opposites attract," so positive and negative ions are drawn to one another. Electricity is the manifestation of this attraction.

There is electricity in the cochlea. The inside of the hair cell has an overabundance of negative ions. Endolymph, which bathes the cilia at the tops of the hair cells, has an excess amount of positive ions. The two groups of ions are kept apart by the insulating membrane that surrounds the cell. Remember that the cilia bend back and forth during sound stimulation. This motion opens and closes miniscule "trap doors" that are thought to exist at the tips of the cilia. When the doors are open, the positive ions rush into the hair cells. Why do the negative ions not flow out of the cell? The current thinking is that the trap doors are too small to allow the larger negative ions to pass through. The influx of positive ions causes the inside of the cell to become depolarized (less negatively charged). The depolarization triggers a reaction at the bottom of the hair cell. Small packets of a chemical substance called neurotransmitter are expelled into fluid-filled space outside the cell. The neurotransmitter makes the short trip across the space where it encounters nerve cells adjacent to the hair cell. The transduction process is complete. The hair cell has converted mechanical (cilia bending) to electrical (neurotransmitter release) energy.

The Auditory Nervous System

Sound is now in an electrochemical form that can be interpreted by the brain. Before this can happen, however, the information must be transmitted from the cochlea to the **auditory nerve**, through the brainstem, then the midbrain, and finally to the auditory cortex. This discussion begins with the auditory nervous system by examining the eighth nerve.

The **eighth nerve** derives its name from the fact that it is cranial nerve VIII. The eighth nerve consists of approximately 30,000 individual cells called **neurons**. Neurons are simple in the sense that they can conduct information in only one direction. Because of this constraint, the eighth nerve contains two neural subsystems. The afferent subsystem transmits messages from the cochlea to the brain, while the efferent subsystem carries messages from the brain back to the cochlea. Approximately 95% of the afferent cells originate at the inner hair cells; the remaining 5% are connected to the outer hair cells. The fact that most of the afferent neurons are connected to the inner hair cells suggests that these cells are the primary ones for carrying information about sound to the brain. If this is the case, then what is the function of the outer hair cells? This question is addressed after a short discussion of the efferent subsystem.

The efferent neurons carry messages from structures in the brain, which have not yet been described, back to the cochlea. Unlike the afferent subsystem, the neurons in the efferent subsystem mostly make connections with the outer hair cells. Remember that outer hair cells are attached to both the basilar membrane and tectorial membrane. Recent evidence indicates that the outer hair cells are capable of rapidly altering their length. These minute movements may affect the traveling wave by either increasing or decreasing its amplitude. A boost in amplitude may enhance hearing, while a reduction may serve a protective function. In either case, more work needs to be done to define the specific role of the outer hair cells.

Besides conducting information in only one direction, neurons are simple in their response properties. Neurons communicate with one another using a simple language based on action potentials. An **action potential** is a brief electrical pulse. A neuron produces a series of action potentials in response to stimulation. All action potentials are identical in duration and amplitude; thus, the rate (i.e., number of action potentials per second) provides a convenient means of quantifying the neural response. It turns out that intensity is the dimension of sound coded by rate. The relation is a direct one—as sound intensity increases, neural rate increases. The neuron, however, is limited in that its rate can vary over only a 30- to 40-dB range. The problem is that human hearing spans a range of at least 120 dB. To provide adequate coverage, the activation level of individual neurons is staggered. To see how this might work, consider three neurons. Neuron 1 responds from 0–40 dB, neuron 2 responds from 40–80 dB, and neuron 3 responds from 80–120 dB. By staggering the activation level, the full 120-dB range can be realized. Moreover, rate and activation level are important mechanisms used by the auditory nerve to code sound intensity.

Two mechanisms exist for coding sound frequency. The first one is based on the idea that the neural site-of-origin and the frequency are related. Conceptualize the eighth nerve as a rope made up of many individual fibers (the neurons). The neurons coming from the apex form the rope's inner core, while those cells coming from the base make up the outer layer. Because the tonotopic organization in the cochlea is maintained in the nerve, it is possible to predict the frequency information carried by a particular neuron. The location-frequency relation is better known as the place mechanism.

A second mechanism for conveying frequency information to the brain relates to a neuron's predisposition for responding at a specific point in the vibratory cycle. For example, an action potential may be generated only when a sound wave reaches its maximum amplitude. If this were to happen repeatedly, an equal time interval or period would occur between each subsequent action potential. As mentioned earlier, frequency and period are inversely related ($f = 1 / p$). It is possible that the brain, too, understands this association and uses neural periodicity to gain information about frequency. Therefore, both place and periodicity are important mechanisms used by the auditory nerve to code sound frequency.

Information about sound is not transmitted directly to the brain by the eighth nerve. Instead, parallel neural pathways run on both sides of the head. This complicated network consists of many individual neurons that begin and end at specific centers called nuclei. Nuclei are situated at various locations throughout the auditory nervous system. For the sake of brevity, the primary nuclei are listed in the order found in the afferent auditory pathway. Keep in mind that a parallel efferent pathway also exists. A schematic diagram of the afferent pathways is shown in Figure 13-6.

The eighth nerve carries messages from the cochlea to the **cochlear nucleus**, which is located in the lower brainstem. Like many areas in the auditory nervous system, the cochlear nucleus is divided into smaller regions. Providing the names of these nuclei, however, is beyond the scope of this introductory chapter. All afferent neurons coming from the hair cells terminate in the cochlear nucleus.

A second group of neurons leaves the cochlear nucleus and extends to the next cluster of nuclei collectively known as the **superior olivary complex**. Actually, a portion of the neurons leaving the cochlear nucleus travels to the superior olivary complex on the same (ipsilateral) side of the head. The other neurons exit the cochlear nucleus, cross the midline, and connect to the superior olivary complex on the opposite (contralateral) side. One reason mammals have two ears is to help locate the source of sound. The superior olivary complex likely plays an important role in sound localization because this is the first place in the afferent pathway where information from the right and left ears is integrated or combined.

A third set of neurons goes from the superior olivary complex to the **lateral lemniscus nucleus**. The lateral lemniscus is large in mammals that live under ground, but relatively small in primates. This suggests that the role of the lateral lemniscus in human hearing may be a minor one.

A fourth group of neurons extends from the lateral lemniscus to the **inferior colliculus nucleus**. A neural pathway connects the inferior colliculus on the right side to

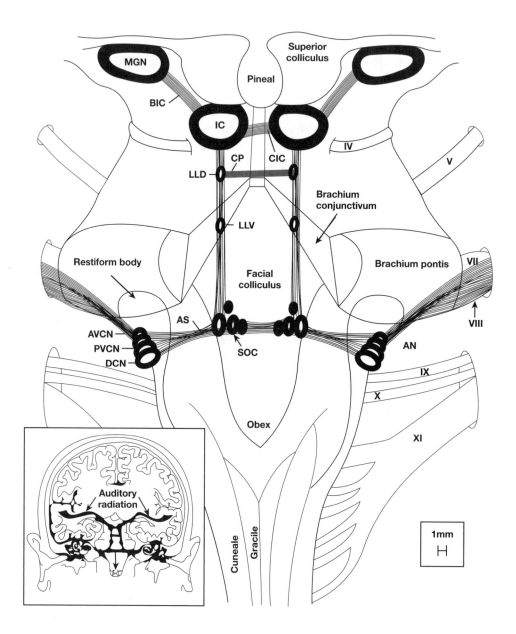

Figure 13-6 Ventral view of the subcortical pathways of the central auditory nervous system. The abbreviations are as follows: VII = cranial nerve 7; VIII = cranial nerve 8; AVCN = anterior ventral cochlear nucleus; PVCN = posterior ventral cochlear nucleus; DCN = dorsal cochlear nucleus; IC = inferior colliculus; LLV = ventral lateral lemniscus; LLD = dorsal lateral lemniscus; MGN = medial geniculate nucleus; SOC = superior olivary complex. *Source:* Hall, J. W., & Mueller, H. G. III (1997). *Audiologists' Desk Reference, Diagnostic Audiology, Principles, Procedures, and Practices* (Vol. 1, p. 36). San Diego, CA: Singular Publishing Group.

the inferior colliculus on the left side. Such interconnecting tracts or **commissures** are found at several levels in the auditory nervous system.

Extending from the inferior colliculus to the midbrain is a fifth set of neurons. These cells terminate in the **medial geniculate body**. The sixth and final set of neurons leaves the medial geniculate body on its way to the **auditory cortex**. Unlike the medial geniculate body, which lies deep within the head, the auditory cortex is found on the surface of the brain. The brain, once the skull is removed, consists of two cerebral hemispheres. A hemisphere is divided into four sections called lobes. The auditory cortex is located in the temporal lobe, which is the thumblike region on the side of each hemisphere. The auditory cortex marks the end of the afferent auditory pathway. From there, connections are made with other areas of the brain that are responsible for important functions such as language, memory, movement, and so on.

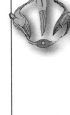

BOX 13-9   Personal Story

As best I can tell, my fascination with sound and hearing emerged during my high school years. I became sincerely interested in music then. As a musician, I played the trombone and the electric guitar. Of the brass instruments the trombone is arguably the toughest to play. Unlike the trumpet or other instruments with valves, the slide of the trombone is moved to a specific position for each musical note. The correct location can be taught in a general sense, e.g., place the slide directly across from the horn's bell. To play in tune, however, requires one to learn the pitch of a given note and then to make fine adjustments in slide position until the note 'sounds right.' The process of matching a musical percept in my brain with a physical position of the trombone slide has been captivating me since those halcyon days of my youth.

While the acoustics of musical instruments is interesting, what attracted me to the study of hearing was what happened when the vibrations of the electric guitar were amplified. It turns out that sounds emitted by a loudspeaker are transmitted through the air and into the inner ear where the sensory cells of hearing are forced to vibrate. These cells are very small and delicate, so it is relatively easy for intense (and loud) sounds to cause damage to the hearing mechanism. Moreover, injury to sensory cells produced by amplified music can lead to temporary or even permanent hearing loss. I played in a rock band. My exposure to intense sounds was frequent and prolonged. One would expect that my hearing would have been negatively impacted by such careless behavior. Curiously, tests revealed that my hearing remained within the normal range. Several of my band mates, however, were not so fortunate. They incurred hearing loss in both ears, and what made matters worse, the more they played, the greater their hearing loss became. All the members of the band received comparable sound exposures, yet we were not equally affected by intense stimulation. Why? What about our ears is apparently different from person to person? This variation in individual susceptibility still captivates me, and I continue to explore these questions in my research. Some day I may find the answers. Perhaps, you will choose to join me in the quest to better understand sound and hearing.

SUMMARY

Sound moves from its source through the medium to the listener. The outer ear of the listener gathers the sound present in the air and directs it to the middle ear. The middle ear is a mechanical system that boosts sound amplitude so that the vibration is transmitted more effectively into the inner ear. The inner ear separates complex sounds into simple ones according to frequency. Additionally, the inner ear converts vibration to electrical impulses. The eighth nerve and the auditory neural pathways carry the impulses to the brain, which attempts to assign meaning to sound.

STUDY QUESTIONS

1. Describe the interplay between the forces of momentum and elasticity during vibration.

2. What four measurable quantities characterize all simple sounds?

3. Sketch the waveform of a simple sound.

4. Name five structures of the middle ear.

5. What are the two functions of the cochlea?

6. Contrast the afferent and efferent pathways of the auditory nervous system.

7. Proceeding from cochlea to brain, list the main structures in the auditory pathway.

8. How are changes in the amplitude and frequency of sound communicated to the brain by the auditory nervous system?

KEY TERMS

Acoustic reflex
Action potential
Amplitude
Auditory cortex
Basilar membrane
Cerumen
Cochlea
Cochlear nucleus
Commissure
Complex sound
Eighth nerve
Elasticity
Endolymph
Eustachian tube
External auditory meatus
   (EAM)
Frequency
Hair cells
Impedance matching

Incus
Inferior colliculus nucleus
Labyrinth
Lateral lemniscus nucleus
Malleus
Mass
Medial geniculate body
Membranous labyrinth
Neuron
Organ of Corti
Osseous labyrinth
Ossicular chain
Oval window
Perilymph
Period
Pinna
Reissner's membrane
Resonance

Round window
Simple sound
Sound generation
Sound propagation
Spectrum
Stapedius muscle
Stapes
Starting phase
Stria vascularis
Superior olivary complex
Tectorial membrane
Temporal bone
Tensor tympani muscle
Tonotopic organization
Transduction
Traveling wave
Tympanic membrane (TM)
Waveform

SUGGESTED READINGS

Gelfand, S.A. (2004). *Hearing: An introduction to psychological and physiological acoustics* (4th ed.). New York: Marcel Dekker.

Seikel, A. J., King, D. W., & Drumwright, D. G. (2005). *Anatomy and physiology for speech, language, and hearing* (3rd ed.). San Diego, CA: Singular.

Speaks, C. E. (1999). *Introduction to sound: Acoustics for the hearing and speech sciences.* San Diego, CA: Singular.

Yost, W. A. (2000). *Fundamentals of hearing: An introduction.* San Diego, CA: Academic Press.

Zemlin, W. R. (1997). *Speech and hearing science: Anatomy and physiology* (4th ed.). Boston: Allyn & Bacon.

chapter *fourteen*

Hearing Disorders

FREDERICK N. MARTIN

LEARNING OBJECTIVES

1. To understand what the profession of audiology is designed to accomplish.

2. To determine what a hearing loss is.

3. To differentiate among different kinds of hearing losses.

4. To understand the causes of hearing loss.

5. To grasp the kinds of difficulties in understanding speech encountered by people with different kinds of hearing loss.

6. To understand the basics of hearing testing.

7. To understand the kinds of instrumentation required for adequate hearing testing.

8. To grasp the concepts of tuning fork tests and their relationships to modern audiometry.

9. To be able to interpret basic hearing test results.

10. To have an insight into auditory evoked potentials and otoacoustic emissions.

The previous chapter describes the anatomy and physiology of the auditory system, that is, how it is constructed and how it works. This chapter introduces the kinds of hearing disorders encountered by audiologists and SLPs, the diagnostic procedures available for making the appropriate appraisals of these disorders, and their effects on the communication process. Although audiologic test procedures are discussed, it is important to realize that the practice of audiology goes far beyond the performance of tests and their interpretation. These tests help to determine the kinds of intervention that are necessary to improve the communication of those with hearing impairment and others with whom they interact. At the conclusion of this chapter, you should be able to interpret the basic tests described, including the audiograms and related procedures using speech stimuli. This chapter assumes a basic knowledge of the anatomy and physiology of the auditory system as described in Chapter 13. An understanding of the principles of this chapter is essential for understanding Chapter 15 on auditory (re)habilitation.

HEARING TESTS

The evolution of hearing tests has been ongoing for centuries. There is no doubt that as long as humans have relied on their hearing for receptive communication, there have been individuals whose hearing has been impaired. Just when informal testing began and how it was carried out are unknown, although a little educated guessing may give insight.

Informal Tests

The early hearing tests, some of which have carried over to modern times, probably included the production of gross sounds and the search for some kind of acknowledgment by cooperative individuals and overt responses from those who could not cooperate. Noncooperative individuals include small children, older adults, the infirm, and those who feel they can benefit by having people believe they have a hearing loss that does not exist.

Sound Pathways

Sound travels through the air as a series of waves, with their respective compressions and rarefactions. The **air-conduction** pathway is the natural way by which most land-living animals hear. Those sounds reaching the head are gathered by the pinna of the outer ear, carried down the external auditory canal, and directed to the tympanic membrane, often called the eardrum. Vibration of the tympanic membrane sets the chain of middle-ear ossicles into motion, which, in turn, disturbs the fluids of the cochlea of the inner ear. The cochlea, acting as a sort of microphone that converts mechanical energy into an electrochemical code, sends information to the brain via the auditory (eighth cranial) nerve. It has been said many times, and it bears repeating here, that people do not hear with their ears but rather with their brains. The ear is a necessary, but not totally efficient means of enabling "hearing."

Sound energy may also reach the inner ear by vibrating the bones of the skull, thereby setting the bony labyrinth into sympathetic vibration and eliciting the same response from the cochlea as is produced by air conduction. This process of bypassing the conductive mechanism (the outer ear and middle ear) and going directly to the sensorineural mechanism (the inner ear and the auditory nerve) has been given the obvious name of **bone conduction**.

Pure-Tone Audiometry

Among the many notable inventions of the 20th century was the pure-tone **audiometer** (see Martin & Clark, 2009, and Figure 14-1). Although improvements in technology have resulted in vastly different circuitry from the early instruments, all pure-tone audiometers have certain things in common. They produce a series of pure tones that can be delivered via earphones to a patient's ears or via a bone-conduction oscillator affixed to the skull. Frequencies are generated that are usually available at octave intervals over a fairly wide frequency range. The usual frequencies found on pure-tone audiometers include 125, 250, 500, 1000, 2000, 4000, and 8000 hertz (Hz) (note the correspondence to the musical C scale). Some midoctave frequencies are typically included such as 750, 1500, 3000, and 6000 Hz.

Pure-tone tests are designed to determine a patient's **threshold of audibility** at a number of different frequencies for each ear. Air conduction is tested by using a pair of earphones held firmly to the head by a headband (Figure 14-2) or, preferably, inserted into the ears (Figure 14-3). Bone-conduction testing is accomplished with a specially designed steel band holding an oscillator against the skull. Many audiologists measure

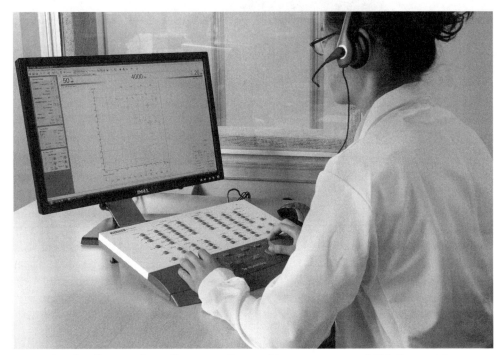

Figure 14-1 An example of a diagnostic audiometer. *Source:* Photo courtesy of GN Otometrics

bone conduction on each **mastoid process** independently to obtain threshold information for both cochleas (Figure 14-4). However, the reality is that it is often impossible to know which cochlea is responding because vibrating the skull from any location usually results in both cochleas being stimulated equally. For this and other reasons the forehead is the preferred testing site (Studebaker, 1962).

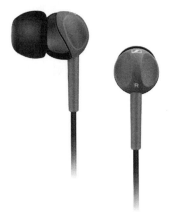

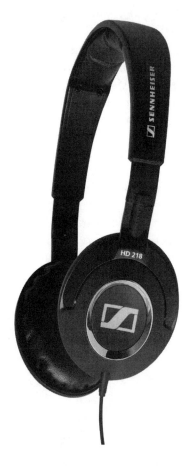

Figure 14-2 (left) Photograph of a pair of supra-aural earphones. *Source:* Photo courtesy of Sennheiser Electronic Corporation

Figure 14-3 (above) Photograph of a pair of insert earphones. *Source:* Photo courtesy of Sennheiser Electronic Corporation

Figure 14-4 (below) Photograph of a bone-conduction oscillator. *Source:* Photo courtesy of GN Otometrics

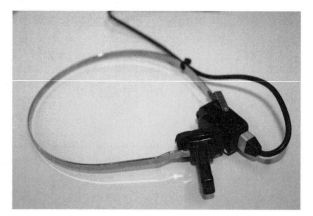

As stated, the frequencies produced by audiometers are measured in cycles per second or Hz. Intensity changes are measured in decibels (dB). Chapter 13 discusses the dB as a unit of sound pressure that is expressed as a logarithmic unit because of the large range of intensities that can be heard by normal-hearing persons. The reference described is specified as sound-pressure level (SPL). The audiometer uses the dB in a different manner, which introduces the concept of **hearing level (HL)**.

Whereas SPL has a specific intensity reference (20 micropascals), HL refers to the intensity necessary to evoke a threshold response from persons with normal hearing. Because the human ear is not equally sensitive at all frequencies, the audiometer produces different SPLs at different frequencies to reach 0 dB HL. Theoretically, a person with normal hearing would show threshold responses at about 0 dB HL at all frequencies tested, even though the SPL required to produce 0 dB HL is different at each frequency. Therefore, audiologists using pure-tone audiometers need to compare the thresholds of their patients to 0 dB HL at each frequency to determine how much hearing loss is present. Although there is some disagreement about this, normal hearing, as described in this book, is said to encompass a range from –10 to 15 dB HL. Any threshold found to be greater than 15 dB HL is considered to demonstrate a hearing loss by air conduction, bone conduction, or both.

Another reference for the decibel is **sensation level (SL)**, which is simply the difference (in dBs) between the level of a signal presented and the threshold of the individual receiving that signal. A tone of 50 dB SL is 50 dB above a listener's threshold, regardless of what that threshold might be. A person with a threshold of 20 dB HL would hear a signal of 50 dB HL at 30 dB SL. It is essential whenever discussing the intensity of a sound that the reference for the dB be specified.

Hearing sensitivity is normally displayed on a graph called an **audiogram**. Unlike most graphs, which show the larger numbers near the top and the smaller numbers near the bottom, audiograms are inverted. The lowest number of dBs is shown near the top of the graph. The number of dBs (HL) is shown to increase going down the page. The different test frequencies are displayed on the horizontal axis of the audiogram, with the lowest test frequency (usually 125 Hz) on the left side and the highest frequency tested (usually 8000 Hz) on the right side of the graph.

A grid is thereby created (e.g., see Figures 14-6 through 14-9). As the patient's hearing is tested, each test signal is raised and lowered in intensity until the sound is so soft that it can be detected only about 50% of the time. This level is called the threshold of audibility and is expressed in dBs with an HL reference. By placing symbols where the horizontal and vertical axes of the audiogram intersect, the audiologist plots the patient's threshold for each frequency for each ear by air conduction and bone conduction. The right ear air-conduction thresholds are usually shown in red using a circle, and the left ear air-conduction thresholds are shown in blue using an X. When bone-conduction thresholds are measured from the mastoid, they are also plotted in red (for the right ear) and blue (for the left ear) using the symbol < for the right and the > for the left.

Speech Audiometry

Pure-tone tests have remained the mainstay of diagnostic audiology for many years. They supply information about hearing sensitivity over a range of frequencies and are helpful in determining the type and degree of hearing loss so that appropriate remediation can be instituted.

However, because pure tones do not exist in nature, they are abstract stimuli. People who seek help for their hearing difficulties, or for the hearing problems of significant other persons, generally do so because of difficulties in hearing speech.

In consideration of that statement, it was only natural that testing devices would be developed to measure different aspects of speech. These include how intense speech must be to be barely audible (the **speech-recognition threshold [SRT]**), and how well speech can be discriminated when it is loud enough to be heard (the **word-recognition score [WRS]**). The degree of hearing loss expressed as an SRT is described in HLs, and it usually approximates the degree of loss by air conduction at the average of the thresholds obtained at 500, 1000, and 2000 Hz. In this way, the SRT, in addition to expressing how much hearing loss a patient has for speech, also lends verification to the pure-tone audiogram. If the two measures disagree by more than about 5 dB, an explanation should be sought, because the accuracy of one or both of these tests is in question.

SRTs are customarily measured using two-syllable words called **spondees**, where both syllables are uttered with the same stress. Examples of spondaic words are *hotdog*, *baseball*, *toothbrush*, and *sidewalk*. Although spondaic stress is not used in English discourse, spondaic words are clinically useful in that they are fairly easy to discriminate, even close to threshold.

The WRS of patients is of clinical interest in that it helps both in determining the cause and possible treatment of their hearing loss. WRS is often a useful predictor of the outcome of audiologic rehabilitation. Most clinicians measure WRS using lists of 50 one-syllable **phonetically balanced** words, so called because they are said to contain all the phonemes of the language with their approximate frequencies in connected discourse. Although this is not necessarily the case, these word lists have been popular for more than half a century. Unlike the tests described earlier, WRSs are measured in percentages, rather than in dBs. When a list of 50 words is presented, the patient is asked to repeat each word. The number of words correctly repeated is multiplied by 2% and the result is the WRS.

People with normal hearing usually have very high WRSs (90% to 100%), as do people with conductive hearing losses, regardless of the degree of impairment. This is because there is little distortion in their auditory systems. In the case of a sensorineural hearing loss, there is almost always some measurable distortion. Therefore, as a general rule, there is a relationship between the degree of sensorineural hearing loss and the drop in WRS. For example, patients with mild sensorineural hearing loss (15 to 30 dB HL) may show WRSs of 80% to 90%, those with moderate losses (30 to 60 dB HL) may show WRSs of 60% to 80%, and those with severe losses (65 to 85 dB HL) may show WRSs of 40% to 60%. Patients with profound hearing losses sometimes have such great difficulties in discriminating speech that the scores are extremely low or not even measurable. It goes without saying that the preceding statement is intended only as a set of examples. Usually, the greater the sensorineural hearing loss, the greater the distortion and the poorer the WRS, but there are many exceptions to these assumptions.

Electrophysiological Tests

The tests just described all require some measure of cooperation from the patient and have been called *subjective tests*. It has long been thought desirable to have tests that can be carried out without direct patient response to a signal. The evolution of these procedures has been most pronounced in the last few decades and is described briefly in the following sections.

Acoustic Immittance

The term **immittance** was coined by the American National Standards Institute (ANSI, 1987) as a combination of *impedance* (the sound energy that is reflected from the tympanic membrane) and *admittance* (the energy that is admitted via the tympanic membrane to the middle ear). Because no system, including the human ear, is totally efficient in sound transmission, there is always some impedance, and thus admittance is never total. The development of immittance meters has introduced a number of procedures that have become standard in clinical audiology. An example of a modern acoustic immittance meter is shown in Figure 14-5.

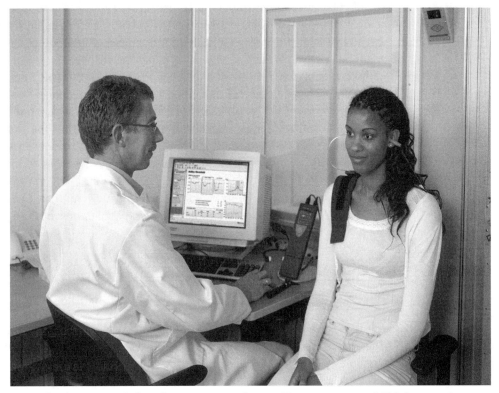

Figure 14-5 Photograph of an acoustic immittance meter. *Source:* Photo courtesy of GN Otometrics

The measurement of the mobility of the tympanic membrane and middle-ear system is called **tympanometry**. This is accomplished by varying the amount of positive and negative air pressure imposed on it. Air pressure changes are applied by a probe placed in the external auditory canal. As the air pressure is varied above and below normal atmospheric pressure, the tympanic membrane becomes stiffer by being gently pushed into the middle ear (with positive pressure) and pulled out into the external auditory canal (with negative pressure). A test sound is introduced into the canal, and the amount of sound energy bouncing back is monitored as the pressure is varied. Tympanometry can reveal such conditions as tympanic membrane perforation, interrupted ossicular chain, fluid in the middle ear, and stiffness of the ossicles.

In addition to tympanometry, audiologists can measure the acoustic reflex, which is the contraction of the middle-ear muscles in response to intense auditory signals (about 85 dB SL for normal hearers). They can glean a great deal of insight from acoustic reflex thresholds that can be obtained at normal sensation levels, high sensation levels (greater than 100 dB), low sensation levels (less than 65 dB), or reflexes that cannot be obtained at all.

Performance of a basic hearing evaluation is demonstrated on the accompanying CD-ROM.

Auditory Evoked Potentials

Whenever a sound is heard, it is recognized as changes in electrical activity by a number of relay sites along the auditory path in the brain. These responses are small in comparison to the ongoing electrical activity that is present in any living brain. As such, they are difficult to observe, but the development of computers has allowed for averaging the signals in such a way as to make the responses recognizable. Within 300 milliseconds of the introduction of a sound (called the *latency period*) the signal has reached the higher centers of the brain. The earlier the response occurs (the shorter the latency), the lower in the auditory system the response is generated. The most widely used diagnostic results are those that are obtained within the first 10 milliseconds. These early responses are called the **auditory brainstem response (ABR)**.

The ABR is presently used for a number of purposes, including testing newborn infants, determination of the site of lesion in the auditory pathway, and measuring hearing in noncooperative individuals such as small children, older adults, and individuals willfully or unconsciously attempting to make their hearing appear worse than it is.

BOX 14-1   A Hearing Evaluation

CD-ROM segment Ch.14.01 is a movie that shows portions of a hearing evaluation. The procedures that are demonstrated include pure-tone air- and bone-conduction audiometry, SRTs, WRSs, and immitance measures.

Otoacoustic Emissions

The scientific community was rocked a little over two and a half decades ago with the realization that the inner ear actually produces some very faint sounds (Kemp, 1978). These sounds have been called spontaneous **otoacoustic emissions (OAE)** and are present in about half of all individuals with normal hearing. For some reasons yet to be explained, spontaneous OAEs are found more often in females than in males and are more often present in right ears than in left ears. It was then learned that an emission could be produced as a kind of "echo," by introducing a signal to the ear and then monitoring the sound that is returned from the tympanic membrane. The sound is mechanically generated by the outer hair cells of the cochlea. These have been called evoked otoacoustic emissions.

OAEs have leapt into clinical prominence since their development, and now devices are used for this purpose that are so small they can be held in one hand. OAEs have taken their rightful place beside acoustic immittance and auditory evoked potentials in the battery of tests available to clinical audiologists.

TYPES OF HEARING LOSS

Hearing status is generally classified as being normal or showing one of three types of hearing loss: conductive, sensorineural, or mixed, as described in the following sections.

Normal Hearing

People with normal hearing sensitivity show auditory thresholds below (less than) 15 dB HL at all frequencies, as shown in Figure 14-6. The patient illustrated here would be expected to have little or no difficulty hearing under most circumstances.

Conductive Hearing Losses

Individuals with **conductive hearing losses** show impairment by air conduction (which measures the total amount of loss they experience), but they have normal hearing by bone conduction. This is because the air-conducted signal must pass through both the outer and middle ears, where the problem presumably resides, and where the sound, coming from the earphone of the audiometer, is attenuated (made weaker). When the test is carried out by bone conduction, which bypasses the conductive system, hearing appears to be normal because the sensorineural system is undamaged in conductive hearing losses. Figure 14-7 shows a moderate conductive hearing loss. Note that there is a loss by air conduction in both ears at each frequency, but that bone conduction is normal throughout.

The degree of hearing loss will vary for air conduction based on the cause and extent of the problem, but bone conduction will always remain within the normal range. The configuration of the audiogram is fairly flat; that is, there is approximately the same degree of loss at each frequency. This is fairly typical of conductive hearing losses, although there is naturally some variation.

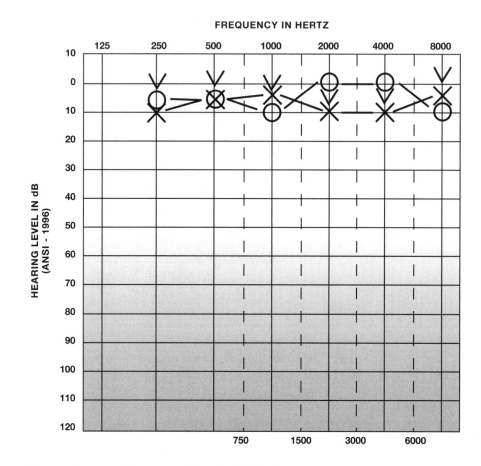

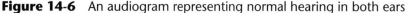

Figure 14-6 An audiogram representing normal hearing in both ears

Causes of Conductive Hearing Loss

Conductive hearing losses are caused by damage to the outer ear or middle ear.

Outer-Ear Hearing Loss

Experts disagree on whether the tympanic membrane should be considered a part of the outer ear or a part of the middle ear because it is the boundary that separates these two cavities. This argument is like asking whether a closed door between the living room and dining room is in one room or the other. It is really a part of both. So it is with the tympanic membrane, but for purposes of this chapter, the tympanic membrane is considered to be a part of the middle ear.

Outer-ear conditions produce hearing losses when the external auditory canal becomes occluded. Although loss of or damage to the pinna is known to effect changes in the acoustics of the external auditory canal, pinna abnormalities do not produce measurable hearing loss when hearing is tested using earphones. Nevertheless, they should be considered when working with people who have pinna abnormalities.

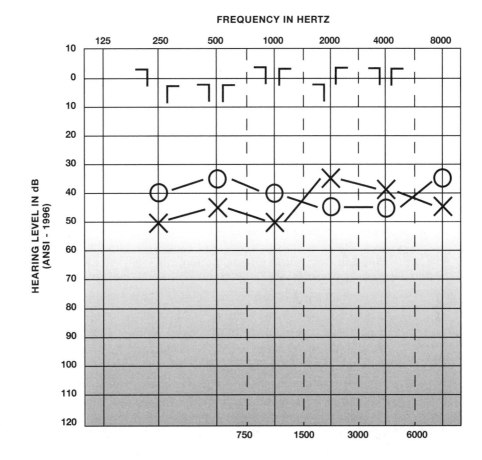

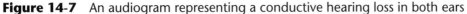

Figure 14-7 An audiogram representing a conductive hearing loss in both ears

The lumen of the external auditory canal can be partially or completely blocked by such things as foreign objects (like pencil erasers), ear wax, the buildup of debris from infection, or swelling of the canal walls because of infection or irritation. Also, conditions such as tumors, burns (which cause the canal to collapse), or congenital partial or complete closure can occlude the canal. All of these conditions require careful scrutiny by an ear specialist before otological or audiological rehabilitation should begin.

When hearing losses occur because of external auditory canal disorders, the hearing loss is of the conductive type, and WRSs are generally excellent. The value afforded by immittance measures is denied to the audiologist because the fact that the external auditory canal is closed makes inserting the immittance probe tip impossible.

Middle-Ear Hearing Loss

The primary cause of hearing loss in the middle ear is infection called **otitis media**. In fact, otitis media is the largest single cause of hearing loss in general. Most people have at least one bout of otitis media in childhood, and although it is most common in children, it can occur at any age. Otitis media causes hearing loss in several ways: The fluid that forms in the middle-ear space secondary to the infection can act as a sound barrier, or the infection may cause thickening or destruction of the tympanic membrane or ossicular chain. Otitis media should be viewed primarily as a medical condition, and treatment should be sought as soon as symptoms appear. Audiologic intervention is indicated if there is any indication that the treatment for hearing loss secondary to otitis media will be prolonged.

Although the term *otitis media* literally means infection of the middle ear, many of these cases do not involve infection per se, but rather the accumulation of sterile fluid because of the negative middle-ear pressure that results from Eustachian tubes that do not function properly. Children and adults who suffer from chronic Eustachian tube dysfunction may have a simple operation called **myringostomy**. A small plastic tube is placed through an incision made in the tympanic membrane, allowing the middle ear to ventilate by the passage of air through the tube from the external auditory canal to the middle ear. These tubes are often worn for periods up to a year or so, at which time they often extrude spontaneously.

Other causes of conductive hearing loss in the middle ear include a variety of congenital disorders. Some occur in isolation and some as one symptom of a syndrome that includes other abnormalities (as of the bones of the cranium and face). Other causes include tumors, trauma, or fixation of the ossicular chain by a condition called **otosclerosis** (most commonly seen in white adult females).

It is now commonly agreed that even very mild conductive hearing losses in young children may interfere with normal language development, and hearing aids are often prescribed at very young ages in these cases. A condition called **minimal auditory deprivation syndrome** may result from the lack of sensory input to the auditory centers of the brain, resulting in what has been referred to as **auditory processing disorder (APD)**.

Sensory/Neural Hearing Loss

Chapter 13 discusses the inner ear as being responsible for the body's balance and equilibrium, as well as its role in hearing. The balance portion, called the **vestibular mechanism** (the utricle, saccule, and semicircular canals), can go awry for a number of reasons, resulting in the disturbing symptom of vertigo, the sensation of whirling or violent turning. Damage to the cochlea produces what is called a **sensory/neural hearing loss**. Sensorineural hearing losses may range from very mild, sometimes showing virtually normal hearing for low frequencies and depressed hearing for higher frequencies, to profound or even total hearing loss

The term *sensory/neural* suggests that the lesion causing the hearing loss is either sensory (in the cochlea) or neural (either in the neural structures of the cochlea or the **auditory [eighth cranial] nerve)**. As shown in Figure 14-8, cochlear hearing losses evince an absence of an air–bone gap (ABG), which is the hallmark of the conductive hearing loss. That is, in sensory/neural hearing loss the thresholds for air-conducted tones are about the same as the thresholds for bone-conducted tones. The WRSs are almost always poorer than those of patients with normal hearing or those with conduc-

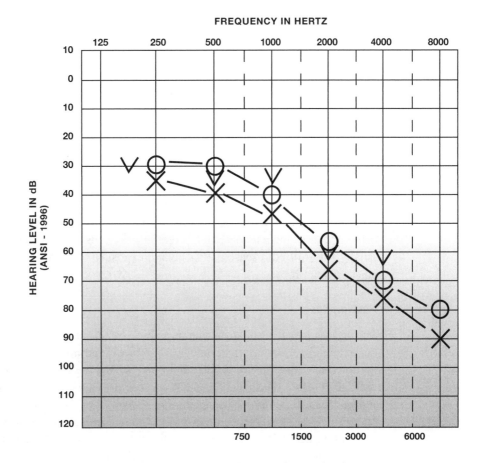

Figure 14-8 An audiogram representing a sensorineural hearing loss in both ears

tive hearing losses, and the degree of speech discrimination difficulty is often linked directly to the degree of hearing loss.

The degree of loss illustrated in Figure 14-8 is moderate. Notice that the audiogram tilts downward, suggesting greater hearing difficulty in the higher frequencies than in the lower frequencies. Although this configuration is typical of sensory/neural hearing loss, there is great variation in the type and severity of these losses. In addition to high-frequency losses, it is common to see flat audiograms, low-frequency losses, and a variety of shapes. The degree of loss may be quite different at different frequencies and may range from mild to profound.

Causes of Sensory/Neural Hearing Loss

Sensorineural hearing losses usually involve damage to the cochlea or the auditory nerve. Like conductive losses, sensorineural hearing losses may occur prenatally (before birth), perinatally (during the birth process), or postnatally (after birth).

Cochlear Hearing Loss

Prenatal cochlear hearing losses may be inherited, either in isolation or as a part of a syndrome. They may be caused by anoxia (oxygen deprivation) of the fetus, trauma, viral infections, fetal alcohol syndrome, or variance between the blood of the mother and the fetus, such as in Rh incompatibility.

Perinatal cochlear hearing losses are usually caused by some disruption in the normal birth process. Complications such as umbilical strangulation or other trauma may affect the cochlea by causing anoxia. Such conditions often affect not only the auditory structures but the brain as well, resulting in conditions such as cerebral palsy and mental retardation.

Postnatal cochlear hearing losses often result secondary to prolonged otitis media, occurring first as conductive, then as mixed, and finally as pure sensorineural losses. Postnatal causes include viral and bacterial infections such as meningitis, a number of sexually transmitted diseases, high fevers, exposure to loud noise, a variety of drugs, and the aging process.

Auditory Nerve Hearing Loss

Hearing losses that result from damage to or irritation of the auditory nerve are usually unilateral (occur in only one ear). The most common cause is **acoustic neuroma**, a tumor that forms on the vestibular branch of the auditory (eighth cranial) nerve. It eventually presses on the cochlear branch, usually causing **tinnitus** (ringing or roaring sounds), then difficulty in discriminating speech, then hearing loss, which progresses either rapidly or slowly from very mild to total. The decision to surgically or radiologically remove acoustic neuromas or to inhibit their growth is based on a number of factors, including the patient's age, general health, and symptoms. There are other causes of eighth nerve hearing losses, but acoustic neuroma or acoustic neuritis (inflammation) are the most common.

Mixed Hearing Loss

As shown in Figure 14-9, a **mixed hearing loss** is a combination of both the conductive and sensory/neural varieties. The amount of sensory/neural impairment is expressed as the difference between 0 dB HL and the bone-conduction threshold at each frequency. The amount of conductive hearing loss is the difference between the bone-conduction threshold and the air-conduction threshold at each frequency (this is called the **air–bone gap [ABG]**). As the sensory/neural component increases, the bone-conduction threshold becomes higher (lower on the audiogram), and as the conductive component becomes greater, the air–bone gap increases. The air-conduction threshold reveals the total amount of hearing loss at each frequency.

Auditory Processing Disorders

Auditory processing disorders (APD) were mentioned earlier as occurring among children suffering from sensory deprivation in the auditory path. Both children and adults may present in the audiology clinic with complaints of difficulty in hearing that do not relate to how loud particular sounds may be. The difficulty appears to be in processing

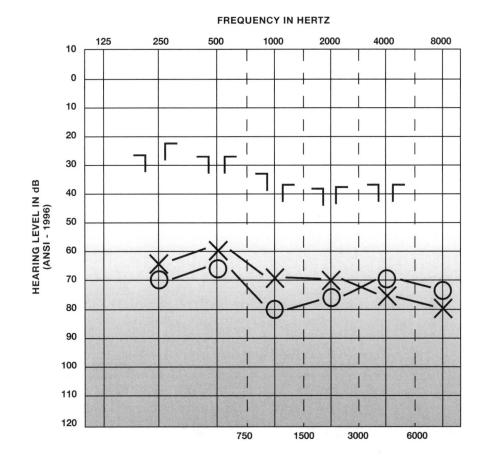

Figure 14-9 An audiogram representing a mixed hearing loss in both ears

or discriminating speech, and the problem is exacerbated in noisy or otherwise untoward listening situations.

For a time, the emphasis was on the diagnosis of central disorders and pinpointing the site of lesion (i.e., brainstem vs. cortex). Since the emergence of modern imaging techniques such as positron emission tomography, magnetic resonance imaging, and computed tomography scanning, the contribution of audiology to these diagnoses has decreased, although some of the recent breakthroughs in evoked-potential testing show great promise.

In seeking to find children who might suffer from APD, the American Academy of Audiology (1992) recommends the following steps:

1. *Identification:* This includes screening children who are at risk for APD.
2. *Assessment:* The performance of routine audiometric procedures and the referral to SLPs of patients considered to be at risk.
3. *Audiometric monitoring:* This involves follow-up audiometry for children who have been identified (step 2). Testing should be performed at the beginning of every school year, even if the child appears asymptomatic.

Specific Tests for APD

Routine audiometric procedures rarely reveal APD in either children or adults. As a matter of fact, because these two conditions should not be considered to be mutually exclusive, the presence of a peripheral hearing loss may actually impede the diagnosis of APD. A wide variety of special diagnostic tests has been developed for APD, which are not reviewed here, but the one enjoying the most popularity today is the SCAN-C (Keith, 2000).

Testing for APD should not be a goal in itself. The important thing, after identification of patients is completed, is to address the problems and seek practical solutions. It is essential to understand the individual's specific difficulties and, after the possibility of a health- or life-threatening lesion has been eliminated, to focus on improving the skills these patients need to cope with their difficulties. These issues are addressed in Chapter 16.

SUMMARY

Audiology has evolved over nearly 60 years from a profession dedicated to the development and performance of accurate diagnostic hearing tests to one that is involved in every aspect of auditory rehabilitation. The diagnostic audiologist must determine the need for medical and nonmedical (rehabilitative or psychological) intervention to improve the quality of life of people with hearing loss. Modern techniques now permit early diagnosis of hearing loss in children so that appropriate education and training may begin. Chapters 15 and 16 delve further into audiologic (re)habilitation, which is one of the primary justifications for diagnostic audiology.

BOX 14-2   **Personal Story**

One of the main goals of audiology is to find hearing loss as early as possible so that medical treatment or audiological (re)habilitation can begin quickly. This is especially true for children whose language development, academic progress, and social futures may be disrupted by hearing loss. It is probably the case that most rehabilitative efforts are successful and patients and their families are benefitted significantly. Unfortunately, this is not always the situation.

The profession of audiology has come a very long way since this audiologist began to practice in a state school for the deaf in the 1950s. Some of the children in that school had never had an actual hearing test and were placed there based on a variety of criteria. This included one child, with a condition called Treacher Collins syndrome, which had not been medically diagnosed but was obvious based on his craniofacial abnormalities. He had no pinnae or external auditory canals and was mildly retarded. When I asked why he had never been tested, I was greeted with surprise and told that there was no point because he had "no ears." I originally observed him in a classroom where the other students were using the newly installed, hard-wired auditory training units. He sat in a corner and was the only one not wearing earphones because he had "no ears." He used a crude signing system and no speech and he was rejected by his peers who taunted him because he was "different."

I was anxious to see this child because children with conductive hearing losses should rarely be educated in a manual environment and often develop language stimulation. When I tested him I found the almost-predictable bilateral 60-dB conductive hearing loss with perfectly normal bone conduction. My efforts at getting a bone-conduction hearing aid on this 12-year-old boy, which could have altered his life dramatically even at this relatively late time in his education, were unsuccessful, and were blocked primarily by his mother. When I spoke with her I was told that if God had wanted her son to hear, he would have given him ears. That was hardly the last time I would hear this sort of thing.

This is a child whose education and potential for a normal life might have been dramatically altered had he been seen by a persuasive audiologist when he was very young. It can only be hoped that this kind of tragic error is encountered less frequently today for, excepting medical or surgical intervention, clinical audiology affords the best opportunity to better the lives of children and adults with hearing loss.

STUDY QUESTIONS

1. List causes for conductive hearing loss caused by damage to the outer ear.

2. List causes for conductive hearing loss caused by damage to the middle ear.

3. List causes for sensory/neural hearing loss caused by damage to the inner ear.

4. List causes for sensory/neural hearing loss caused by damage to the auditory nerve.

5. What are the principal features of conductive hearing loss in terms of the relationships between air conduction and bone conduction? What is typical in the way of word-recognition scores?

6. Answer question 5 in terms of sensory/neural hearing loss.

7. What is a mixed hearing loss?

8. What is otitis media?

9. Why, and in what ways, are word-recognition scores different between patients with conductive and sensory/neural hearing losses?

10. Explain why a child might have difficulty in processing speech although he or she has normal hearing sensitivity.

KEY TERMS

Acoustic neuroma
Air conduction
Air–bone gap (ABG)
Audiogram
Audiometer
Auditory brainstem response (ABR)
Auditory nerve
Auditory processing disorder (APD)
Bone conduction
Conductive hearing loss

Hearing level (HL)
Immittance
Mastoid process
Minimal auditory deprivation syndrome
Mixed hearing loss
Myringostomy
Otitis media
Otoacoustic emission (OAE)
Otosclerosis
Phonetically balanced

Sensation level (SL)
Sensory/neural hearing loss
Speech-recognition threshold (SRT)
Spondee
Threshold of audibility
Tinnitus
Tympanometry
Vestibular mechanism
Word-recognition score (WRS)

REFERENCES

American Academy of Audiology. (1992). Position statement. Public meeting on clinical practice guidelines for the diagnosis and treatment of otitis media in children. *Audiology Today. 4*, 3–24.

American National Standards Institute. (1987). *American national standard specifications for instruments to measure aural acoustic impedance and admittance (aural acoustic immittance).* ANSI S3.39-1987. New York: Author.

Johnson, E. W. (1970). Tuning forks to audiometers and back again. *Laryngoscope, 80,* 49–68.

Keith, R. W. (2000). *SCAN-C. A test for auditory processing disorders in children—Revised.* San Antonio, TX: Psychological Corporation.

Kemp, D. T. (1978). Simulated acoustic emissions from within the human auditory system. *Journal of the Acoustical Society of America, 64,* 1386–1391.

Martin, F. N., & Clark, J. G. (2009). *Introduction to audiology* (10th ed.) Boston: Allyn & Bacon.

Studebaker, G. A. (1962). Placement of vibrator in bone conduction testing. *Journal of Speech and Hearing Research, 5,* 321–331.

SUGGESTED READINGS

Clark, J. G., & English, K. E. (2004). *Audiologic counseling: Helping patients and families adjust to hearing loss.* Boston: Allyn & Bacon.

Katz, J. (Ed.). *Handbook of clinical audiology* (4th ed.). Baltimore, MD: Williams & Wilkins.

Martin, F. N., & Clark, J. G. (1996). *Hearing care for children.* Boston: Allyn & Bacon.

Stach, B. A. (1998). *Clinical audiology: An introduction.* San Diego, CA: Singular.

chapter fifteen

Audiologic Rehabilitation

MARGARET S. DEAN AND JOHN A. NELSON

LEARNING OBJECTIVES

1. To understand the basic components and benefits of personal amplification systems, including hearing aids and cochlear implants.

2. To understand what makes some listening environments more difficult than others and how assistive listening devices might be helpful in these situations.

3. To understand the basic aural habilitation services for children who have hearing loss.

4. To understand how to empower adults who have hearing losses through aural rehabilitation.

> **BOX 15-1   Overview of the CD-ROM Segments**
>
> The CD-ROM segments that supplement this chapter contain both pictures and video demonstrations. There are five sections: hearing aids, taking an ear impression, cochlear implants, personal frequency modulation (FM) systems, and assistive listening devices (ALDs). The segments show many of the devices associated with audiologic rehabilitation as well as how some of them benefit the listeners.

Many different professionals employ techniques and provide services to empower individuals who have hearing losses. In many instances, the services are provided by a team of professionals. For example, audiologists fit hearing aids, teach patients how to use them, and provide information about effective communication strategies. Speech-language pathologists teach individuals with hearing impairments how to listen for important speech sounds, how to make their language more informative and complex, and how to produce intelligible speech. Educators of children who are deaf adapt traditional teaching techniques for children with hearing impairments. Psychologists and social workers assist in dealing with the psychological effects of hearing impairment on adults and children along with their caregivers. School administrators advocate and coordinate services for children.

The services that these professionals deliver are usually divided into two categories: **audiologic habilitation** and **audiologic rehabilitation**. Audiologic habilitation services are provided to children who are learning to listen and to use speech and language skills for the first time. Audiologic rehabilitation services are provided to adults who need to modify their communication style as a result of their acquired hearing impairments.

The first step in audiologic rehabilitation is to increase the individual's ability to hear sounds, usually using amplification. The extent of necessary services following amplification varies from individual to individual. Although follow-up services are beneficial, they are not always provided, which is unfortunate.

PERSONAL HEARING DEVICES

Hearing is an essential part of normal communication. People rely on hearing for such things as safety, communication, and pleasure. Thus, inventors and researchers have been trying for centuries to help people to hear better. The discovery of electricity was an important milestone for the development of hearing aids because it led to the invention of the electrical amplifier.

Nonelectrical Hearing Devices

Many things can be done to increase the intensity of sound to make people hear better. For example, an individual can cup a hand behind his or her ear. The hand helps to direct sound into the outer ear, leading to a perception of increased loudness. Horns and tubes provided an additional increase in audibility. Acoustic horns were used to direct sound from a large area into a small area. The effectiveness of the acoustic horn is dependent on its physical properties of size and shape, which can be altered to increase the energy applied to the smaller area, the outer ear. Unfortunately, it was awkward to speak into an acoustic horn placed at someone's ear. To rectify this problem, an acoustic horn was attached to a tube, which was then directed to the ear. With this instrument, speakers did not have to talk directly into the listener's ear.

For cosmetic reasons, these devices took many forms. The acoustic horn and tube device, often called the "ear trumpet," was often decorated with paintings or jewels. Sometimes the device was hidden in another object. The listening stick was a walking cane that was hollowed out to provide a tube for directing sound. The listening chair had hollowed tubes in the arms and back to direct sound to the listener's ear. Although modern hearing aids use electrical circuits, the physical properties of horns and tubes are still incorporated into their design.

Hearing Aids

With the discovery of electricity, amplification systems changed dramatically. The original electrical devices were quite large and required a direct line to a power source, for example, an electrical outlet. Thus, these devices were not portable. New developments in technology such as the vacuum tube and then the transistor and integrated circuit have provided miniaturization of the electrical circuits as well as decreased power requirements. These devices are now referred to as hearing aids, which require four basic components: a microphone, an amplifier, a receiver, and a battery.

A microphone converts acoustic signals into electrical signals. The changes in the electrical voltage are the same as the changes in the sound pressure of the acoustic signal. The electrical impulses are passed to the amplifier, which increases the amplitude of the electrical signal. The hearing aid does not amplify all frequencies by the same amount. The amount of amplification provided is dependent on the type and extent of the individual's hearing loss. The amplified electrical signal is then sent to a receiver, which converts the amplified electrical signal back into an acoustic signal. The acoustic signal is now more intense than its original input to the microphone. The receiver can be thought of as a small loudspeaker.

These three components require energy, which is provided by a battery. Currently, there are five sizes of hearing aid batteries. Only one battery size will work for a given hearing aid. Each battery has a positive side and a negative side and thus must be inserted in the correct direction for the device to operate.

In addition to the four basic components, there are many controls on a hearing aid (see Figure 15-1). The simplest is the on-off control, which might require flipping a switch, rotating the volume control wheel, or opening the battery door. Another user control is the volume control wheel, which allows the hearing aid user to change the intensity of the signal that reaches the ear. Some modern hearing aids do not have a volume control. Instead, advanced signal-processing systems within the instrument control the volume automatically.

Another common option on hearing aids is a **telecoil switch (t-switch)**. Telephones emit electromagnetic energy that fluctuates in the same pattern as the original acoustic

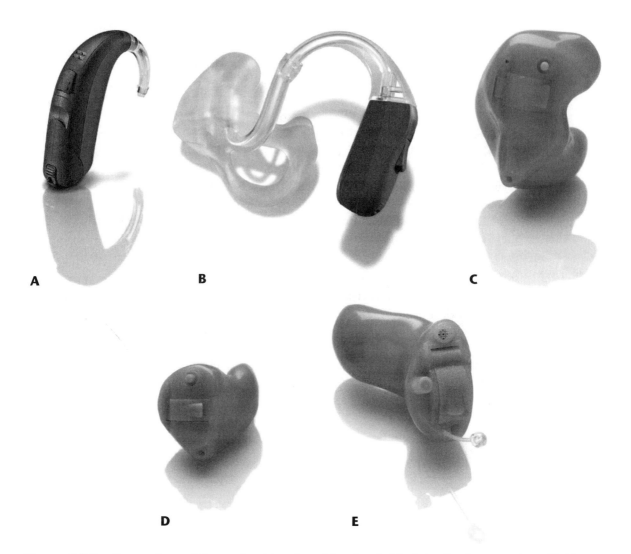

Figure 15-1 Comparison of the ear-level hearing aid styles: Behind-the-Ear (large and small) (**A, B**), In-the-Ear (**C**), In-the-Canal (**D**), and Completely-in-the-Canal (**E**). *Source:* Courtesy of Sonic Innovations, Inc.

signal. When the user flips the t-switch into the telecoil position, the hearing aid microphone is turned off, and the telecoil inside the hearing aid picks up the electromagnetic energy. The telecoil converts this energy to an electrical signal that is delivered to the amplifier. An advantage to using the telecoil mode is that it reduces feedback when using the telephone. Feedback is the whistling sound produced from a hearing aid when an object, such as a hand or telephone handset, is placed next to it. By turning the hearing aid microphone off, the hearing aid will not feed back. Additionally, because the microphone is turned off in the telecoil mode, the acoustic signal (noise) in the room will not be amplified. Imagine talking on the phone in a noisy restaurant and being able to "turn off" the background noise. The t-switch makes telephone conversations easier.

Hearing aids are available in many different styles. The body type hearing aid was the first mass-produced portable device and, as its name suggests, it is worn on the body (see Figure 15-2). The device consists of a small metal box, which contains the microphone, amplifier, battery, and user controls. Attached to the body aid is an electrical cord that extends to the ear and attaches to a button receiver that actually looks like a thick button. The button receiver is attached to an **earmold**, which directs sound into the outer ear. The earmold is either vinyl or acrylic material that is custom fit to fill a part of the outer ear. It has a bore or hole to direct sound from the button receiver down the ear canal toward the tympanic membrane.

The main disadvantage of the body hearing aid involves the microphone. Because the microphone is worn on the chest, body hearing aid users "hear" from their chests instead of their ears. This also makes the microphone susceptible to unwanted noise when clothing rubs against it. One advantage of the device is that it allows for large controls, which is beneficial for individuals with limited dexterity, such as those who are elderly. The original body-worn device was necessary to house the large electronics and battery. With the miniaturization of electronic circuitry and batteries, the housing requirements were also reduced. Therefore, body hearing aids are no longer commonly used.

The behind-the-ear hearing aid (BTE), as its name suggests, is worn behind the pinna (see Figure 15-3). The microphone is in the top of the device and is aimed toward

Figure 15-2 (right)   A Body-worn hearing aid. *Source:* Photograph courtesy of Beltone.

Figure 15-3 (below)   External parts of the BTE and ITE style hearing aids. *Source:* Photograph courtesy of Sonic Innovations, Inc.

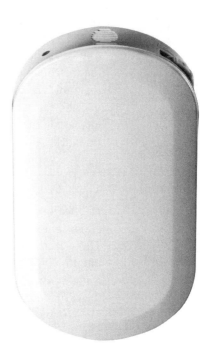

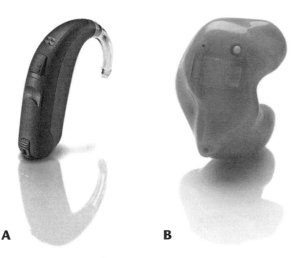

A   **B**

the front of the user where the top of the pinna attaches to the head. The device houses the microphone, amplifier, receiver, and battery in one case. The amplified acoustic energy exits the hearing aid at the top and is directed into an earhook, a curved, hard plastic tube that directs sound out of the BTE to a flexible tube that is inserted into the earmold. The earhook also helps to hold the BTE hearing aid on the ear. The BTE hearing aid is relatively large compared to the other current styles, allowing for more circuitry and signal processing options. Although part of the BTE hearing aid is hidden behind the ear, many people feel it is not cosmetically acceptable.

One variation of the BTE hearing aid is the eyeglass device. Individuals who need glasses and hearing aids but want to wear only one prosthetic device find the eyeglass hearing aid to be an acceptable option. The bows of the glasses, the sidepieces, were hollowed out and hearing aid components inserted. The portion of the bow that reaches behind the ear is the most common place because this area could easily be enlarged to encase the hearing aid components. Tubing from the glasses' bow was directed to an earmold. As might be imagined, the device required a rather large pair of glasses. Although an admirable idea, the device caused many problems for the people who were responsible for fitting both hearing aids and glasses. People fitting hearing aids usually did not know much about adjusting glasses, and people fitting glasses usually did not know much about adjusting hearing aids. Further, if one aspect of the device needed repair, the benefits of both prosthetic devices were made unavailable until the complete system was fixed. Today, these devices are rarely seen. Fortunately, with smaller glasses and hearing aids, both devices can be comfortably worn together.

More recent variations of the BTE include the mini-BTE and the receiver-in-the-ear (RITE) hearing aids. The mini-BTE is a smaller version of the original BTE and is designed to be less visible to be more appealing to those with cosmetic concerns. The RITE hearing aid is similar to the mini-BTE in that the small case that houses the microphone, amplifier, and battery fits behind the pinna. The RITE differs from the mini-BTE in that the receiver is located in the end of the long thin tubing that fits into the ear canal, maximizing the distance between the microphone and receiver. The increased separation between the microphone and receiver decreases the occurrence of feedback. A soft plastic dome is attached to the end of the receiver to hold the receiver in place within the canal.

The next smaller hearing aid is the in-the-ear hearing aid (ITE) (see Figure 15-3). All of the components are placed in a plastic shell that is custom fit to the user. The ITE hearing aid fills up the concha as well as part of the external ear canal. The microphone, battery door, and volume control are located on the faceplate of the hearing aid. The receiver is located in the canal portion of the aid and delivers the amplified sound into the lower portion of the ear canal. The microphone is located in the concha where sound normally arrives. Also, the hearing aid is now contained in a single unit because the earmold and the hearing aid are both part of one device.

The in-the-canal hearing aid (ITC) is even smaller than the ITE and completely fills the outer part of the external ear canal. This hearing aid is custom fit for an individual user. Currently, there are some options that are unavailable with ITC hearing aids. For example, a telecoil will not fit within this device. Also, as hearing aids

---

BOX 15-2   Hearing Aids

In segment Ch.15.01, you can see every angle of BTE, ITE, ITC, and CIC hearing aids. After opening the file, click on one style of hearing aid to activate the movie. Then, click and drag to rotate the hearing aid to different viewing angles—all 360°! In that segment, the hearing aids are not at the relative scale. To see a size comparison of the ear-level hearing aids, open segment Ch.15.02. Segment Ch.15.03 is an example of a body-worn hearing aid, with an appropriate earmold. The major parts of a hearing aid are labeled for a BTE and an ITE hearing aid in segments Ch.15.04 and Ch.15.05, respectively. The segment Ch.15.06 shows a variety of earmold styles and colors.

---

become smaller and smaller, the batteries, which will fit in the aid, also need to be smaller. Less energy can be stored by smaller batteries, and thus, the battery life is decreased. For those who are concerned about cosmetic issues, the ITC is less noticeable than is the ITE hearing aid.

A recent advancement in hearing aids is the completely in-the-canal hearing aid (CIC), which fits deep in the ear canal and must be custom fit to the individual user. The hearing aid is removed by pulling on a piece of plastic that is similar to a short length of fishing line. Because of this deep fit, a volume control wheel is not an option. As might be expected, the device is very difficult to see when in place, making it very desirable by those who are the most concerned about cosmetics. The obstacles to fitting this device are twofold. First, the individual must have an average to large external ear canal to accommodate the device. Second, as with all aids, as they become smaller, the amplification that can be provided is increasingly limited. CIC hearing aids are appropriate only for individuals with mild and moderate degrees of hearing loss.

The bone-conduction hearing aid is a special device used for individuals with substantial conductive losses, such as individuals who do not have an external ear canal or those who have constant drainage from the canal as a result of infection. The bone-conduction hearing aid consists of a microphone, amplifier, battery, and a bone oscillator. The bone oscillator replaces the air-conduction receiver and is usually placed behind the pinna on the mastoid process.

Traditional hearing aids are called analog devices because the output signal that is emitted from the speaker is analogous to the input signal that enters the microphone, but is increased in intensity. The newest generation of devices is digital and, like tiny computers, are capable of processing, operating on, storing, transmitting, and displaying data (in this case sound waves) in the form of numerical digits. Digital hearing aids have almost replaced analog devices. The digital processing provides benefits in many listening situations. Digital hearing aids are available at a range of prices. The basic devices are similar to the analog amplifiers and the high-end devices incorporate advanced signal processing that can benefit some individuals in some situations. A

BOX 15-3 **Taking an Ear Impression**

You can watch an abbreviated video of an audiologist taking an ear impression in segment Ch.15.16. The first step in taking an ear impression is for the clinician to perform an otoscopic examination looking at the size and shape of the ear canal. It is also important for the clinician to look for cerumen and objects in the canal. The second step is for the clinician to place an oto-block in the ear canal to ensure that the impression material does not reach the tympanic membrane. The clinician mixes the impression material and uses a syringe to direct it into the ear canal. After the material cures, the clinician removes it, and then repeats the otoscopic examination. Note: This video clip has no audio.

recent advancement of some digital hearing aids is Bluetooth capability, which allows the aid to be linked to various electronic devices including the television, MP3 players, and the telephone, as well as cell phones.

Hearing Aid Fitting

The first step in fitting a hearing aid is to obtain an ear impression of the individual. The process consists of placing soft plastic material into the ear following the insertion of a cotton or foam block into the ear canal so that the material does not come in contact with the tympanic membrane. After a few minutes, the material hardens and is removed. If the individual is going to use a body or BTE style hearing aid, the ear impression is sent to a laboratory for fabrication of an earmold. If the individual is going to use an ITE, ITC, or CIC style hearing aid, the ear impression is sent to the hearing aid manufacturer to make the custom-fit case that holds the hearing aid components.

There are two main goals in fitting an amplification system. The first is to provide audibility for sounds that cannot be heard because of the hearing loss. This is accomplished by the amplifier and is measured in acoustic **gain**. Gain is calculated by subtracting the intensity of sound entering the microphone of the hearing aid (input) from the intensity of sound exiting the earmold (output). The unit used for measuring hearing aid gain is the decibel (dB). Thus, if the input intensity is 65 dB sound-pressure level (SPL) and the output intensity is 85 dB SPL, the gain is 20 dB.

Fitting hearing aids is not like fitting glasses, where the goal is to achieve 20/20 vision. The audiologist is not trying to achieve hearing thresholds within normal limits. Research has shown that providing gain values that are equal to the hearing loss are often unacceptable to the listener. Therefore, instead of providing enough gain for the individual to hear at 0 dB HL, most audiologists try to achieve gain values that are between one third and two thirds of the hearing loss. The gain at each frequency depends on the shape of the hearing loss. A plot of the gain across frequencies is called the frequency response of the hearing aid.

The second goal in fitting hearing aids is to ensure that the **output** of the device does not reach intensities that cause discomfort or damage. High-intensity sounds can harm the ear and can be perceived as unacceptably loud. It is important to verify that the maximum output of the hearing aid, independent of the input signal, never reaches a level of discomfort. Thresholds of discomfort can be measured with an audiometer and applied to the fitting of the hearing aid. The setting of the maximum output of the hearing aid is commonly verified by producing an intense input signal, like speaking loudly into the hearing aid microphone. This activity provides the hearing aid user an opportunity to comment on the loudness and annoyance of intense inputs. Because intense sounds can damage the auditory system without being uncomfortable, it is also important to measure the output of the hearing aid in the individual's ear.

The physical measurements of gain and output of a hearing aid can be accomplished in two ways. One way is to obtain behavioral thresholds with and without the hearing aid. The difference between the aided and unaided thresholds is referred to as **functional gain**. A disadvantage of this technique is that it involves a time-consuming process.

The alternative to functional gain measures is to obtain real-ear probe-microphone measurements. These measurements allow audiologists to determine the intensity of sound in the ear canal. A small flexible tube is placed in the external ear canal with the end near the tympanic membrane. The other end of the tube is connected to a small microphone. The **real-ear gain** is the difference between the intensity at the tympanic membrane measured with and without the hearing aid. This whole procedure takes only a few minutes and yields very useful data.

Hearing aid research laboratories around the world are continually investigating new signal processing techniques. Hopefully, these techniques will increase the quality of life for individuals who wear hearing aids. One common goal is to increase the ability of the patient to understand speech in the presence of background noise. Although signal processing techniques used in hearing aids have had some success, the most desirable way is to decrease the level of background noise before it enters the microphone. This is usually accomplished with **assistive listening devices (ALDs)**, which are discussed later in this chapter.

Hearing Aid Maintenance

Hearing aids need to be checked daily. First, it is critical that the hearing aid battery has sufficient voltage to power the aid. This can be ascertained with a battery tester. The outer part of the hearing aid should be cleaned of debris, including removal of cerumen (ear wax) from the hearing aid receiver. Any part of the hearing aid that has electronic controls cannot be washed with water. Only the earmold of a body or BTE hearing aid can be cleaned with water after it is removed from the aid. If a hearing aid does not amplify with a charged battery, sounds distorted, has intermittent sound, does not make sounds audible, or is uncomfortably loud, the device should be taken to an audiologist to have it checked. The audiologist has tools necessary to fix many problems, but there are times when the hearing aid must be returned to the factory for repair.

Tactile Aids

Tactile aids are used by individuals who cannot benefit from traditional amplification. These devices contain a microphone that picks up the acoustic signal. The signal is amplified and converted to a vibration that is delivered to the skin. The vibrotactile stimulation is often delivered to the individual's chest, back, or arm. As might be suspected, the sensitivity of the skin to tactile vibrations is not as precise as the sensitivity of the ear to acoustic vibrations. Therefore, one important disadvantage of these devices is the limited frequency resolution that they can provide to the listener. In the normal auditory system, very small changes in frequency can be perceived across a large frequency range. The tactile aid is usually limited to coding 10 different frequency bands. This means that less than 10 different "pitches" can be perceived and used for coding speech. Most individuals have experienced difficulty understanding speech with a tactile aid unless it is supplemented with visual and contextual cues.

Cochlear Implants

For individuals with severe to profound sensory/neural hearing losses, traditional hearing aid amplification provides limited or no benefit because of damage within the cochlea. As discussed by Dr. Champlin in Chapter 13, the ear converts an acoustic pressure wave to a mechanical force at the tympanic membrane, which is then delivered to the oval window and results in vibration of the basilar membrane within the cochlea. The basilar membrane movement causes a shearing action of the hair cells and resulting electrical activity that can generate action potentials on the auditory nerve. Direct electrical stimulation of the auditory nerve generates action potentials that are perceived by the brain as auditory stimuli. Most individuals with severe to profound sensory/neural hearing losses have damage within the cochlea.

In 1972, after decades of research and product development, the first human received a **cochlear implant**. At first, cochlear implants were only available to adults with profound acquired hearing loss. After many years of clinical investigation, the devices are now available for infants, children, and adults. It is important to understand that cochlear implants are not appropriate for every child with a severe hearing impairment. The Food and Drug Administration imposes guidelines regarding candidacy for implants.

The implant consists of a microphone, a signal processor, a transmitter, a receiver, and an electrode array see Figure 15-4). The microphone picks up the acoustic signal and delivers it to the signal processor. The electronics of the cochlear implant limit the frequency resolution that can be delivered to the cochlea. The first devices were single-channel, and only the presence or absence of a signal was delivered to the user. Today more than 20 channels are available for stimulating the cochlea. The signal processor analyzes the input signal and determines how to stimulate the cochlea.

Information about the input signal is coded and delivered to the external transmitting device that is worn behind the ear. (See Figures 15-4 and 15-5.) The transmitting device is held in place by a magnetic force between it and the receiving device that was surgically placed under the skin. The signal is transmitted to the receiver through the skin by means of a radio frequency. The internal receiver delivers the electrical signal to an electrode array within the scala tympani of the cochlea (see Figure 15-5). The electrode array sends electrical currents through different regions of the cochlea. This causes the generation of action potentials on the auditory nerve that are perceived by the brain as sounds.

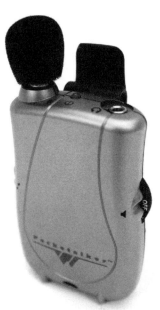

Figure 15-4 A body-worn speech processor and internal components of a cochlear implant. Courtesy of Williams Sound Corporation

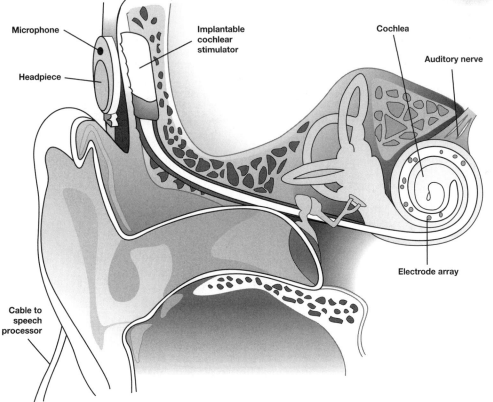

Figure 15-5 A diagram of where the cochlear implant is located in the cochlea. *Source:* Clar, J. G., & Dowell, R. C. (1997). *Cochlear Implants for Infants and Children* (p. 510). San Diego, CA: Singular Publishing Group.

As mentioned earlier, the Food and Drug Administration has specific guidelines for determining candidacy for cochlear implants. (See Table 15-1.) These guidelines continue to change with advancements in research and technology. Some of the guidelines include an absence of medical contraindications, bilateral profound hearing loss for young children ages 12 months to 2 years or a severe to profound loss for children ages 2 to 17 years and adults who lost their hearing after language acquisition, little to no benefit from traditional amplification, a desire to communicate in an auditory mode, high motivation, and realistic expectations. Infants must be approximately 12 months old before they can become candidates for surgery.

There are many reasons why an individual might not wish to obtain a cochlear implant. Not wanting to undergo the surgery is a major reason, especially for parents of very young infants. Also, individuals who are deaf might not feel that hearing is critically important to their quality of life. Many deaf individuals live happy, fulfilled lives without hearing. Professionals should respect these personal beliefs, and the rehabilitation team should assist the individual and family members in deciding whether a cochlear implant is an appropriate option.

Table 15-1   Guidelines for Candidacy to Obtain a Cochlear Implant

Young Children: 12 months to 2 years

Bilateral profound sensory/neural hearing loss

Limited or no useful benefit from hearing aids

No medical contraindications

High motivation and realistic expectations of both child and caregivers

Educational placement that emphasizes auditory skill development

At least 12 months of age

Children: 2 to 17 years

Bilateral severe to profound sensory/neural hearing loss

Little or no benefit from hearing aids

Lack of progress with respect to auditory skills

High motivation and realistic expectations of both child and caregivers

Adults: 18 years and older

Bilateral profound sensory/neural hearing loss or bilateral severe to profound sensory/neural hearing loss if acquired after the acquisition of language

Limited or no useful benefit from hearing aids

No medical contraindications

At least 17 years of age

BOX 15-4   Cochlear Implants

See segment Ch.15.08 for an example of an early speech processor and segment Ch.15.09[1] for examples of more recent models. The device that is implanted in the cochlea is shown with a gloved hand in segment Ch.15.10.[2] This particular device has an electrode array that is placed in the cochlea and a second electrode that is placed outside of the cochlea. Finally, the placement of the ear-level speech processor and external transmitter is shown in segment Ch.15.11.[3]

---

1. Courtesy of MED-EL
2. Courtesy of Cochlear Americas
3. Courtesy of MED-EL

Most individuals who receive cochlear implants demonstrate a significant increase in their speech perception ability. With the more recent devices, it is common for these individuals to understand speech even without visual cues, such as on the telephone. Individuals with cochlear implants often report that nonspeech stimuli, such as music, are also pleasurable. Rehabilitation is necessary for the patient to understand how to hear with a cochlear implant signal, and many hours of intensive therapy are usually needed to develop speech and language skills, especially for individuals who have not heard before. Even with intensive therapy, not all children with cochlear implants develop intelligible speech.

DIFFICULT LISTENING ENVIRONMENTS

The main goal of hearing aids is to increase the audibility of the speech signal. Many individuals have difficulty hearing and understanding speech in situations that involve a lot of background noise and reverberation. Reverberations are the sound reflections from hard surfaces. A room, such as a bathroom, with tile walls and a tile floor, has considerable reverberation. A living room with carpeting, drapes, and soft furniture has much less reverberation. Reflections of sound interact and interfere with the original signal and make understanding speech difficult. These characteristics of a room are measured as **reverberation time**, which is determined by calculating the amount of time it takes for an intense sound to decrease by 60 dB after it is turned off. Most classrooms typically have reverberation times between 0.4 second and 1.2 seconds (Crandell & Smaldino, 1995). Children with hearing loss should be placed in classrooms that have reverberation times no greater than 0.4 second (Crandell & Smaldino, 1995). Thus, many classrooms need to be acoustically modified to reduce reverberation.

Listening environments can also be described in terms of **signal-to-noise ratio (SNR)**. The SNR is the signal intensity minus the noise intensity. Positive SNRs indicate that the signal is more intense than the noise; negative SNRs indicate that the noise is more intense than the signal. Talking with a friend in a living room would be an example of a positive SNR; talking to a friend with the fire alarm going off would be an example of a negative SNR. The more positive the SNR, the better the listening situation. Typical SNRs for classrooms have been reported in the range of +5 to –7 dB (Crandell & Smaldino, 1995). Children with hearing loss should be placed in classrooms in which the SNR is greater than +15 dB (Crandell & Smaldino, 1995). As is clearly evident, most public school classrooms are atrocious listening settings for instruction, especially for children with hearing impairments.

To improve speech discrimination, it is ideal to reduce the levels of background noise and reverberation. Unfortunately, this is not always possible. For example, in a restaurant it is difficult to have all the other customers sit silently. Or in a school gymnasium that is also used as an auditorium, carpeting on the floor would not be an option. A way to compensate for background noise and reverberation is to increase the intensity of the speaker's voice. The disadvantage of this solution is that a classroom teacher experiences more vocal strain, and listeners near the teacher are in positions of greater intensities compared to listeners who are farther away.

A better way to increase the SNR is to use an ALD. These devices pick up the sound at its source and transmit it directly to the listener without sending intense sound waves through the air. FM systems constitute one example of an ALD that is often used in school settings. (See Figure 15-6.) Teachers wear a microphone that is attached to an FM transmitter (see Figure 15-6). The transmitter acts as a miniature radio station. It broadcasts the FM signal to an FM receiver that is worn by a student. The receiver converts the FM signal back into an acoustic signal with the help of devices such as headsets or personal hearing aids. Wherever the student is in the classroom, he or she can listen to sounds that come directly from the microphone worn by the teacher and the signal intensity and SNR are both increased.

Other ALDs use different technology to deliver a signal across distances. For example, the signal might be transmitted by infrared or light frequencies that cannot be seen by the human eye. The benefit of such systems is that the signal cannot travel outside of

BOX 15-5 Personal FM System

A picture of a personal FM system is shown in segment Ch.15.12. The transmitter is connected to a head-worn boom microphone; the receiver is connected to BTE microphones that direct the sound into an earmold. The four video clips demonstrate the advantages of listening with an FM system. Segments Ch.15.13 and Ch.15.14 describe the listening environment. The audio was recorded from the back of the classroom using ear simulators. You can see that the signal is more intense and clear with the FM system (Ch.15.13) than without the FM system (Ch.15.14). The second pair of movies, segments Ch.15.15 and Ch.15.16, demonstrate not only the decrease in intensity, but also when the students are making a variety of distracting noises. It is important to note that I was speaking at a normal conversational level. If I were to increase my voice for the size of the room, I could experience vocal fatigue and possibly abuse.

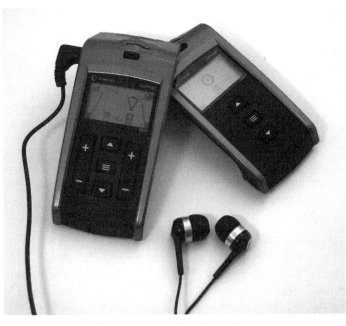

Figure 15-6 An example of an FM system. In this situation, the transmitting unit is connected to a head-worn boom microphone and the receiving device is connected to BTE-microphones that direct sound to an earmold. *Source:* Courtesy of Comfort Audio, Inc.

a room, thereby denying the signals to unintended listeners. FM broadcasts can travel through walls just like FM radio signals.

Another way to transmit signals is by electromagnetic fields. Electromagnetic fields can be generated by telephone handsets, and a hearing aid in the telecoil mode can pick up these signals. Electromagnetic fields can also be produced by running electricity through a special cable. The cable is placed around the section of room where the electromagnetic field is desired. This is referred to as "looping" a room. The talker speaks into the microphone of the ALD, the signal is delivered through the "loop," and an electromagnetic field is generated. Hearing aid users can set their hearing aids to the telecoil position to pick up the speaker's voice.

These examples of ALDs require that the individual with a hearing loss has a receiving device or a hearing aid to pick up the signal. Some systems support multiple users. For example, various individuals using FM receivers can tune to the same transmission frequency, or they can all use hearing aids in the telecoil position. Some of these systems can be adapted to benefit every individual in a room. In group amplification systems, the speaker wears a microphone and the signal is transmitted, amplified, and delivered to loudspeakers placed around the room, such as in public address (PA) systems. These systems are beneficial in places like classrooms because the teacher's voice can be heard above the noises of the room. This results in an improved SNR and less vocal strain for the teachers.

ALERTING DEVICES

Alerting devices help individuals hear important sounds such as fire alarms, a baby's cry, the telephone, or an alarm clock. Alerting devices have the ability to increase the intensity of a signal or alter its frequency range so that it is in the audible range of the listener; for example, using a low-frequency telephone ringer for an individual with a high-frequency hearing loss. Another way to alert someone who has difficulty hearing is to use flashing lights or vibrotactile stimulation. In this case, an alarm clock might be hooked up to cause lights to flash or a bed to shake. In some instances, dogs are trained to inform the individual of a sound. These wonderful, dedicated animals are called "hearing dogs."

AUDIOLOGIC HABILITATION

Audiologic habilitation services are provided to individuals who have not mastered oral communication. The first step in audiologic habilitation is the diagnosis of a hearing loss. Until recently, it was difficult to identify hearing loss in young children because testing results were based on limited behavioral reactions to sound. Many times the hearing loss was not documented until several years into the child's life. Normal language development begins at birth and a number of major milestones are accomplished by the first year of life. Infants with hearing losses might not hear the speech of their caregivers or even their own attempts at babbling. If this is the case, the development of speech and language skills will be delayed. Sometimes these delays are never overcome and children do not reach their full spoken language potential.

Fortunately, auditory brainstem response (ABR) and otoacoustic emission (OAE) testing, as discussed by Dr. Martin in Chapter 14, have decreased the delay in documenting the hearing sensitivity of infants. In previous decades, successful early identification of hearing loss was measured in years; today it can be measured in days. This allows infants to be fitted with hearing aids as early as 1 month of age. Part of the success of early identification is a result of infant hearing screening programs that are encouraged or mandated in many states. It is estimated that hundreds of thousands of dollars can be saved by early amplification and intervention. If a child can hear during the early years of speech and language development, that child might not need as many services to "catch up" later.

BOX 15-6   Assistive Listening Device

The segment Ch.15.17 demonstrates a doorknocker assistive listening device. The vibrations of the door caused by knocking cause a light on the back of the door to flash. To enhance this experience, there is no sound in this video.

Hearing Aids for Children

There are many special considerations when amplifying the hearing of infants. The primary considerations regard the main two goals of amplification: gain and output. When fitting hearing aids, it is helpful to know the threshold of hearing at each frequency. The hearing threshold for each frequency is then used in calculating the hearing aid gain. ABR and OAE testing provide estimates of hearing thresholds, but these estimates are not always specific in the degree of hearing loss at particular frequencies. Therefore, the hearing aid gain used with an infant may not be adjusted to the optimal setting. The child may need to visit the audiologist multiple times for more diagnostic testing to specifically define the hearing loss and to adjust the hearing aid appropriately.

The second goal of fitting hearing aids in children is appropriate output. Because an infant cannot directly convey when a hearing aid is too loud, it is difficult to ensure that the maximum output of the hearing aid will not cause discomfort. One way that the infant might express loudness discomfort with the hearing aid is by crying. However, infants use this expression for many reasons, and it may be difficult to differentiate the meaning of the cry. Therefore, it is important that the caregiver reports the infant's reactions to the hearing aid to the audiologist. Another reason to check the maximum output levels of a hearing aid is to avoid causing additional hearing loss from exposure to intense sounds.

When fitting hearing aids on infants, there are special considerations in addition to gain and output. As infants grow, so do their ear canals, conchae, and pinnae. Thus, the hearing aid will need physical modifications to continue to fit the ear. If an ITE, ITC, or CIC style hearing aid is used with an infant, it must be sent back to the manufacturer to be recased for the growing ear. Thus, the infant would be without hearing aids during those few weeks. With a BTE style hearing aid, a new earmold can be ordered when necessary and replaced in the audiologist's office. Thus, the infant is not deprived of amplification. Further, a new earmold is a less expensive option than is recasing a hearing aid. For the first few years of life, a child outgrows an earmold almost every 6 months.

The BTE style hearing aid allows the most flexibility for necessary changes in gain and output because the hearing loss is documented more precisely. The BTE aid is also the most flexible device to be used with ALDs. The BTE style hearing aid decreases expenses and duration without amplification and allows the most flexibility in amplification procedures.

Caregivers of children with hearing losses are responsible for ensuring that the child's hearing aids are functioning and worn properly. Because infants cannot voice their concerns about the functioning of their hearing aids, the caregiver must check the battery, listen for clarity of the output signal, and clean the hearing aids. It is often a major task just to keep the hearing aid on an infant. Caregivers have come up with many ways to accomplish this. Sometimes a soft rubber ring is attached to the BTE hearing aid and is wrapped around the pinna. Another option is to use toupee tape to adhere the hearing aid to the skin with minimal irritation upon removal. As children grow older, their responsibility for their hearing aid care should increase. During the school-age years, teachers, school nurses, principals, and speech-language pathologists might assist children with hearing aids during the daytime hours. These individuals require training in hearing aid care as well as ALD care and maintenance.

Communication Mode

The communication mode is another choice that must be made for the child with hearing loss. There are three communication modes: oral, manual, and total communication. The decision about communication mode can be difficult to make. Many parents want their children to communicate in a mode that they feel proficient in using. When hearing parents have children with severe or profound hearing losses, it is difficult for them to change from speaking to signing. It is important for parents and hearing professionals to decide on a communication mode early to initiate the learning process. If one mode does not prove successful, caregivers can reevaluate their decisions.

An oral communication mode uses only auditory signals for the transfer of messages. The underlying assumption of oral communication training is that children will communicate in an auditory world and with individuals with normal hearing. To be able to communicate with the most people, children need to be able to hear and speak messages. In oral communication education settings, children with hearing impairments are taught to rely on only auditory signals. The facial cues and visual speech movements are eliminated from the message during therapy to force the child to listen more carefully. Although this therapy technique is not an accurate representation of communication, it forces children to maximize their residual hearing to understand auditory signals. Oral communication becomes more difficult with increased amounts of hearing loss.

A manual communication mode uses hand shapes and movements to communicate a message. (See Figure 15-7.) In this mode, no auditory message is communicated. American Sign Language, total communication, fingerspelling, Signed Exact English, Cued Speech, and Total Communication are all examples of manual communication. The subject of manual communication and the deaf culture is covered in greater detail by Dr. Bernstein in Chapter 16.

Learning to Hear

For most individuals, learning to hear requires minimal effort. Hearing and the knowledge of sounds are matters that individuals with normal hearing take for granted. Learning to hear with an impaired auditory system is a complicated process. Three levels of auditory processing must be obtained before auditory comprehension can take place.

The first level is **detection**. This level is fairly simple to understand. If a sound is not heard, it cannot be processed by the auditory system. Thus, the first step in audiologic habilitation is to document the softest sound that is audible with and without amplification.

The second level of auditory processing is **discrimination**, which is the ability to determine whether two or more sounds are the same or different. This level of auditory processing can often be learned. It is important to realize that the impaired auditory system might not be able to code some sounds. Two sounds that are inadequately

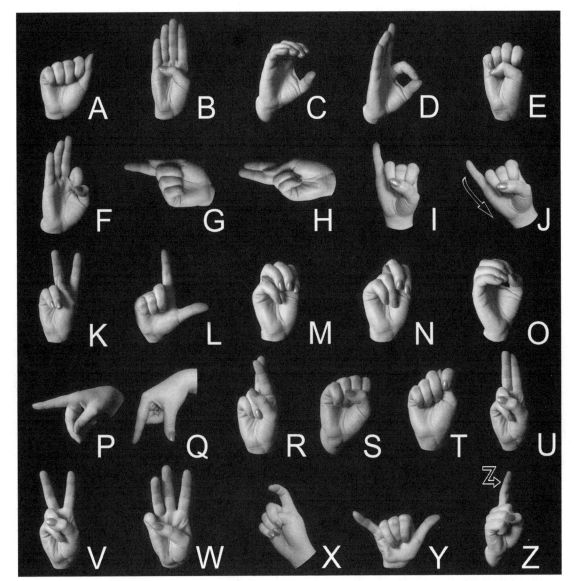

Figure 15-7 There are twenty-six hand shapes, which correspond to each letter in the English alphabet. *Source:* © Tammy Mcallister/Dreamstime.com

coded might sound the same. Children who cannot discriminate between two important sounds cannot advance to higher levels of auditory processing. When this is the case, the use of nonauditory cues, such as visual cues, becomes critical.

If children can detect a sound and discriminate it from other sounds, they can begin to identify the sound. **Identification**, the third level of auditory processing, occurs after the child has learned a symbolic representation for the sound. Here, *representation* means categorization within the auditory system. If all four phonemes of the word *dogs* have been coded and processed as a meaningful unit, the child can begin to comprehend *dogs* as multiple, four-legged animals that bark. This subject is discussed in greater detail by Drs. Gillam, Bedore, and Davis in Chapter 2.

It is critical to ensure that each level of auditory processing is accomplished before expecting the child to reach higher processing levels successfully. Consider a child who cannot hear the sound /s/. Instead of hearing *dogs*, the child would hear "dog." This problem with detection would interfere with the child's ability to learn the plural morpheme in English. Children might use nonauditory cues in this situation. For example, the placement of the lips might provide a visual cue of an /s/ at the end of a word. Contextual cues also become important for the child. If contextual cues were understood, the phrase "five dogs" would allow the child to "fill-in" the undetectable /s/ sound at the cortical level.

Educational Environments

Audiologic habilitation services are provided in various settings. The diagnostic evaluation and hearing aid fitting are usually done in an audiologist's office. Some audiologists operate their own private practices in medical or professional buildings. Other audiologists see clients in hospitals or provide services as part of a team working out of a physician's office. Sometimes, the audiologist might provide these services in a quiet room in a school. In 1975, Public Law 94-142, the Individuals with Disabilities Education Act, was the first of many laws requiring that children be educated in the "least restrictive environment" following amplification. The concept of a least restrictive environment is discussed in more detail by Drs. Gillam and Petersen in Chapter 11. The educational environment that should be the most beneficial for the child is determined by the caregivers and the habilitation team.

Success of audiologic habilitation is achieved when children have integrated what they have learned into their daily lives. Therefore, although services are usually provided in a classroom setting, these skills must also be reinforced outside the school. Parents, grandparents, siblings, babysitters, and other caregivers need to be included in the process. They need to know how to reinforce effective communication as well as to understand realistic expectations.

AUDIOLOGIC REHABILITATION

Audiologic rehabilitation is provided to individuals who need to modify their communication style because of acquired hearing loss. Hearing loss is often difficult for individuals to accept. To many people, a hearing loss represents getting older. It is often difficult to get adults to undergo a hearing test and to understand the results. Sometimes, a great deal of encouragement is required before an individual will try hearing aids. Fortunately, many people realize the benefits of audiologic rehabilitation. It is rewarding to be told by a new hearing aid user, "I can hear my grandchildren," "I enjoy the symphony again," or even "I had a great conversation with my spouse at dinner last night." These individuals are benefiting from amplification.

Communication Breakdown

The main speech communication loop consists of speakers who produce acoustic signals and listeners who receive those signals. When an individual has a hearing loss, part of that entire acoustic signal may be inaudible and therefore unavailable for auditory perception. One way to compensate for hearing loss is to have people speak louder. In some situations, speakers might find themselves shouting to be heard. Although the message might be heard, shouting also carries a message, often perceived as anger. The message "Good morning" has a different tone when shouted into someone's face. These communication situations can cause tremendous distress in a relationship.

Imagine a couple who have been married for many years. Over the years, either one or both of the individuals have developed hearing losses as a result of the normal aging process. A simple whisper in one's ear of "I love you" might receive a response of "What?" A few repetitions with each getting louder might result in "Never mind" or "You don't have to yell at me!" These situations can cause emotional strain in a relationship. Further strain might also occur as a result of one person not responding because he or she did not hear the other. This can be internalized by the speaker as being ignored.

A hearing loss might also cause miscommunication. For example, if someone does not hear a grocery list correctly, he or she would not get the items requested. These errors might be interpreted as the loss of cognitive ability and memory. Because this type of hearing loss usually progresses slowly, individuals might not realize that they are experiencing hearing loss and not memory loss. If a person cannot hear a message, he or she certainly cannot remember it. Paranoia can also develop from these miscommunications.

When each of a couple's hearing is not similar, other problems can occur. For example, the person with a greater hearing loss might want the television or radio set at a higher volume. One spouse might consider this volume setting comfortable while the other considers it too loud. These topics are often addressed within an adult rehabilitation group. Adult rehabilitation should include more than fitting amplification and should address communication difficulties.

Aural Rehabilitation Groups

Aural rehabilitation groups are designed to empower individuals who have hearing losses. The discussions are tailored for adults with hearing losses and their significant others to learn more about hearing loss. Group sessions usually focus on understanding the hearing mechanism, types of hearing aids, communication strategies, and ALDs. Some of this information will have been presented during the audiologic evaluation and the hearing aid fitting, but the group sessions allow for further clarification.

The Hearing Mechanism

Many individuals with hearing losses do not understand how signals travel from the mouth of the speaker to the brain of the listener. Thus, the first topic for an aural rehabilitation group is the nature of the communication channel. When group members understand the concept of how signals travel through a normal auditory system, the discussions turn to understanding the impaired auditory system. The different types of hearing losses are discussed and the audiogram is explained. Finally, group members learn to interpret their own audiograms. At this point, individuals should begin to understand why they are having difficulty communicating.

Hearing Aids

Another session of an aural rehabilitation group might focus on how hearing aids work. The group can review the components of the hearing aid as well as how to care for them. Tips on how to fix a hearing aid problem are also provided. During these sessions, it is important that the group discusses realistic benefits from amplification. Many individuals have difficulty accepting that hearing aids do not fix a hearing loss. Questions also arise concerning hearing aid advertisements and modern technology. Advertisements often stir hope of better hearing aids, and this might not always be feasible.

Communication

Because amplification is only the first step in rehabilitation, effective communication using hearing aids must be discussed. Most individuals develop poor communication strategies during the years prior to amplification. Often they do not try to seek clarification of a misunderstood message because it might be too difficult or perceived as weakness. Assertiveness training is often beneficial. Assertive interactions allow for each individual's needs to be met while respecting the feelings of others.

For example, an individual with a hearing aid might say, "I have difficulty understanding you when I cannot see your face. It would be helpful if you would get my attention before speaking." In this situation, the individual has stated the problem and requested, but not demanded, a solution. It is also important during communication to realize that it is not the sole responsibility of one person to set up ideal listening situations. Both participants need to actively use effective communication strategies. It is not effective when people communicate between different rooms. They need to decide together how they are going to get to the same room. These are a few of many possible improvements that can be made in communication styles.

Assistive Listening Devices

Group sessions are good opportunities to demonstrate and practice using ALDs. Because many of these systems are available, the hearing aid user might become overwhelmed when investigating them without assistance. Adults often find benefit from infrared systems, which are used in connection with their televisions. These systems increase the intensity of the sound to the listener without requiring the television volume to be increased. Individuals also benefit from ALDs available at public theaters. The Americans with Disabilities Act (1990) requires public theaters to have ALDs available. The FM system is most commonly used in these settings. Group sessions increase the awareness of these systems and teach participants how to use them.

Empowerment

The aural rehabilitation group is one way to empower individuals with hearing losses. These sessions might be held during one afternoon or occur one evening a week. Although aural rehabilitation groups are important in the rehabilitation process, the individual might need some extra assistance. For example, individuals with severe hearing impairment might require individual sessions to work on monitoring articulation, nasality, or vocal intensity. These individual sessions would also be helpful for adults who have recently obtained a cochlear implant.

SUMMARY

Audiologic habilitation and rehabilitation services are critical to effective communication for individuals with hearing impairments. These services can be divided into two areas: amplification devices and communication strategies. Amplification devices include hearing aids, tactile aids, cochlear implants, and ALDs, which assist individuals to hear. Communication strategies teach individuals how to decrease the obstacles resulting from a hearing loss. Although devices and counseling are quite different, both are necessary to empower individuals with hearing impairments. Most important, audiologists should make sure that individuals with hearing impairment and the significant people in their lives play an active role in decision-making processes.

BOX 15-7 Personal Story

As a student clinician, I often had the opportunity to complete a hearing evaluation and subsequent hearing aid fitting on elderly patients. I was always amazed at the range of reception and acceptance of hearing aids, from very negative to very positive. It was also evident that isolation was the most common and most painful effect of hearing loss that my patients were experiencing, especially with regards to their immediate family and caregivers.

One very elderly gentleman will forever motivate me to encourage people with hearing loss, or those with family members who have hearing loss, to explore the benefits of amplification. I refer to my elderly gentleman patient as Sam, and his caregiver as Joe. Both names are fictitious. Sam was from a nearby nursing home and Joe had escorted Sam, who was in a wheelchair, to our clinic to be fitted with just one hearing aid. I happened to pass through the waiting room on my way to see another patient, and I overheard Sam say quietly as he looked down at the floor, "I don't know where I am and I don't know why I am here." He was not talking to Joe or anyone specifically. I thought that must be the saddest and most vulnerable feeling a person could experience.

Joe wheeled Sam back to the audiologic suites, and we talked at length to Joe with respect to hearing aid fitting, care, and so forth. Sam never looked up and neither did he participate in the conversation. As I placed the hearing aid on Sam's ear, there was no immediate reaction in response to my inserting the earmold into his ear canal and the BTE behind his ear. He still continued to look quietly at the floor. As I turned the hearing aid on, I instructed Joe on where to set the volume control wheel. As I turned the volume up, Joe was saying that he was hoping that Sam's new hearing aid would benefit him. At the sound of Joe's voice, Sam's face changed from sullen, with no emotion, to bright and smiling and he looked up for the first time and said, "Hey, Joe, how are you doing!" as though he had not seen Joe in years. We all choked back tears as Sam and Joe became reacquainted while I completed the hearing aid fitting process. Sam went on to very successful hearing aid use.

Hearing loss can result in the isolation of people of any age, but most tragically it affects the very young and the very old because of their dependency on others for their well-being. For these individuals, amplification can not only be a benefit, but can be life changing.

STUDY QUESTIONS

1. Hearing aids have decreased in size because of what developments?

2. What is signal-to-noise ratio?

3. Name the circuit in a hearing aid that is useful in talking on the telephone.

4. List the electroacoustic properties of hearing aids.

5. What is acoustic feedback in hearing aids and how can it be reduced?

6. What is a vibrotactile aid?

7. What are the responsibilities of educational audiologists in a school setting?

8. List some forms of manual communication.

9. List the different types of hearing aids.

10. Who are candidates for cochlear implants?

KEY TERMS

Alerting devices
Assistive listening device (ALD)
Audiologic habilitation
Audiologic rehabilitation
Cochlear implant
Detection

Discrimination
Earmold
Functional gain
Gain
Identification

Output
Real-ear gain
Reverberation time
Signal-to-noise ratio (SNR)
Telecoil switch (t-switch)

REFERENCES

Americans with Disabilities Act of 1990. (Public Law 101-336). USC Sec. 12101.

Crandell, C. C., & Smaldino, J. J. (1995). Classroom acoustics. In R. J. Roeser & M. P. Downs (Eds.), *Auditory disorders in school children* (3rd ed., pp. 217–234). New York: Thieme.

SUGGESTED READINGS

Alpiner, J. G., & McCarthy, P. A. (Eds.). (2000). *Rehabilitative audiology* (3rd ed.). Baltimore, MD: Williams & Wilkins.

Clark, J. G., & English, K. E. (2004). *Audiologic counseling: Helping patients and families adjust to hearing loss.* Boston: Allyn & Bacon.

Dillon, H. (2001). *Hearing aids.* New York: Thieme.

Roeser, R. J., & Downs, M. P. (1995). *Auditory disorders in school children* (3rd ed.). New York: Thieme.

Ross, M. (Ed.). (1992). *FM auditory training systems: Characteristics, selection, and use.* Timonium, MD: York Press.

Sanders, D. A. (1993). *Management of hearing handicap: Infants to elderly* (3rd ed.). Englewood Cliffs, NJ: Prentice Hall.

Sandlin, R. E. (2000). *Textbook of hearing aid amplification: Technical and clinical considerations* (2nd ed.). San Diego, CA: Singular.

Show, R. L., & Nerbonne, M. A. (1996). *Introduction to audiologic rehabilitation* (3rd ed.). Boston: Allyn & Bacon.

Tye-Murry, N. (1998). *Foundations of aural rehabilitation: Children, adults, and their family members.* San Diego, CA: Singular.

Tyler, R. S. (Ed.). (1993). *Cochlear implants: Audiological foundations.* San Diego, CA: Singular.

Wayner, D. S., & Abrahamson, J. E. (1996). *Learning to hear again: An audiologic rehabilitation curriculum guide.* Austin, TX: Hear Again.

chapter sixteen

sixteen

The Habilitation of Children With Severe to Profound Hearing Loss

MARK E. BERNSTEIN

LEARNING OBJECTIVES

1. To understand and describe the possible developmental consequences of prelinguistic severe to profound deafness.

2. To differentiate communication development in deaf children who have parents who are deaf from those with parents who have normal hearing.

3. To learn about speech and language development in children with hearing impairments.

4. To learn about the communication options available for children with hearing impairments, including the use of speech, listening, writing, and sign communication.

5. To understand and describe the concept of "bilingual-bicultural" education for children who are deaf.

6. To learn about approaches to assessment and intervention in speech and language for children with hearing impairments.

Sally always sits in the front of her second-grade classroom and watches the teacher intently. Her hearing aids are barely visible beneath her hair, and almost no one in the class pays attention to them. Sally is just one of the kids. When the boy next to her starts a conversation with their neighbor, she turns to him and says, "Shush, it's hard for me to listen!"

David watches his algebra teacher demonstrate how to work an equation on the board. The teacher never utters a word; his hands do the communicating, showing how to move elements of the fractions and group them. David isn't sure about something, so he raises his hand, and in the spatial eloquence of the sign language he learned growing up, asks his question.

Wendy sits near the front of Ms. Smith's classroom, her gaze following Julie, the Signed English interpreter. Julie converts Ms. Smith's spoken words into manual gestures so that Wendy can listen to Ms. Smith and also "see" her words. Wendy and Julie have become close because Julie accompanies Wendy throughout the school day.

Ricky stands up in front of the class and takes the microphone proffered by his teacher. He reads his poem to his classmates, and they watch closely and listen carefully through the miniature radio receivers that pick up Ricky's speech. Ricky's speech is somewhat strange sounding, but intelligible. His deaf classmates watch his face, "read" his lips, listen to his voice, and enjoy the poem.

Katie's teacher accompanies her speech with manual signs as she discusses the types of birds found in the nearby park. Katie has a question about blue jays, so she, too, uses her speech and signs. Her five other classmates are also deaf and use sign and speech simultaneously in the classroom. At play in her neighborhood, Katie mostly talks with her friends; in the school cafeteria she will sign with her classmates. If her friend Jan, who hears normally, comes over, she'll start to talk, too.

The previous examples depict a few children in school with hearing impairment. The life experiences of such children vary tremendously, as do their educational experiences. This chapter explores the relationship between serious hearing impairment and a child's development and education and introduces the range of possibilities for educational intervention. Despite a long history of striving, educators are still challenged to provide a completely effective education for all children with hearing impairment.

As noted in Chapter 14, there is tremendous variation in type and degree of hearing impairment. Many children with mild to severe hearing impairment benefit greatly from personal amplification systems such as conventional hearing aids. With a modicum of special attention, these children can function socially and educationally essentially as if they have normal hearing. This is true primarily for children whose hearing impairment was detected early (within the first 2 years or so) or whose hearing loss occurred after the development of speech and language. Such a child might be like Sally, who must sit near the teacher, and must listen very carefully, but who otherwise differs little from her peers with normal hearing.

This chapter focuses on children like David, Wendy, Ricky, and Katie, whose hearing impairment has a much greater impact on their lives and who present the biggest challenge to educators, audiologists, and speech-language pathologists (SLPs). These children have severe to profound hearing losses, typically of a sensory/neural nature.

This is not to suggest that children with less severe hearing losses require little or no intervention. On the contrary, such children (and their families) may require a fair amount of attention, especially with regard to management of hearing aids, speech training, and the like, to ensure optimum growth and development. Most of these children's needs will be met by the procedures discussed in Chapter 15. But severe to profound hearing loss typically represents a quantum leap in developmental consequences and professional intervention, and children with such losses are those most typically served in special education programs for the "deaf" or "auditorily impaired." In this chapter, such children are referred to as "deaf" with the caveat that these children represent a variety of hearing levels and communication abilities.

This chapter takes up, in turn, the impact of deafness on a child's development and family; communication choices; and assessment and intervention, including speech, language, and literacy development. The habilitation of most deaf children is by no means a simple matter.

HEARING IMPAIRMENT AND DEVELOPMENT

Hearing loss is one of the most common disabilities in young children that can impede the development of spoken language. It is for this reason that early detection of hearing impairment in newborns is of paramount importance.

Communication Development

When asked whether they would choose to be been born deaf or blind (not that they have this choice!), most people would respond that they would rather be born deaf. People find it difficult to imagine life without sight, unable to read, to drive, and so on.

But those familiar with deaf children might disagree sharply, for the primary consequence of prelinguistic deafness is that it prevents the normal, spontaneous acquisition of speech and language skills in the early childhood years, the so-called **critical period** for language acquisition. It is not hard to imagine how this might affect a child's growth, development, and socialization.

It is generally accepted that more than 90% of deaf children are born to parents who have normal hearing (the remaining children are born into families in which at least one parent is deaf; these children are discussed later in this chapter). Prelinguistic deafness is a relatively low incidence condition (various estimates put it at no more than 2 to 3 per thousand children). Although many cases are caught by the growing use of newborn screenings, a significant number of babies may pass the screening but, unknown to the parents, acquire a serious hearing impairment later. As a result, the assumption is usually made that an infant has normal hearing, and parents do not worry about it until given some reason to do so. This is made easier, of course, by the fact that in most ways, infants who are deaf act no differently from those who have normal hearing. Although it is true that they may not respond appropriately to environmental sounds (or voices), this may not be readily apparent to hearing parents who have no reason to suspect a problem with their child's hearing.

It might not be until the child is 12 to 18 months old that many hearing parents would even suspect a problem, usually because most children with normal hearing begin to use recognizable words at this time, but the child with a significant hearing loss will not. There may in fact be a protracted period of parental suspicion, and then perhaps some denial ("He's just a late talker"), and then only belatedly a hearing assessment and diagnosis. It is not unusual for a deaf child to be as much as 2 to 3 years of age upon diagnosis.

This, of course, is highly significant because until that time the deaf child of hearing parents typically has had only minimal (if any) stimulation of the speech and language components of his or her cognitive system (see Chapter 2). Parents and others in the child's environment may interact with the child; they may talk with him or her. But little or no language-related input actually "gets into" the child's system because the child cannot hear it; in effect, throughout much of the critical period for language and speech acquisition, the system lies essentially dormant. It simply does not receive the "linguistic data" that are required for it to undergo normal development. A child in this situation, if left untreated, may end up with profound delay and deviance in language and speech acquisition to the extent that there is effectively no functional communication method other than idiosyncratic gesture for basic needs, if that. This may result in profound consequences for social and academic development because an effective communication system in the early years provides a critical foundation for both (see Schirmer, 2001, for a thorough review). The key to intervention with deaf children, then, is to establish, as early as possible, a functional communication system for the child and the parents.

Components of Communication Systems Used With Deaf Children

Approaches to communication with deaf children can be distinguished by the extent to which the emphasis is placed on **audition** and speech or on the use of **manual systems** for communication. In most cases, there is general agreement that it is highly desirable to attempt to optimize the child's use of **residual hearing**.

Use of Hearing

The primary goal of any communication intervention is to help the child gain access to linguistic (and other) "data" so that the child's own cognitive system can go to work.

For many children, this involves the use of modern technologies such as hearing aids, wireless frequency modulated assistive listening systems, and cochlear implants. These are more fully described in Chapter 15. Tremendous strides have been made in the technology of assistive listening devices in recent years, enabling many children (particularly those with considerable residual hearing) to function quite well by relying on their hearing alone.

Oral-Auditory Methods

The use of residual hearing is the cornerstone of the group of communication approaches known collectively as the **oral method**. Within this general group, some advocates emphasize the use of listening skills almost exclusively (hence the term *oral-auditory*), while others encourage children to follow the speaker's facial and mouth movements as well (now termed **speechreading**, an update of the older term *lip-reading*). Regardless of their relative emphasis on audition, all oral approaches incorporate intensive speech training and rely exclusively on oral speech for all communication with deaf children.

Oralism, as it is sometimes called, has been deemed a philosophy rather than merely a method of communicating with deaf children (see Mulholland, 1981). The idea is that because this is a world of hearing people, it is critical for deaf children to learn to communicate using the methods used by virtually all others, namely, the spoken language of the culture. Oral advocates do not accept the use of sign language, believing that it perpetuates a separate subculture of deaf people and inhibits the deaf person's success in the "hearing world." Further, oral proponents believe that the use of sign language in any form will interfere with the child's development of speech and listening skills; because signing is seen as "easier" for the child, the fear is that the child will take the easy road when communicating and not work hard enough at the mastery of speech. The oral approach maintains that although it is quite difficult, most deaf children can develop functional speech and listening skills, if given appropriate support and consistency of teaching. If provided appropriate intervention, it is said, deaf children can "catch up" linguistically, socially, and academically. In this view, there is no *need* for sign language for most deaf children, and the overall goal would be integration into the mainstream "hearing" society, having overcome the barrier posed by the hearing impairment.

This approach to communication with deaf children, understandably quite attractive to many hearing parents, has been in existence for many hundreds of years and has indeed been successful for a number of children (e.g., young Ricky from earlier in the chapter). Clearly, the success of oral methods is directly correlated with, among other things, the amount and quality of residual hearing.

One enhancement to oral methods, with a small but devoted following, is the use of **Cued Speech** (Cornett & Daisey, 1992). Cued Speech uses a system of hand gestures that are displayed near the face (see CD-ROM segment Ch.16.01). These gestures serve to distinguish (cue) phonemic distinctions that would otherwise be difficult or impossible to perceive by reading a speaker's lip movements (*m*an vs. *p*an).

As of this writing, oral methods are in use in numerous day classes in public schools around the United States and in several well-known private schools. There has been renewed interest in oralism with the growing use of cochlear implants in children.

BOX 16-1 Cued Speech and Oral Communication Techniques

CD-ROM segment Ch.16.01 is a demonstration of Cued Speech and oral communication techniques. Note how the cueing is coordinated with the speech; the user of Cued Speech must be highly aware of the phonemic structure of the words being uttered. Cueing must be performed in accompaniment to speech; it cannot be done in isolation. Cues themselves carry no meaning; what they do is signal (cue) which phoneme is being produced as it is said. A single gesture, however, is used to cue the presence of more than one phoneme. Which one depends on which particular lip configuration the cue is paired with.

Speech Development

The use of residual hearing is often not sufficient for speech development to occur spontaneously, so additional intervention is typically necessary. The most widely used approach to speech development is the method developed by Ling (1976, 1989). Ling outlines a sequence of developmental steps in the acquisition of specific speech skills, working from the bases of vocalization through the production of consonant clusters, in a highly specific developmental hierarchy that uses primarily drill and practice skill development through the use of isolated nonmeaningful syllables (combinations of target sounds with those already acquired). Ling's approach is relatively easy to use and is spelled out clearly in his books. Research in the area of speech development of deaf children is notoriously difficult to do well, and despite more than 25 years of practice, it is unclear whether the Ling approach is significantly more effective than any other.

Alternative approaches to speech development are more holistic or top-down in nature, with the goal being to stimulate the child's own speech development system (the lack of hearing does not automatically mean that the child has no intrinsic cognitive system devoted to speech development). One influential example of such an approach would be that of Calvert and Silverman (1983), in which the primary method for early speech development work is the provision of a rich interactive communication environment to stimulate the child's own system. Calvert and Silverman also offer a

BOX 16-2   The Ling Method

As CD-ROM segment Ch.16.04 demonstrates, the Ling method focuses on the child's development of individual phonemes in isolated syllables, working toward fluency by extensive practice producing the target in single syllables, repeated syllables, and in syllables alternated with another target. Ling claims that mastery at this, the "phonetic" level, will lead, with relatively little direct instruction, to the use of the speech skill in communicative speech (the "phonological" level).

BOX 16-3   Conversational Interaction

Quite different from the Ling (1976, 1989) approach to speech development is the method proposed by Calvert and Silverman (1983), which suggests that speech development is best achieved through extensive meaningful conversational interaction based on the child's interests, rather than in exercises involving isolated syllables. Note in Segment Ch.16.05 how the clinician focuses the communication interaction in such a way as to engage the child's interest and how she makes sure the child is able to receive the input both auditorily and visually. Approaches such as this use a multisensory approach and attempt to ensure that speech development work takes place only in meaningful contexts.

somewhat more structured component in their approach, to be used with children for whom the general stimulation approach does not seem to be as effective as it should be. This multisensory syllable unit approach, though, is still grounded in communicative interaction, in that the syllables used for specific intervention and practice are derived directly from words the child is using (or attempting to use).

English Language Development

The relatively few deaf children who grow up with deaf parents who use **American Sign Language (ASL)** acquire that language naturally and spontaneously, much as any child with normal hearing acquires his or her first language. Most deaf children, however, will need intervention to acquire their first language.

Some approaches to language teaching have been highly analytic and structured, such as the Fitzgerald Key (Fitzgerald, 1929; still in use in some programs), and the Rhode Island method (Blackwell, Engen, Fischgrund, & Zarcadoolas, 1978). Other approaches are devoted to providing a rich interactive communication environment for the child in which his or her natural language development system may be activated and do much of the work on its own. Obviously, for any such effort to succeed, a fully effective communication system must be in use, whether oral, signed, or in some combination. Easterbrooks and Baker (2002), Stewart and Kluwin (2001), and Paul (2009) present comprehensive reviews of language teaching strategies.

Sign Language and Sign Systems

For as long as there have been partisans of oral approaches, there have also been those who have challenged the oral philosophy by advocating the use of manual communication with deaf children (see Moores [1987] for a historical review). These approaches generally fall into two major categories: those that use one or another form of **manual codes** for English, usually performed simultaneously with spoken English, and those advocating the use of ASL (usually as part of an overall **bilingual-bicultural** philosophy, to be examined shortly).

The basic premise of any of the manually oriented approaches is that the oralists' insistence on the exclusive use of speech is not effective for most deaf children with severe to profound hearing losses and is simply inappropriate for most such children. Rather than attempt to communicate with (and educate) deaf children using their "weakest" channels (hearing and speech), the idea would be to use the modes that are (for most deaf children) readily accessible and quite effective, that is, vision and manual gestures.

Total Communication

Total Communication (see Schlesinger, 1986) became fairly widespread in the early 1970s because of concerns that for many children oral methods do not provide sufficient information in usable form for the child's system to develop adequately.

The basic idea of the most common form of Total Communication is to encourage parents, teachers, and children to use whatever communication method works best.

This would include the use of oral modes, ASL if appropriate, and most important, manual forms of English. The core idea behind manually coded English is to simultaneously *supplement* the information provided in the auditory-speech channel with a redundantly coded version of the same information in the manual-visual channel. This is accomplished by the use of one or another system of "signed" English (or whatever the language of the culture) in which manual signs are produced for each morpheme of the spoken utterances. The specific signs used in most systems are based to some extent on the sign vocabulary of ASL, although the signs are placed in English word order because they accompany English.

Proponents of Total Communication suggest that parents can learn fairly quickly to pair sign gestures with their speech and can use this as a means for multisensory production–reception of English. The deaf child would be provided with a more adequate input and output because of the multichannel redundancy and thus would have several avenues for stimulation of his or her language and speech learning centers. As in oralism, English would be the language the child is exposed to and developing, which has obvious facilitative value for literacy development. In Total Communication, audition and speech are very much part of the communication mix; the use of sign does not replace oral modes as much as it supplements them in a kind of partnership. As many as 90% of the severe to profoundly deaf children in the United States are educated in Total Communication programs (*American Annals of the Deaf*, 1998).

American Sign Language and Bilingual-Bicultural Programs

Since the early 1990s, interest has been growing, particularly in residential schools for the deaf, in what is generically known as bilingual-bicultural approaches to communication and education of deaf children. These philosophies typically involve either an ASL first, English as a second language approach, or a more concurrent bilingualism approach utilizing both ASL and English.

ASL is a manual-visual language utilizing gestures created by the hands, face, head, and body to communicate. ASL is a natural language that, in its general form, appears

---

BOX 16-4 Signing Exact English

Signing Exact English (SEE II) is perhaps the most widely used of the "exact" systems for representing English manually. In SEE II, as in all such techniques, the communicator is required to produce a manual sign for each English morpheme that is spoken, while maintaining normal speech speed and rhythm. Segment Ch.16.02 presents an experienced user of SEE II communicating material that might be found in a high school class of students who are deaf. Notice how there may be numerous gestures accompanying a relatively short English word. Why does this happen? What might be some of the difficulties encountered in trying to use SEE II in some communication situations?

to have evolved from a combination of French Sign Language and an indigenous sign language used by deaf people in the United States at the beginning of the 19th century.

The grammar of ASL is quite unlike that of English, making effective use of the three-dimensional space in which it is created, particularly in case assignment and complex verb inflection processes (see CD-ROM segment Ch.16.03). It is not possible to sign ASL simultaneously with English speech because of the vast differences between the grammars. (To sign along with speech, an individual can use ASL *signs* for English lexical items, but not the grammar.)

Critical to the bilingual-bicultural philosophy is the firm belief that it is important for most deaf children to develop a first language that is best suited to their sensory capabilities (i.e., one that uses the visual-manual modality), coupled with the belief that it is crucial that this signed language be a "natural" sign language (such as ASL) rather than one of the artificial manual coding systems for English used in Total Communication. In addition, proponents of the bilingual-bicultural philosophy explicitly acknowledge the likelihood that the child will eventually become a fully actuated Deaf adult, that is, one who is a member of the Deaf community and shares in its language (ASL), culture, and mores. (The capitalization of the first letter in *Deaf* is a convention signifying a reference to the cultural identity, in contrast to the more common use of the term *deaf* in reference to serious hearing loss in the audiologic sense only.)

This *cultural* aspect of the bilingual-bicultural educational philosophy revolves around the recognition that there is a distinct community and culture of Deaf people within a larger society in which the vast majority of people have normal speech and hearing skills. Descriptions of this community and its culture have emerged in recent years (see, for example, Lane, Hoffmeister, & Bahan, 1996; Padden & Humphries, 1988, 2005). Central to Deaf culture and community is the idea that deafness should not be viewed as a "defect" or pathology, but rather, as a *difference* (some have deemed it akin to ethnicity). In this view, to be Deaf is to have a personal identity *as a Deaf person*, not as a person with impaired hearing. It is less a matter of one's actual level of hearing (in audiologic terms) than it is the belief system and behaviors one demonstrates. "Being" Deaf includes the use of ASL for most daily communication; extensive

BOX 16-5   American Sign Language

CD-ROM segment Ch.16.03 demonstrates the way ASL grammar utilizes the three-dimensional space in which the articulators (hands, arms, body, face, head) operate to produce grammatical utterances. The signer locates points in space (called "index points" by sign language linguists) that serve as pronouns. Verbs can be inflected for direction, number, and other features through changes of direction or modification of the hand shapes used to form the sign utterances. In the early stages of sign language linguistics, researchers had a difficult time figuring out what to even look for because the grammar of ASL is so different from that of English or other languages that have been studied extensively.

social networking with other Deaf individuals; and shared patterns of beliefs, values, and rules for social interaction. It has been suggested that there is a characteristic Deaf worldview (although it would be prudent to be cautious about the stark "either-or" character of some of the descriptions). One major aim of bilingual-bicultural education of deaf children, then, is to help them to learn about and participate in this special community and culture.

The keystone of any bilingual-bicultural program is the early and consistent use of ASL as a medium of communication with the child (and for all academic instruction, once the child gets to school), keeping it separate from the use of English. Some bilingual-bicultural advocates reject outright the notion that a deaf child should develop oral speech skills, while others disagree. In one influential version of the ESL approach (Johnson, Liddell, & Erting, 1989), there is no attempt to use English "through the air" at all; face-to-face communication takes place only in ASL, and English instruction is provided solely in the form of reading and writing, and only once the child has mastered the "first" language (ASL), say, around the age of 6 or 7 years. Other, more concurrent approaches allow for natural code switching, using both ASL and English (in simultaneous manually coded form as well as print).

Bilingual-bicultural methodology is still so new that there is little evidence bearing on its effectiveness. Unfortunately, many programs have been started but without much attention to efficacy research, so it is difficult to tell what, if any, long-term educational impact this approach may have.

The Future of Communication With Deaf Children

Recently, some have advocated the goal of **multimodalism** (see Paul, 1998, 2009; Stewart & Kluwin, 2001). The objective of such intervention efforts would be to help each child to develop, to the extent possible, skills in both oral and sign communication and full English literacy.

Unfortunately, there is no reliable way to tell which approach is best for any particular child. This can lead to some real problems. For example, some educators advocate starting all children off using oral methods only, in the hopes that the children will respond well and not require the use of manual communication. But what of those for whom it doesn't work well? These children will have lost valuable time during the critical period, and it may not be possible to make up that deficit. On the other hand, the more radical proponents of bilingual-bicultural approaches tend to alienate those—including the vast majority of parents—who do see much value in helping deaf children to integrate into the mainstream of society. The middle ground, that is, the use of Total Communication methods including various forms of signed English, tends not to satisfy partisans of both extremes and may represent some compromises that undercut their effectiveness. Andrews, Leigh, and Weiner (2004) present an in-depth discussion of these issues.

Assessment and Team Approaches to Intervention

This chapter would not be complete without a consideration of assessment of communicative functioning, which is best carried out in a collaborative team approach. As discussed, the habilitation of a deaf child is a multidimensional challenge; it is imperative that there be close cooperation among the audiologist, SLP, teacher, and parents, in addition to such professionals as counselors, occupational and physical therapists, and others as required.

The audiologist is the individual most responsible for management of the child's use of his or her hearing, from assessment of residual hearing and fitting of hearing aids, to consultation with regular school personnel on optimizing the acoustic environment. The SLP may take primary responsibility for assessment of the child's speech and language development. Depending on the academic setting, the SLP may take the lead role in development activities (often, if the child is in a mainstream setting) or will work closely with the classroom teacher of the deaf in jointly implementing an approach to speech and language development.

The use of standard speech and language assessment instruments, for example, must be considered quite carefully because deaf children's developmental ages often lag considerably behind their chronological ages. Some speech assessment instruments are simply unsuitable for children with limited vocabularies and/or relatively unintelligible speech, often found among deaf students. Some of the approaches used in assessment of individuals with different cultural backgrounds have been found useful.

Among the standard tests, many have found the various levels of the Grammatical Analysis of Elicited Language (Moog & Geers, 1985) to be valuable. Other approaches to language assessment are presented in Easterbrooks and Baker (2002). In the speech domain, it may be useful to go beyond such commonly used instruments as Ling's (1976) phonetic and phonological analyses of deaf children's speech. Standard articulation testing (e.g., Goldman & Fristoe, 1986), phonological process analysis (e.g., Hodson, 1986), and intelligibility (Monsen, 1981) and suprasegmental measures (Subtelny, Orlando, & Whitehead, 1981) can be combined with the information provided by Ling's instruments to provide a full picture of the child's emerging speech capabilities.

SUMMARY

Serious hearing impairment can have a profound impact on the early development of deaf children. Prevention of negative consequences depends in large part on the establishment of an effective communication system as early as possible. This chapter discusses several major approaches to communication with deaf children, including oral and manual methods. Regardless of the communication method chosen, issues involved in speech and language development are discussed in terms of their relation to the child's naturally operating system.

There is no question that great strides have been made in habilitation and education of deaf children over the years, but there is still quite a bit of work to be done. It is incumbent on all communication disorders professionals to work closely with parents in as professional and empathetic a manner as possible to help them make the choices that are most appropriate for their individual children.

BOX 16-6 Personal Story

Nothing quite prepared me for my first day as a teacher with a class of 6 second-graders in a day school for the deaf in a large city on the East Coast in 1972. I had just completed my master's degree training as a teacher of the deaf, steeped in state-of-the-art oral methods, and I was eager to put my skills to work with that inimitable mixture of enthusiasm and trepidation of the new teacher.

Things got off to a very bad start, as my attempts to break the ice with some conversation met with blank stares. My students, all profoundly deaf, had virtually no oral skills. They could neither understand me nor make themselves understood. To this day I have no idea how their previous teacher managed. To make matters more difficult, the students were not familiar with the techniques I had learned to model and elicit speech and language. I'll never forget the look on one child's face that said, eloquently, "Why are you holding that microphone in front of my mouth?"

These children were unfortunately textbook examples of what can happen to profoundly deaf children if they receive little or no intervention and support in their early childhood years. Late diagnosed, with families that had not benefited from counseling and training in how to communicate with their child and foster their development, these children, almost to a one, were grossly delayed in their speech and language development, and consequently, cognitively and educationally severely at risk. They communicated with each other in a mixture of American Sign Language and homegrown signs, but that was about it.

Somehow we muddled through, but not particularly effectively, until the school developed a pilot Total Communication program. The additional channel of the sign gestures helped greatly, and we saw a blossoming of the students' communication and literacy skills over the next few years, although for none of them was speech ever a particularly useful modality. And all of these children remained behind academically, and never really caught up fully.

If these children were in school today, it is likely that they would be much more successful, whether using oral-only, Total Communication, or bilingual-bicultural approaches—because of the early intervention programs now in place, and the advances in technology over the past decades. What I draw from this episode is a vivid reminder of the importance of early communication intervention with deaf children.

STUDY QUESTIONS

1. What are the primary consequences of prelinguistic deafness if left "untreated"?

2. Explain the ways in which prelinguistic deafness affects the parent–child relationship.

3. What are some of the differences between deaf children who have deaf parents and those with normal-hearing parents? What would be the key educational consequences of these differences?

4. Why do deaf children still require special intervention for speech and language development despite the great advances in amplification system technology over the past few decades?

5. Compare and contrast the oral and Total Communication approaches to communication development with deaf children. On what factors might one base a decision to follow one path or the other with a particular child?

6. What is the relationship between bilingual-bicultural approaches and other communication philosophies used in deaf education?

7. What are some of the special considerations for assessment of deaf children's speech and language?

KEY TERMS

American Sign Language (ASL)
Audition
Bilingual-bicultural

Critical period
Cued Speech Manual codes, manual systems
Multimodalism

Oral method Residual hearing
Speechreading
Total Communication

REFERENCES

American Annals of the Deaf. (1998). Reference Issue. *143*, 2.

Andrews, J. F., Leigh, I. W., & Weiner, M. T. (2004). *Deaf people: Evolving perspectives from psychology, education, and sociology*. Boston: Pearson.

Blackwell, P., Engen, E., Fischgrund, J., & Zarcadoolas, C. (1978). *Sentences and other systems*. Washington, DC: Alexander Graham Bell Association for the Deaf.

Calvert, D., & Silverman, S. R. (1983). *Speech and deafness* (2nd ed.). Washington, DC: Alexander Graham Bell Association for the Deaf.

Cornett, R. O., & Daisey, M. E. (1992). *The Cued Speech resource book*. Raleigh, NC: National Cued Speech Association.

Easterbrooks, S. R., & Baker, S. (2002). *Language learning in children who are deaf and hard of hearing*. Boston: Allyn & Bacon.

Fitzgerald, E. (1929). *Straight language for the deaf*. Staunton, VA: McClure.

Goldman, R., & Fristoe, M. (1986). *Goldman-Fristoe Test of Articulation*. Circle Pines, MN: American Guidance Service.

Hodson, B. (1986). *Assessment of Phonological Processes—Revised*. Austin, TX: Pro-Ed.

Johnson, R., Liddell, S., & Erting, C. (1989). *Unlocking the curriculum: Principles for achieving access in deaf education.* Washington, DC: Gallaudet Research Institute Working Paper.

Lane, H., Hoffmeister, R., & Bahan, B. (1996). *Journey into the deaf-world.* San Diego, CA: Dawn-Sign Press.

Ling, D. (1976). *Speech and the hearing impaired child.* Washington, DC: Alexander Graham Bell Association for the Deaf.

Ling, D. (1989). *Foundations of spoken language for hearing-impaired children.* Washington, DC: Alexander Graham Bell Association for the Deaf.

Monsen, R. (1981). A usable test for the speech intelligibility of deaf talkers. *American Annals of the Deaf, 126*(7), 845–852.

Moog, J., & Geers, A. (1985). *Grammatical analysis of elicited language.* St. Louis, MO: Central Institute for the Deaf.

Moores, D. F. (1987). *Educating the deaf* (3rd ed.). Boston: Houghton Mifflin.

Mulholland, A. (Ed.). (1981). *Oral education today and tomorrow.* Washington, DC: Alexander Graham Bell Association for the Deaf.

Padden, C., & Humphries, T. (1988). *Deaf in America: Voices from a culture.* Cambridge, MA: Harvard University Press.

Padden, C., & Humphries, T. (2005). *Inside Deaf culture.* Cambridge, MA: Harvard University Press.

Paul, P. V. (1998). *Literacy and deafness.* Boston: Allyn & Bacon.

Paul, P. V. (2009). *Language and deafness* (4th ed.). Sudbury, MA: Jones and Bartlett.

Schirmer, B. R. (2001). *Psychological, social, and educational dimensions of deafness.* Boston: Allyn & Bacon.

Schlesinger, H. (1986). Total communication in perspective. In D. Luterman (Ed.), *Deafness in perspective.* San Diego, CA: College-Hill Press.

Stewart, D. A., & Kluwin, T. N. (2001). *Teaching deaf and hard of hearing students.* Boston: Allyn & Bacon.

Subtelny, J., Orlando, N., & Whitehead, R. (1981). *Speech and voice characteristics of the deaf.* Washington, DC: Alexander Graham Bell Association for the Deaf.

SUGGESTED READINGS

Luetke-Stahlman, B., & Luckner, J. (1991). *Effectively educating students with hearing impairments.* New York: Longman.

Luterman, D. (1987). *Deafness in the family.* Boston: College-Hill Press.

Moores, D. F., & Martin, D. S. (Eds.). (2006). *Deaf learners: Developments in curriculum and instruction.* Boston: Houghton Mifflin.

Ross, M. (Ed.). (1990). *Hearing-impaired children in the mainstream.* Parkton, MD: York Press.

Yoshinaga-Itano, C. (1999). *Language development of deaf and hard of hearing children.* San Diego, CA: Singular.

Glossary

Abduction Vocal fold movement away from each other.

Accent A particular nonnative stress on syllables in words, which connotes the influence of a second language.

Accreditation A procedure that recognizes educational institutions or facilities providing services to the public as maintaining and conforming to necessary standards.

Acculturation The process of learning a second culture.

Acoustic neuroma A tumor arising on the auditory (eighth cranial) nerve.

Acoustic reflex The contraction of the middle ear muscles in response to an intense sound. The contraction limits the amount of sound energy passing through the middle ear, thus protecting the delicate structures in the inner ear.

Acquired (or neurogenic) stuttering Stuttering that typically occurs suddenly in adulthood after trauma to the brain.

Acquired disorders Disorders that occur after speech and language skills have been acquired.

Action potential A brief electrical voltage generated by a neuron, typically following stimulation.

Adaptation The percentage of decrease in stuttering when a passage is read multiple times in succession. The percentage of reduction is calculated for each repeated reading.

Adduction Movement toward the midline; vocal fold movement toward each other.

Afferent Axonal fibers that conduct impulses toward the central nervous system; nerve impulses carried from the periphery to the brain.

Agrammatism Language characterized by predominance of content words (nouns, verbs) and absence of functors (articles, prepositions); characteristic of Broca's aphasia.

Air conduction The pathway of sounds that includes the outer ear, middle ear, inner ear, and the structures beyond.

Air–bone gap (ABG) The difference, in decibels, between the air-conduction threshold and the bone-conduction threshold.

Alerting devices Devices that change auditory alerting signals that are inaudible for individuals with hearing losses into audible-acoustic, visual, or vibrotactile stimuli.

Allophone A variant of a phoneme that does not change meaning.

American Sign Language (ASL) The language of the Deaf community in the United States. ASL has its own set of phonological, morphological, semantic, syntactic, and pragmatic conventions that differ from those of English. It is produced in three-dimensional space by the hands, arms, face, and body, and has a complex grammar quite different from that of English.

Amplitude The distance an object moves from its resting position during vibration.

Aneurysm Bulge in the wall of an artery resulting from weakness.

Anoxia A lack of oxygen.

Aphasia Language disorder affecting phonology, grammar, semantics, and pragmatics as well as reading and writing caused by focal brain damage.

Aphonia Loss of voice.

Articulation The physical ability to produce speech sounds. A speaker needs to be able to manipulate the articulators including the tongue, lips, and velum to produce all of the required place and manner distinctions.

Articulation disorder Difficulty producing speech sounds and speech sound sequences.

Aspiration The presence of food or liquid in the airway below the level of the true vocal folds.

Assistive listening device (ALD) Devices that transfer an acoustic message over distance so that the listener can hear the signal with greater intensity and signal-to-noise ratio.

Ataxia (ataxic) Neuromuscular disorder characterized by errors in the direction, force, and timing of movements resulting from cerebellar damage.

Athetosis (athetoid) Congenital neuromuscular disorder characterized by writhing involuntary movement caused by extrapyramidal tract damage.

Atrophy Withering or wasting away of tissues or organs.

Attempt In an episode, information about the actions that the main character takes to achieve his or her goal.

Audiogram A graph depicting the threshold of audibility (in decibels) as a function of different frequencies.

Audiologic habilitation Amplification, auditory training, and speech-language services provided to children with a hearing loss.

Audiologic rehabilitation Amplification and coping strategies.

Audiometer A device used for the measurement of hearing.

Audition Related to the power of hearing.

Auditory brainstem response (ABR) Measurable responses in the brainstem to a series of acoustic stimuli.

Auditory cortex An area in the temporal lobe of the brain that is responsible for hearing.

Auditory nerve The eighth cranial nerve that carries information from the inner ear to the brain about hearing and balance.

Auditory processing disorder (APD) Difficulty in discriminating speech, often in the presence of background noise, and frequently in the absence of the loss of hearing sensitivity.

Babbling Prespeech vocalizations.

Basal ganglia A group of subcortical structures that include the putamen, globus pallidus, and caudate that contribute to control of motor behavior.

Basic interpersonal communication skills (BICS) Language proficiency at a level that requires low cognitive load in situations that are highly contextualized.

Basilar membrane A ribbon-like tissue in the cochlea that separates scala media (above) from scale tympani (below). It provides the foundation on which rests the organ of Corti.

Bernoulli effect As the velocity of airflow increases, pressure decreases with total energy remaining constant.

Bifid Divided into two parts.

Bilateral Pertaining to two sides.

Bilateral hearing loss Hearing loss in both the right and the left ears.

Bilingual Use and comprehension of two languages; speakers with some competence speaking one or more secondary languages, but a different primary language. Level of proficiency in each language may be different across situations, communicative demands, and over time.

Bilingual-bicultural A general term to describe a number of related yet distinct approaches to help deaf children acquire communication facility in both sign language and spoken language, while also helping them to discover their cultural identities in both the hearing and Deaf communities.

Bolus A term used to describe food after it has been chewed and mixed with saliva.

Bone conduction The pathway of sound that bypasses the conductive mechanisms of the outer and middle ears by vibrating the skull and stimulating the cochlea of the inner ear.

Bound morpheme A morpheme that cannot stand alone as a separate word.

Brainstem A portion of the brain containing the midbrain, the pons, and the medulla.

Breathy Vocal production in which the vocal folds do not completely touch each other during vibration, resulting in excess air escaping through the glottis.

Broca's area Brodmann's area 44 located on the third frontal gyrus anterior to the precentral face area. Functions to program speech movements.

Cancellation A speech modification technique in which individuals who stutter are taught to stop as soon as a stuttered word is completed, to pause, and to say the word again in an easy, relaxed manner.

Canonical babbling Around the age of 7 months, infants start to use their voice to make syllable-like strings.

Cerebral hemispheres Two major parts of the cerebrum joined by the corpus callosum.

Cerebrovascular accident (CVA) A stroke. Interruption of blood supply to an area of the brain.

Certificate of Clinical Competence (CCC) A certificate issued by the American Speech-Language-Hearing Association in either speech-language pathology or audiology that affirms the individual has met the minimal standards for practice in the profession.

Certification A procedure by which an individual is affirmed as meeting an educational and professional standard. In speech-language pathology and audiology, certification is administered by the American Speech-Language Hearing Association.

Cerumen A tacky yellow or brown substance secreted by oil glands in the external auditory meatus. This substance is commonly known as earwax.

Chelioplasty Surgical repair of a lip defect.

Child-centered approaches Approaches in which the clinician follows the child's lead with respect to the activities, the topics of discussion, and the toys that are played with.

Chronic stuttering Stuttering that continues into adulthood.

Chronological age The use of years and months (e.g., 2;3 means 2 years, 3 months) to determine a child's age and to compare him or her to other children of the same age.

Chronological age referencing The diagnosis of language disorder is accomplished by comparing a child's language ability to the language abilities that are expected for children his or her chronological age.

Circumlocution A circuitous description of a word that cannot be recalled.

Circumstantial bilingual Someone who becomes bilingual as a result of living in a bilingual environment. May come about because of forced migration or for economic reasons such as traveling to another country to find work.

Classroom collaboration Speech-language pathologists and classroom teachers work together to provide language intervention within the regular classroom setting.

Clinician-centered approaches Approaches in which the clinician controls the intervention context, goals, and materials.

Cluttering A fluency disorder that is characterized by very rapid bursts of disrhythmic, unintelligible speech.

Coarticulation Overlapping of articulatory and acoustic patterns of speech production caused by anticipation or retention of a speech feature.

Cochlea The coiled tube in the inner ear that houses the sensory cells for hearing; a structure in the inner ear that converts the mechanical energy received from the middle ear into an electrochemical code for transmission to the brain.

Cochlear implant A device that is surgically placed in the cochlea and provides auditory stimulation for individuals with severe to profound hearing loss.

Cochlear nucleus A way station in the lower brainstem that communicates with the cochlea via the eighth nerve.

Code switching The alternating use of two languages at the word, phrase, and sentence levels with a complete break between languages in phonology. In African American English (AAE), code switching refers to alternations in intonation, prosody, and specific grammatical features determined by the situational context. More formal settings typically result in "switches" toward Standard American English, and more informal situations typically yield switches toward AAE grammatical and intonational patterns.

Cognitive academic language proficiency (CALP) Language proficiency at a level that requires high cognitive load in situations that are decontextualized.

Commissure A group of neurons that cross the midline, from one side of the brain to the other.

Communication Any exchange of meaning, whether intended or unintended.

Communication differences Communicative abilities that differ from those of other individuals in the same environment in the absence of an impairment.

Communication disorder Sometimes used as a synonym for impairment, and other times as a synonym for disability.

Communication sciences and disorders (CSD) A discipline that consists of two professions (speech-language pathology and audiology). The professions are composed of people who study the nature of communication and communication disorders and who assess and treat individuals with communication disorders.

Communicative demand The expectations of a specific language interaction.

Compensatory articulations Production of a sound utilizing alternative placement of the articulators rather than the usual placement.

Complex sound A sound composed of at least two, but usually many more, frequency components.

Comprehension The ability to understand language (the opposite of expression).

Conductive hearing loss A loss of hearing sensitivity caused by damage to the outer and/or middle ear.

Consequence In a narrative episode, information about the outcomes of the main character's actions in relationship to the initiating event.

Consistency The percentage of stuttered words from the first to the second repeated reading of the same passage.

Consonant cluster Two or more consonants spoken together without an intervening vowel (e.g., *sp*oon, *tr*ee, *bl*ue, *str*ing).

Content Language content refers to the meaning of language (semantics).

Continuing education units (CEUs) Documentation that affirms a professional person has engaged in new learning related to his or her area of practice that is often required for renewal of a license.

Contusions Injuries causes by a blow from a hard object that do not break the skin but do cause hemorrhaging below the skin.

Corpus callosum Fiber pathways joining the cerebral hemispheres.

Criterion-referenced assessment Nonstandardized approaches to assessment that provide descriptive information about tasks children routinely encounter in their environment. Unlike norm-referenced measures, scores on criterion-referenced measures are not compared to the average scores of same-age peers.

Critical period The idea that some biological events (e.g., hemispheric specialization) must occur by a certain time in order for language to develop normally.

Cued Speech A gestural system, unrelated to sign language, used to signal (cue) distinctions among spoken phonemes by use of particular hand configurations and positions that accompany speech. Cued Speech is often accepted as a gestural supplement to oral communication methods with deaf children.

Culture The set of beliefs and assumptions shared by a group of people that guide how individuals in that group think, act, and interact on a daily basis.

Deaf education Deaf educators teaching academic subjects to children and adults with severe to profound hearing impairments.

Decoding The ability to read single words.

Decontextualized language Refers to a language learning environment devoid of significant nonverbal or contextual cues to assist meaning.

Dementia Deterioration of intellectual abilities such as memory, concentration, reasoning, and judgment resulting from organic disease or brain damage. Emotional disturbances and personality changes often accompany the intellectual deterioration.

Detection The ability to hear whether a sound exists; the first level in auditory processing.

Developmental age The child's level of development in a given area, in this case language. The developmental age is the age of most typically developing children at the time their language is similar to the language of the child being tested.

Developmental disorders Speech and language disorders that occur after birth (during childhood).

Developmental language disorder When a child has problems acquiring language even though there is no obvious cause. *See also* Specific language impairment.

Dialect Variation of a language that is understood by all speakers of the "mother" language. May include sound, vocabulary, and grammatical variations.

Diffuse axonal injury Damage to nerve cells in the connecting fibers of the brain.

Diplophonia A "two-toned" voice resulting from simultaneous vibration of two structures with differing vibratory frequencies.

Disability A reduced ability to meet daily living needs.

Discipline A unique field of study that is supplemented by research.

Discrepancy modeling The determination of a learning disability is based on a significant discrepancy between a child's IQ score (a measure of ability) and his or her scores on measures of achievement in the areas of speaking, listening, reading, writing, reasoning, and/or mathematics.

Discrimination The ability to hear differences between sounds; the second level in auditory processing.

Disfluency The flow and ease of speech is disrupted by repetitions, interjections, pauses, and revisions.

Distinctive features A system of the component features of sounds (e.g., +/– continuant, +/– voicing, +/– anterior, etc.) that is used for describing the differences between phonemes in a language.

Distortion A sound is termed "distorted" when the speaker does not achieve the intended articulatory target and the resulting production is not a recognizable phoneme in the child's native language.

Dysarthria Neuromuscular speech disorder.

Dyslexia A language-based disorder characterized by difficulties in decoding words during reading. The child's reading problems usually reflect insufficient phonological processing.

Dysphagia Difficulty in swallowing or an inability to swallow.

Dysphonia Disturbed muscle tone; disturbed phonation

Dyspnea Difficult or labored breathing; a shortness of breath.

Earmold Vinyl or acrylic material that is custom-fit to fill part of the outer ear. A hole in the earmold directs sound from the receiver to the ear canal. When fitted properly, the earmold prevents feedback.

Edema Accumulation of an excessive amount of fluid in cells, tissues, or serous cavities; usually results in a swelling of the tissues.

Efferent Conduction away from a central structure; nerve impulses carried from the brain to the periphery.

Efficacy Research showing that a therapy procedure is helpful.

Eighth nerve The cranial nerve (VIII) devoted to carrying information about hearing and balance to and from the auditory nervous system. The eighth nerve in humans is made up of about 30,000 individual neurons.

Elasticity The property that enables an object to return to its original shape after being deformed.

Elective bilingual Refers to someone who learns a second language by choice.

Embolus A moving clot from another part of the body that may lodge and interrupt the blood supply.

Ending In a narrative episode, the moral of the story or final statements that bring the episode to a close.

Endolymph The fluid found within the membranous labyrinth.

Endoscopy Examination of the interior of a canal or hollow space; the insertion of a flexible scope through the nose to look at the anatomy of the pharynx and to observe the pharynx and larynx before and after swallowing.

Episode A part of a story that consists of an initiating event, attempt, and consequence. Episodes may also contain internal responses, plans, and reactions/endings.

Esophageal speech A laryngeal speech in which the air supply for phonation originates in the upper portion of the esophagus, with the pharyngoesophageal segment functioning as a neoglottis.

Ethics The principles of conduct that govern an individual or a group. The American Speech-Language-Hearing Association has an official code of ethics, and members can be censured or they can lose their membership in the association for ethical violations.

Eustachian tube The canal that connects the middle ear cavity to the back of the throat. The Eustachian tube opens briefly to equalize pressure in the middle ear.

Evidence-based practice Making assessment and treatment decisions by integrating the best research evidence with clinical expertise and patient values.

Expository texts The language of academic textbooks. This type of language is used to teach or explain new information.

Expression The ability to produce language (the opposite of comprehension).

Expressive jargon Babbling in an adult-like intonation pattern. Sequences of syllables sound like statements or questions, but they contain few real words.

External auditory meatus (EAM) The canal that directs sound from the pinna to the tympanic membrane.

Extrapyramidal tract Indirect motor pathway made up of networks of neurons.

Extrinsic laryngeal muscles Muscles originating or acting from outside of the part where they are located.

Family-centered practice Services that incorporate families into the assessment and treatment process. This construct is designed to recognize the importance of connections with family members in communication development.

Fluency Speech that is easy, rhythmical, and evenly flowing.

Fluency disorder Unusual disruptions in the rhythm and rate of speech. These disruptions are often characterized by repetitions or prolongations of sounds or syllables plus excessive tension.

Fluency shaping A therapy approach in which the clinician teaches the person who stutters a new way of talking that is designed to reduce the likelihood of stuttering.

Form The structure of language including syntax, morphology, and phonology.

Formant A resonance of the vocal tract.

Free morpheme A morpheme that can stand alone as a word.

Frequency The number of cycles of vibration completed in 1 second, measured in hertz (Hz).

Functional disorder A disorder with no known physical cause; the cause of difficulties with speech development cannot be determined precisely.

Functional gain The increase in sound intensity provided by a hearing aid (in decibels) calculated by subtracting behavioral thresholds without a hearing aid from behavioral thresholds with a hearing aid.

Fundamental frequency (F0) The lowest frequency (first harmonic) of a complex periodic waveform.

Gain The increase in sound intensity provided by an amplification system and measured in decibels.

Gastric tube (G-tube) A feeding tube that is placed directly into the stomach through an incision in the skin.

Genre A literary style (narration, description, persuasion, mystery, horror, fairy tale, etc.).

Glial cells Support cells of the nervous system.

Glottal stops A plosive sound made by stopping and releasing the breath stream at the level of the glottis; may be a compensatory behavior in the presence of inadequate velopharyngeal closure.

Glottis The opening or space between the vocal folds.

Grammatical patterns Rule-governed organization of words in sentences.

Gyri Folds of the cerebral cortex.

Hair cells The sensory cells of hearing and balance that convert sound energy from one form to another.

Handicap A social, educational, or occupational disadvantage that is related to an impairment or disability. This disadvantage is often affected by the nature of the person's impairment and by the attitudes and biases that may be present in the person's environment.

Harmonic An integer multiple of the fundamental frequency.

Harsh Phonation with excessive muscle tension. The vocal folds are pressed together tightly with a quick release during each cycle of vibration; the walls of the throat are tightened to amplify the high-frequency components of the voice.

Hearing level (HL) The reference that uses normal hearing in the scale of decibels.

Hematoma Encapsulated blood from a broken blood vessel.

Hemiplegia Paralysis or weakness on one side of the body. Typically the side affected is opposite the side of the brain injury.

Hemorrhage Bleeding from a broken artery or vein.

Hoarse Phonation that sounds both harsh and breathy. Hoarseness results from irregular vocal fold vibrations.

Homonymous hemianopsia Loss of vision in part of the visual field caused by brain injury.

Hybrid approaches Hybrid approaches focus on one or two specific language goals. The clinician selects the activities and materials rather than following the child's lead and responds to the child's communication to model and highlight the specific forms that are being targeted for intervention.

Hyperfunction Excessive forcing and straining, usually at the level of the vocal folds, but which may occur at various points along the vocal tract.

Hypernasality Excessively undesirable amount of perceived nasal cavity resonance during phonation.

Hyperreflexia Abnormally increased reflexes resulting from nervous system damage.

Hypertonicity Abnormally increased background activity of a muscle resulting from nervous system damage.

Hypofunction Reduced vocal capacity resulting from prolonged overuse, muscle fatigue, tissue irritation, or general laryngeal or specific problems relating to the opening and closing of the glottis, characterized by air loss and sometimes hoarseness and pitch breaks.

Hyponasal (denasal) Lack of nasal resonance for the three phonemes /m/, /n/, and /ng/ resulting from a partial or complete obstruction in the nasal tract.

Hypotonicity Abnormally decreased background activity of a muscle resulting from nervous system damage.

Identification The ability to associate a sound with a symbolic representation; the third level in auditory processing.

Idiom An expression that can have both a literal and a figurative interpretation (e.g., skating on thin ice).

Immittance Measurement of the impedance of the tympanic membrane or admittance of sound to the middle ear.

Impairment Any loss or abnormality of psychological, physiological, or anatomic structure or function.

Impedance matching A technique that helps energy move from one medium to another with minimal loss. The ossicles in the middle ear perform this function.

Incidence lifetime risk The percentage of individuals in a given population who report that they have, at one time or another, exhibited a particular disorder or condition. Number of individuals who experience a disorder during their lifetime.

Incus Middle bone in the ossicular chain, attached at either end to the malleus and stapes, respectively.

Individualized education program (IEP) A document that describes a child's disability and the scope of services that will be provided to help the child receive an appropriate education in the least restrictive environment.

Individuals with Disabilities Education Act (IDEA) The federal law that provides federal funding for special education and regulates special education procedures.

Infarct An area of dead tissue resulting from interruption of the blood supply.

Inferior colliculus nucleus A way station in the midbrain that lies between the lateral lemniscus nucleus and the medial geniculate body.

Initiating event Background information about the event that propels the main character into action. The initiating event is usually a problem.

Intelligibility The ability to understand the words that someone else is producing.

Interactive assessment A form of assessment that allows speech-language pathologists to test beyond the limits of the behaviors the child displays in nonteaching (e.g., testing) situations. This type of testing helps clinicians decide whether poor test performance is caused by language learning difficulties, lack of understanding of the test task, or limited exposure to the types of questions that are being asked.

Internal response Information about the main character's thoughts or feelings about the initiating event.

Intracerebral Refers to injuries or structures within the brain.

Intravenous (IV) A needle that is placed into a vein through which liquid nutrition or medication can be given.

Jargon aphasia Meaningless words typical of Wernicke's aphasia.

Jim Crow segregation The legalized segregation (from about 1900 through the 1960s) barring African Americans from public and social interaction with whites.

Labyrinth A system of canals connecting portions of the inner ear. The larger osseous labyrinth contains perilymph and the smaller membranous labyrinth contains endolymph.

Lacerations Torn tissue caused by blunt trauma.

Language A standardized set of symbols and the conventions for combining those symbols into words, phrases, sentences, and texts for the purpose of communicating thoughts and feelings.

Language content The meaning of an utterance or word. Content relates to the linguistic system of semantics.

Language disorder An impairment or deviant development of the form, content, or use of language. The impairments can impact language comprehension, production, or both.

Language form The structure of language. Form relates to the linguistic systems of phonology, morphology, and syntax.

Language use Choices that speakers, signers, and writers make about the words and sentence structures that will best express their intended meanings. These choices are made with respect to the formality of the speaking situation. Language use relates to the linguistic system of pragmatics.

Laryngectomee One who has undergone a laryngectomy.

Laryngectomy Surgical removal of the larynx.

Lateral lemniscus nucleus A way station in the brainstem that lies between the superior olivary complex and the inferior colliculus nuclei.

Learning disability A significant difficulty with the acquisition and use of one or more of the following abilities: listening, speaking, reading, writing, reasoning, mathematical computation, or mathematical problem solving.

Lexicon A mental dictionary of words.

Licensure A procedure that grants legal permission for an individual to practice in a specific area, usually a profession, and affirms that standards have been met.

Literal paraphasia Sounds and syllables of a word are articulated correctly but are substituted or transposed (i.e., *bork* for *fork*).

Literature-based language intervention An approach to language intervention in which all the language therapy activities are related to a children's book.

Malleus The outermost bone in the ossicular chain. One end is attached to the tympanic membrane; the other end is connected to the incus.

Manner of articulation The amount and type (i.e., oral vs. nasal) of constriction during the production of phonemes.

Manual codes, manual systems Systems of manual gestures (often adapted from existing sign languages) that are used simultaneously with speech to present a redundant representation of the spoken signal in another mode. These are typically used in the practice of Total Communication. Manual codes are not sign languages; the codes merely offer a way to make the spoken language more accessible to the deaf "listener" as it is produced, and the grammar is still that of the spoken language. *See also* Total Communication.

Mass The amount of matter an object has.

Mastoid process The bony protrusion behind the pinna.

Maze A repetition, a false start, or a reformulation of a sentence.

Medial geniculate body A way station in the brainstem that lies between the superior olivary complex and the inferior colliculus nuclei.

Medulla The lower part of the brainstem that contains many of the motor nuclei important for swallowing.

Membranous labyrinth A flexible sac found within the osseous labyrinth that houses the structures of the inner ear.

Meninges Tissue coverings overlying the central nervous system.

Mental graphemic representations (MGRs) Cognitive images of written letters.

Metacognitive strategies Effortful actions that are used to learn new information (e.g., reading something twice, highlighting information in a textbook, making outlines that coincide with notes from class, etc.).

Metastasize To spread or invade by metastasis, usually from cancer.

Minimal auditory deprivation syndrome (MADS) Difficulty in processing speech because of a central auditory disorder thought to be caused by very mild hearing loss.

Mismatch Refers to the mismatch between child socialization and expectations for home language interactions and school language interactions.

Mixed hearing loss A combination of conductive and sensorineural hearing loss in the same ear.

Modified barium swallow (MBS) A moving X-ray picture of a swallow.

Morphology The part of grammar that concerns the study of morphemes (the smallest units of meaning).

Multidisciplinary assessment Members of an assessment team conduct their own independent assessments of the child's abilities that relate to their own interest areas (i.e., speech-language pathologists evaluate speech and language only, physical therapists evaluate motor abilities only, etc.). In a summary meeting, each member of the team shares his or her findings and recommends treatment. The emphasis is on the parts of the child rather than the whole child.

Multimodalism The approach to communication that supports the deaf person's development of a variety of speech, sign, and writing methods for communication, depending on the communication demands of the situation, rather than being restricted to one mode only.

Myelin White fatty covering of an axon.

Myopathy An abnormal condition or disease of muscle.

Myringostomy Incision into the tympanic membrane with insertion of a small ventilating tube.

Nasal emission Airflow through the nose, usually measurable or audible and heard most frequently during the production of voiceless plosives and fricatives; usually indicative of an incomplete seal between the nasal and oral cavities.

Nasogastric tube (NG tube) A feeding tube that goes through the nose, through the pharynx, and into the stomach.

Nasometer An instrument used to measure the acoustic correlate of nasality.

Nasopharynx That part of the pharynx above the level of the soft palate that opens anteriorly into the nasal cavity.

Neoglottis Vibratory segment or area that functions for vocal phonation in the absence of the glottis following surgical removal of the larynx. *See also* Pseudoglottis.

Neologism A new word that may be meaningless.

Neoplasm (tumor) A new growth.

Neural plasticity The idea that neurological structures and pathways reorganize themselves.

Neuron A specialized cell that conducts bioelectrical messages in the nervous system.

Neurotransmitters Chemical messengers of the nervous system; a substance released by hair cells or neurons that affects neighboring neurons.

Neutralist approach An approach to identifying language disorders in which clinicians base their diagnostic decisions on test scores without taking social norms into consideration.

No Child Left Behind Act (NCLB) A Congressional act that requires stronger accountability for academic achievement. The act states that all schools must make adequate yearly progress in raising the percentage of students who are proficient in math and reading.

Non-stuttering-like disfluencies Phrase repetitions, interjections, or revisions.

Normativist approach An approach to identifying language disorders in which clinicians account for social norms and potential social, educational, vocational, and economic consequences of the child's language abilities in the decision-making process.

Omission An articulation error in which a child leaves out a speech sound (*tip* is produced as "ti").

Oral method The approach to communication with deaf individuals that fosters the exclusive use of speech, speechreading, and hearing; sign language is not permitted.

Oral-peripheral evaluation When the clinician examines the structures used to produce speech sounds and assesses adequacy of movement of those structures for speech production.

Organ of Corti A collection of sensory and supporting cells that extends from the base of the cochlea to its apex.

Organic Disorders that have a physical cause.

Osseous labyrinth A hollowed out portion of the temporal bone that encases the inner ear.

Ossicular chain The three interconnected bones in the middle ear that conduct vibration from the tympanic membrane to the cochlea.

Otitis media Infection of the middle ear.

Otoacoustic emission (OAE) Either spontaneous or evoked sounds emanating from the inner ear.

Otology The medical specialty that deals with ear disease and the peripheral hearing mechanism.

Otosclerosis A hearing loss caused by bony fixation of the stapes in the oval window.

Output The intensity of the acoustic signal produced by an amplification system.

Oval window The opening between the middle ear and scala vestibuli of the cochlea. The stapes footplate seals the opening.

Palatoplasty Surgical repair of a palatal defect.

Paramedian Near the middle line.

Perilymph The fluid found within the bony labyrinth.

Period The amount of time needed to complete one cycle of vibration.

Peristalsis The contraction of smooth muscles to propel food through the digestive tract.

Person-first language When describing a person with a communication disorder, professionals should refer to the individual first, and then the disorder that the person presents. For example, it is better to say "children with autism" than "autistic children." Similarly, "He has aphasia" is preferred over "He is an aphasic."

Pharyngeal flap surgery Surgical procedure to aid in achieving velopharyngeal closure. A flap of skin is used to close most of the opening between the velum and the nasopharynx.

Pharyngeal fricatives Fricative sounds produced by approximating the back of the tongue and the posterior pharyngeal wall and forcing air through the resultant constriction.

Pharyngeal stops Plosive sounds produced by contacting the back of the tongue to the posterior pharyngeal wall, building up air pressure behind that obstruction and rapidly releasing it to produce a popping or (ex)plosive sound.

Pharyngeal-esophageal (PE) segment Pharyngoesophageal junction; another name for the neoglottis.

Phonatory disorders Abnormalities in the pitch, loudness, or quality of the voice.

Phoneme A speech sound that can change meaning (e.g., *pan* – *f*an).

Phonetically balanced (PB) word lists Lists of 50 words that are supposed to contain all the phonetic elements of English speech. These lists are used for testing word recognition.

Phonological awareness A type of metalinguistic awareness. Knowledge of the sequence of sounds that make up words (*soup* starts with an *s*). The ability to identify the phoneme structure of words (e.g., *ball* begins with a /b/).

Phonological disorder Difficulty understanding and implementing the language conventions for producing speech sounds and speech sound sequences.

Phonological processes Simplifications of adult-like productions of words. Some of the more common processes are weak syllable deletion, final consonant deletion, and velar fronting (substitution of a /t/ or /d/ for a /k/ or /g/). Descriptions of variations in the way sounds are produced when they co-occur with other sounds. For example, vowels become more nasal when they are followed by a nasal consonant in words.

Phonology The study of the organization of sounds; language rules that govern how sounds are combined to create words.

Pinna The cartilaginous flap of skin attached to the side of the head around the opening to the external auditory meatus.

Place of articulation The place of construction during the production of phonemes.

Plan In a narrative episode, information about what the main character intends to do and why.

Posterior pharyngeal wall (PPW) Back of the throat.

Pragmatics Conventions related to the use of language in various speaking situations.

Prelinguistic communication Communication that occurs before children use words; includes gestures and nonword vocalizations.

Preparatory set A technique in therapy for stuttering in which persons who stutter ease their way into words they thought they would stutter on.

Prevalence Percentage of individuals in a population who demonstrates a disorder at a given point in time.

Primary stuttering behaviors Stuttering-like disfluencies (i.e., repetitions, prolongations, and blocks) that are sometimes referred to as "core behaviors."

Production The use of speech or writing to express meaning.

Profession An area of practice requiring specialized knowledge and academic preparation.

Prolongations A type of dysfluency in which a sound is held out or prolonged for an unusually long time.

Prosody Changes in pitch, stress, intensity, and duration of sounds during connected speech; the intonation and rhythm of a spoken language.

Pseudoglottis Vibratory segment or area that functions for vocal phonation in the absence of the glottis; neoglottis.

Public Law 94-142, the Education of All Handicapped Children Act of 1975 The first law that guaranteed a free appropriate public education in the least restrictive environment to all children with disabilities and that provided funding for special education activities.

Pull-out A therapy strategy for stuttering in which persons who stutter are taught to ease their way out of repetitions, prolongations, and blocks.

Pyramidal tract Major motor pathway from cerebral cortex to brainstem and spinal cord.

Reaction In an episode, information about the main character's thoughts or feelings about the consequence.

Real-ear gain The increase in sound intensity provided by a hearing aid (in decibels) calculated by subtracting the intensity at the tympanic membrane without the hearing aid from the intensity at the tympanic membrane with the hearing aid, by using a probe microphone.

Reduplicated babbling Babbled sequences in which the same syllable is repeated.

Reissner's membrane The thin layer of tissue that separates scala vestibuli from scala media.

Residual hearing Hearing that remains after a hearing loss.

Resonance The frequency at which an object vibrates best.

Resonance disorders Abnormalities in the use of the nasal cavity during speaking. Individuals can be hypernasal (excessive nasality) or denasal (insufficient nasality).

Response to intervention (RTI) A method for identifying children with learning disabilities in which a child receives increasingly more intensive levels, or "tiers," of instruction until his or her response to that intervention is acceptable.

Resting expiratory level Mechanically neutral position of the respiratory system.

Reverberation Time the amount of time (in seconds) it takes a signal that was abruptly turned off to decrease in intensity by 60 dB.

Rigidity (rigid) Balanced hypertonicity that results in resistance to movement.

Rolandic fissure Fissure that divides posterior frontal lobe from anterior parietal lobe.

Round window The opening between the middle ear and scala tympani of the cochlea. The round window membrane covers the opening.

Secondary stuttering behaviors Adaptations that stutterers make as they try to get through primary stuttering behaviors or to avoid them altogether. The most common secondary stuttering behaviors are eye blinks, lip pursing, arm movements, and head nods.

Section 504 A law passed in 1973 that prohibited public schools from discriminating against children with disabilities in any way.

Semantics The meaning of individual words (lexical semantics) or the meanings that are expressed when words are joined together (relational semantics).

Sensation level (SL) The number of decibels above the auditory threshold of an individual.

Sensorineural hearing loss Hearing loss caused by damage to the inner ear and/or auditory nerve.

Sequential bilingual A second language is introduced after the primary language is established.

Setting In a narrative, background information about the characters, the place where the story occurs, or the time of the story.

Signal-to-noise ratio (SNR) A representation of the signal intensity compared to the background noise intensity calculated by subtracting the intensity of the noise from the intensity of the signal (in decibels).

Simple sound A sound composed of a single frequency component.

Simple view of reading The idea that reading is comprised of two components: language comprehension and word recognition.

Simultaneous bilingual Two languages are acquired early in development.

Single-word articulation test A test consists of pictures of words. The pictured words usually sample all of the consonants at the initial, medial, and final positions of words. Children are asked to say the name of the object when they see it.

Socialization The degree to which an individual is able to interact with others following appropriate social norms.

Socioeconomic status A family's status based on family income, parental education level, parental occupation, and social status in the community.

Sound generation The process where an object is set into motion through the application of an external force.

Sound propagation The movement of vibration through a medium brought about by collisions between neighboring particles.

Source-filter theory An acoustic theory of speech production that states a sound energy source is modified by the filter characteristics of the vocal tract.

Spasticity (spastic) Abnormal muscle tone, primarily in antigravity muscles, resulting from upper motor neuron damage.

Specific language impairment Difficulties acquiring language in the absence of any other mental, sensory, motoric, emotional, or experiential deficits.

Specific learning disability A disorder in the psychological processes involved in learning that may manifest itself in an imperfect ability to listen, think, speak, read, write, spell, or do mathematical calculations.

Spectrum A graph that shows the amplitude or phase as a function of frequency.

Speech delay Articulation errors or phonological processes that are often seen in younger, normally developing children.

Speech disorder Articulation errors or phonological processes that are rarely seen in normally developing children.

Speech-recognition threshold (SRT) The lowest intensity at which speech can barely be heard.

Speechreading Sometimes called "lip-reading," speechreading is a method used by people with hearing impairments to "read" the movements of a speaker's face and mouth to understand what he or she is saying. Speechreading is an art not easily acquired by all deaf individuals and at best is notoriously unreliable.

Spondee A two-syllable word pronounced with equal emphasis on both syllables. Used in testing the SRT.

Spontaneous recovery Recovery from stroke resulting from physiological and reorganizational changes in the brain and not attributable to rehabilitation.

Spontaneous speech and language sample When the clinician gathers a sample of the individual's speech and language in a communication situation that is considered to be the normal way in which the individual communicates using voice, gestures, and nonvocal communication.

Standardized assessment Administration of formal tests to determine how a child's performance on an aspect of language compares to the average performance of children who are the same chronological age.

Stapedius muscle A middle ear muscle that is attached to the stapes. This muscle contracts in response to intense sound.

Stapes The innermost bone in the ossicular chain. One end is attached to the incus; the other end, or footplate, occupies the oval window.

Starting phase The position occupied by an object at a particular time within one cycle of vibration. Starting phase may be measured in degrees or radians.

Stoma A small opening, such as the mouth; an artificial opening between cavities or canals, or between such and the surface of the body.

Story grammar Conventions for the ways in which meanings are sequenced to form a story (e.g., initiating event, internal response, plan, attempt, consequence, reaction/ending).

Stria vascularis A collection of blood vessels that is found within the scala media. The stria vascularis delivers nutrients and removes waste from cells in the organ of Corti.

Stroboscopy A slow-motion video image of vocal fold vibration.

Stuttering An unusual amount of tense, within-word disfluencies that interfere with the continuity of speech.

Stuttering modification A therapy approach in which the clinician teaches the client to alter the way he or she stutters.

Stuttering-like disfluencies Single-syllable-word repetitions, syllable repetitions, sound repetitions, prolongations, and blocks.

Substitution A speech error in which the child substitutes one sound (usually a sound that is developmentally earlier than the target) for the target sound. Common substitutions are /t/ for /s/ and /w/ for /r/.

Sulci Furrows of the cerebral cortex.

Superior olivary complex A way station in the brainstem that lies between the cochlear nuclei and the lateral lemniscus nucleus.

Superior sphincter pharyngoplasty Surgical procedure to aid in achieving velopharyngeal closure; the posterior faucial pillars are raised and used to form a bulge that reduces the size of opening between the velum and the nasopharynx.

Syllable A basic unit of speech production that must contain a vowel.

Sylvian fissure Horizontal fissure superior to the temporal lobe.

Syntax Conventions related to the way words are ordered to create sentences.

Tectorial membrane A gelatinous substance that is attached at one edge to the spiral limbus. The bottom of the tectorial membrane is connected to the cilia of the hair cells.

Telecoil switch (t-switch) An option on a hearing aid to use electromagnetic energy as the input instead of the microphone.

Temporal bone One of the seven bones that form the skull. The temporal bone contains the middle and inner ears.

Tensor tympani muscle A middle ear muscle that is attached to the malleus. This muscle contracts in response to intense sound and to tactile stimulation of the face.

Thalamus Structure located at either side of the third ventricle; responsible for sensorimotor integration and sensory projection to the cerebral cortex.

Threshold of audibility The lowest intensity at which a signal can barely be heard.

Thrombosis Accumulation of material within an artery. When complete, it causes a stroke.

Tinnitus Ringing, roaring, or other sounds heard in the absence of an external sound.

Tonotopic organization An arrangement where one of a structure's dimensions is systematically laid out according to frequency.

Total Communication A philosophy of communication with deaf children and adults that advocates the use of multimodalism, including speech, sign, writing, and anything else that would facilitate the communication process. In practice, Total Communication typically involves the use of speech accompanied by one of the manual codes for English.

Transcript A written record of the language that was used during a language sample.

Transdisciplinary assessment When a team of professionals works together to evaluate a child. Members of the team are not limited to the evaluation of any single area of development.

Transduction The process where energy is converted from one form to another. The hair cells change mechanical energy to electrical energy.

Transient ischemic attack (TIA) Temporary interruption of blood flow to an area of the brain. The effects typically resolve within 24 hours.

Traveling wave The displacement pattern of the basilar membrane brought about by stimulation with sound.

Tremor Rhythmic involuntary movements resulting from basal ganglia disease/damage.

Tympanic membrane (TM) The cone-shaped layer of tissue that separates the external auditory meatus from the middle ear cavity. The malleus is connected to the inner surface of the tympanic membrane.

Tympanometry A pressure/compliance function that reveals the status of the middle ear.

Unilateral Pertaining to or restricted to one side of the body.

Unilateral hearing loss A hearing loss in the right or left ear, but not both.

Use Language use refers to the social aspects of language, which are also called pragmatics.

Uvula Small cone-shaped process hanging from the lower border of the soft palate at midline.

Variegated babbling Babbled sequences in which the syllable content varies.

Verbal paraphasia Unintended substitution of one word for another, usually from the same category (e.g., *horse* for *cow*).

Vestibular mechanism That part of the inner ear responsible for reporting balance and equilibrium to the brain.

Video endoscopy An instrument called an endoscope is passed into the pharynx so that a fiberoptic camera can project greatly magnified images of the vocal folds onto a video screen.

Visipitch An instrument used by speech-language pathologists that displays pitch, amplitude, and spectral characteristics of speech production.

Voicing Vibration of the vocal folds during the production of a phoneme.

Waveform A graph that shows the amplitude as a function of time.

Wernicke's area Posterior part of first temporal gyrus important for auditory processing and comprehension.

Whisper Soft speech in which there is little or no vibration of the vocal folds.

Word recognition The ability to identify a written word without having to sound it out.

Word-recognition score (WRS) The score, in percent, that reveals the ability to discriminate among the sounds of speech.

Index

Page numbers in **bold type** refer to glossary references. Page numbers followed by *f* and *t* refer to figures and tables, respectively.